T0259237

Sports-related Injuries of the Hip

Guest Editor

BRIAN D. BUSCONI, MD

CLINICS IN
SPORTS MEDICINE

www.sportsmed.theclinics.com

Consulting Editor
MARK D. MILLER, MD

April 2011 • Volume 30 • Number 2

SAUNDERS an imprint of ELSEVIER, Inc.

W.B. SAUNDERS COMPANY

A Division of Elsevier Inc.

1600 John F. Kennedy Blvd. • Suite 1800 • Philadelphia, Pennsylvania 19103

http://www.theclinics.com

CLINICS IN SPORTS MEDICINE Volume 30, Number 2
April 2011 ISSN 0278-5919, ISBN-13: 978-1-4557-0507-8

Editor: Jessica Demetriou

Clinics in Sports Medicine (ISSN 0278-5919) is published quarterly by Elsevier Inc., 360 Park Avenue South, New York, NY 10010-1710. Months of issue are January, April, July, and October. Business and Editorial Offices: 1600 John F. Kennedy Blvd., Ste. 1800, Philadelphia, PA 19103-2899. Customer Service Office: 3251 Riverport Lane, Maryland Heights, MO 63043. Periodicals postage paid at New York, NY and additional mailing offices. Subscription prices are $297.00 per year (US individuals), $466.00 per year (US institutions), $147.00 per year (US students), $337.00 per year (Canadian individuals), $563.00 per year (Canadian institutions), $205.00 (Canadian students), $409.00 per year (foreign individuals), $563.00 per year (foreign institutions), and $205.00 per year (foreign students). Foreign air speed delivery is included in all *Clinics* subscription prices. All prices are subject to change without notice. **POSTMASTER:** Send address changes to *Clinics in Sports Medicine*, Elsevier Health Sciences Division, Subscription Customer Service, 3251 Riverport Lane, Maryland Heights, MO 63043. Customer Service (orders, claims, online, change of address): Elsevier Health Sciences Division, Subscription Customer Service, 3251 Riverport Lane, Maryland Heights, MO 63043. Tel: 1-800-654-2452 (U.S. and Canada); 314-447-8871 (outside U.S. and Canada). Fax: 314-447-8029. E-mail: journalscustomerservice-usa@elsevier.com (for print support); journalsonlinesupport-usa@elsevier.com (for online support).

Reprints. For copies of 100 or more of articles in this publication, please contact the Commercial Reprints Department, Elsevier Inc., 360 Park Avenue South, New York, NY 10010-1710. Tel.: 212-633-3812; Fax: 212-462-1935; E-mail: reprints@elsevier.com.

Clinics in Sports Medicine is covered in *MEDLINE/PubMed (Index Medicus) Current Contents/Clinical Medicine, Excerpta Medica,* and *ISI/Biomed.*

Printed and bound by CPI Group (UK) Ltd, Croydon, CR0 4YY

Transferred to Digital Print 2011

Contributors

CONSULTING EDITOR

MARK D. MILLER, MD
S. Ward Casscells Professor of Orthopaedic Surgery, University of Virginia, Charlottesville, Virginia; Team Physician, James Madison University, Harrisonburg, Virginia

GUEST EDITOR

BRIAN D. BUSCONI, MD
Associate Professor, Department of Orthopedics and Physical Rehabilitation; Chief of Sports Medicine and Arthroscopy, University of Massachusetts Medical School, Worcester, Massachusetts

AUTHORS

JAMES R. BOYLE, MD
Orthopedic Sports Medicine Fellow, Department of Orthopedics, Division of Sports Medicine, University of Massachusetts Memorial Medical Center, Worcester, Massachusetts

JAMES A. BROWNE, MD
Assistant Professor, Department of Orthopaedic Surgery, University of Virginia, Charlottesville, Virginia

BRIAN D. BUSCONI, MD
Associate Professor, Department of Orthopedics and Physical Rehabilitation; Chief of Sports Medicine and Arthroscopy, University of Massachusetts Medical School, Worcester, Massachusetts

JAVIER CAMACHO-GALINDO, MD
Attendant Surgeon of Adult Hip and Knee Reconstruction, National Rehabilitation Institute of Mexico; Assistant Professor of Hip and Knee Surgery, Universidad Nacional Autónoma de México, Mexico City, Mexico

MICHAEL B. CROSS, MD
Orthopaedic Surgery Resident, Hospital for Special Surgery, New York, New York

LEANDRO EJNISMAN, MD
Visiting Scholar, Steadman Philippon Research Institute, Vail, Colorado

PETER D. FABRICANT, MD
Orthopaedic Surgery Resident, Hospital for Special Surgery, New York, New York

MICHAEL T. FREEHILL, MD
Fellow of Orthopaedic Sports Medicine and Sports Orthopaedic Surgery, Department of Orthopaedic Surgery, Stanford University, Redwood City, California

YARI LIZETTE GONZALEZ IBARRA, MD
National Rehabilitation Institute of Mexico; Orthopaedic Surgery Resident, Universidad Nacional Autónoma de México, Mexico City, Mexico

VICTOR M. ILIZALITURRI Jr, MD
Chief of Adult Hip and Knee Reconstruction, National Rehabilitation Institute of Mexico, Professor of Hip and Knee Surgery, Universidad Nacional Autónoma de México, Mexico City, Mexico

LEAH JACOBY, BS
Medical Student, Duke University School of Medicine, Durham, North Carolina

BRYAN T. KELLY, MD
Assistant Professor of Orthopaedic Surgery, Hospital for Special Surgery, New York, New York

MININDER S. KOCHER, MD, MPH
Associate Director, Department of Orthopaedic Surgery, Division of Sports Medicine, Children's Hospital Boston; Associate Professor, Harvard Medical School, Boston, Massachusetts

JO-ANN LEE, MS
Board Certified Registered Nurse Practitioner, Department of Orthopaedics, Massachusetts General Hospital, Boston; Kaplan Center for Joint Reconstructive Surgery, Newton Wellesley Hospital, Newton, Massachusetts

PISIT LERTWANICH, MD
Steadman Philippon Research Institute, Vail, Colorado

DEMETRIUS E.M. LITWIN, MD
Professor and Chairman, Department of Surgery, University of Massachusetts Memorial Medical Center, University of Massachusetts Medical School, Worcester, Massachusetts

TRAVIS G. MAAK, MD
Orthopaedic Surgery Resident, Hospital for Special Surgery, New York, New York

JOSEPH C. MCCARTHY, MD
Vice Chairman, Department of Orthopaedics, Massachusetts General Hospital, Boston; Director, Kaplan Center for Joint Reconstructive Surgery, Newton Wellesley Hospital, Newton, Massachusetts

PATRICK M. MCENANEY, MD
Assistant Professor, Department of Surgery, Milford Hospital, University of Massachusetts Medical School, Worcester, Massachusetts

SEAN MC MILLAN, DO
Orthopedic Sports Medicine Fellow, Department of Orthopedics, Division of Sports Medicine, University of Massachusetts Memorial Medical Center, Worcester, Massachusetts

KETAN PATEL, MD
Attending Radiologist, Shields Healthcare Group, Brockton, Massachusetts; Associate Professor, Department of Radiology, University of Massachusetts Medical Center, University Campus, Worcester, Massachusetts

MARC J. PHILIPPON, MD
Director of Hip Research, Steadman Philippon Research Institute, Orthopaedic Surgeon, Steadman Clinic, Vail, Colorado (Managing Partner); Associate Clinical Professor, Department of Surgery, Faculty of Health Sciences, McMaster University, Hamilton, Ontario, Canada

MATTHEW PLANTE, MD
Attending Orthopedic Surgeon, The Miriam Hospital, Providence, Rode Island

ALBERTO NAYIB EVIA RAMIREZ, MD
National Rehabilitation Institute of Mexico; Hip and Knee Surgery Research Fellow, Universidad Nacional Autónoma de México, Mexico City, Mexico

MARK RYAN, MS, ATC, CSCS
Howard Head Sports Medicine, Vail, Colorado

MARC R. SAFRAN, MD
Professor of Orthopaedic Surgery, Director, Orthopaedic Sports Medicine, Fellowship, Associate Director of Sports Medicine, Department of Orthopaedic Surgery, Stanford University, Redwood City, California

THOMAS G. SAMPSON, MD
Medical Director of Hip Arthroscopy, Post Street Surgery Center; President Elect, International Society for Hip Arthroscopy (ISHA 2011), Former Associate Clinical Professor of Orthopaedics, University of California, San Francisco, San Francisco, California

BEATRICE SHU, MD
Resident, Department of Orthopaedic Surgery, Stanford Hospital and Clinics, Stanford, California

JASON A. SILVA, MD
Orthopedic Resident, Department of Orthopedics, University of Massachusetts Memorial Medical Center, Worcester, Massachusetts

ERICA B. SNEIDER, MD
Department of Surgery, University of Massachusetts Memorial Medical Center, University of Massachusetts Medical School, Worcester, Massachusetts

MICHAEL WAHOFF, PT, SCS
Howard Head Sports Medicine, Vail, Colorado

ROXANNE WALLACE, MD
Sports Medicine Fellow, Department of Orthopedic Surgery, University of Massachusetts, Worcester, Massachusetts

YEN YI-MENG, MD, PhD
Medical Staff, Department of Orthopaedic Surgery, Children's Hospital Boston; Instructor, Harvard Medical School, Boston, Massachusetts

Contents

> Hip arthroscopy began with resection of pathologies and later progressed
> to repair of different tissues. There is an increasing impetus for reconstruc-
> tion of biologic joints; although this has occurred with other joints, hip
> arthroscopic procedures are now headed in this direction. Thus, despite
> considerable initial challenges, multiple opportunities are now available
> in this fertile field.

> This article reviews the evaluation of the hip including the clinical history
> and physical examination. As our understanding of hip pathology evolves,
> and arthroscopic and other minimally invasive operative techniques im-
> prove, the focus is shifting toward earlier identification of hip pathology.
> Risk factors for the development of arthritis are now well established
> and include femoral acetabular impingement, labral tearing, developmen-
> tal dysplasia, and slipped capital femoral epiphysis. Emerging treatment
> options may address these conditions in the early stages and prevent or
> slow the progression of hip degeneration. It is vitally important to elucidate
> intra-articular versus extra-articular pathology of hip pain in every step of
> the patient encounter: history, physical examination, and imaging.

> Hip and groin pain are a common complaint among athletes of all ages,
> and may result from an acute injury or from chronic, repetitive trauma.
> Hip injuries can be intraarticular, extraarticular, or both. Labral abnormal-
> ities may occur in asymptomatic patients as well as in those with incapa-
> citating symptoms and signs. Athletic hip injury leading to disabling
> intraarticular hip pain most commonly involves labral tear. The extraarti-
> cular causes are usually the result of overuse activity, leading to inflamma-
> tion, tendonitis, or bursitis. In clinical practice, the term athletic pubalgia is
> used to describe exertional pubic or groin pain.

> In this article, the concepts important for hip arthroscopy are reviewed.
> Room setup, necessary equipment, and the basics of patient positioning

are detailed, and the benefits of lateral versus supine positions are evaluated. The placement of common arthroscopic portals and the authors' preferred position and technique for hip arthroscopy are discussed. Also, the potential complications encountered are discussed.

The treatment of labral pathologic condition of the hip has become a topic of increasing interest. In patients undergoing hip arthroscopy, tears of the acetabular labrum are the most commonly found pathologic condition and most common cause of mechanical symptoms. Although a labral tear may occur with a single traumatic event, often another underlying cause may be already present, predisposing the individual to injury. This article discusses the structure and function of the acetabular labrum, the diagnosis of labral injury through physical examination and imaging modalities, and the current treatment options, including labrectomy, labral repair, and reconstruction.

Labral tears are an important cause of hip pain in the athlete. Knowledge of labral function is now better understood. The labrum acts as a suction seal stabilizing the hip joint. After a detailed history and physical examination, imaging workup is done to achieve an accurate diagnosis. Hip arthroscopy can be performed to treat labral tears in a minimally invasive manner. This article describes operative techniques to treat labral tears, including a method for labral reconstruction using the iliotibial band autograft.

Arthroscopic treatment of chondral lesions of the hip is challenging. Understanding the etiology is paramount not only in treating hip chondral damage but also in mitigating the cause, using arthroscopic means. This article addresses chondral lesions of the hip caused by either injury or morphologic conflicts such as seen in femoroacetabular impingement. Fractures, aseptic necrosis, and metabolic or immunologic damage are not addressed. Methods using arthroscopic surgery for the treatment of chondral lesions are presented.

Hip instability is uncommon because of the substantial conformity of the osseous femoral head and acetabulum. It can be defined as extraphysiologic hip motion that causes pain with or without the symptom of hip joint unsteadiness. The cause can be traumatic or atraumatic, and is related to both bony and soft tissue abnormality. Gross instability caused by trauma or iatrogenic injury has been shown to improve with surgical correction of the underlying deficiency. Subtle microinstability, particularly from microtraumatic or atraumatic causes, is an evolving concept with early surgical treatment results that are promising.

Femoroacetabular impingement is an abnormal conflict of the acetabular rim and the femoral head-neck junction. This condition causes labral and cartilage damage and leads to early osteoarthritis of the hip. Femoral osteoplasty is performed to restore normal femoral head-neck offset while the amount of bony resection is monitored by periodic examination. Dynamic examination of the area of impingement, which cannot be performed in open treatment of cam impingement, confirms adequate resection and labral seal through hip range of motion.

Rim impingement lesions vary based on the underlying pathology. In general, rim impingement occurs with anterosuperior overhang, coxa profunda, protrusio acetabuli, and acetabular retroversion. The method for addressing these pathologic lesions depends on location and size of the impingement lesion, the underlying pathology, and the degree of labral damage. The ultimate goals of surgical management include accurate localization of the rim impingement lesion, adequate removal of the bony impingement lesion, and preservation and refixation of the viable labral tissue. If the surgeon feels that these goals cannot be accomplished safely and effectively by arthroscopic methods, alternative procedures should be considered.

Snapping hip syndromes have been treated with open surgery for many years. Recently, endoscopic techniques have been developed for treatment of snapping hip syndromes with results that are at least comparable if not better than those reported for open procedures. The greater trochanteric pain syndrome is well known by orthopedic surgeons. However, deep understanding of the pathologic conditions generating pain in the greater trochanteric region and endoscopic access to it has only recently been described. Although evidence regarding endoscopic techniques for the treatment of the greater trochanteric pain syndrome is mainly anecdotal, early published reports are encouraging.

Athletic pubalgia or sports hernia is a syndrome of chronic lower abdomen and groin pain that may occur in athletes and nonathletes. Because the differential diagnosis of chronic lower abdomen and groin pain is so broad, only a small number of patients with chronic lower abdomen and groin pain fulfill the diagnostic criteria of athletic pubalgia (sports hernia). The literature published to date regarding the cause, pathogenesis, diagnosis, and treatment of sports hernias is confusing. This article summarizes the current information and our present approach to this chronic lower abdomen and groin pain syndrome.

Injuries of the hip and pelvis in pediatric athletes are receiving increased attention, which may be due, in part, to the increased participation in competitive sports and focusing on a single sport at younger ages. With the advent of hip arthroscopy and the development of more advanced imaging of the hip through magnetic resonance imaging, internal derangements of the hip such as labral tears, loose bodies, femoroacetabular impingement, and chondral injuries are being diagnosed and treated with increased frequency. This article reviews the more common injuries of the hip and pelvis in pediatric athletes.

Degenerative arthritis of the hip is a common finding in the mature athlete and can have a significant impact on the quality of life of these patients. This chapter reviews the treatment modalities for early arthritis of the hip with a special focus on the current evidence for the role of hip arthroscopy in the care of these patients.

Hip arthroscopic techniques to repair labral tears and address femoroacetabular impingement (FAI) are evolving. This article discusses the different phases of rehabilitation and the rehabilitation protocol. Although there is evidence to support arthroscopic procedures to address labral tears and FAI, there are few published evidence-based rehabilitation studies dedicated to postoperative rehabilitative care. It is thought that by following the restrictions set by the physician while performing early circumduction, using the minimal criteria to advance through each subsequent phase, and allowing patients to perform functional sport progressions throughout the rehabilitation athletes will be able to return to sport smoothly and effectively.

RELATED INTEREST

Radiologic Clinics of North America, November 2010 (Volume 48, Issue 6)
Sports Medicine Imaging
Michael J. Tuite, MD, *Guest Editor*
Available at: http://www.radiologic.theclinics.com/

VISIT THE CLINICS ONLINE!

Access your subscription at:
www.theclinics.com

Foreword

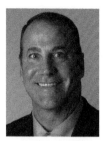

Mark D. Miller, MD
Consulting Editor

Hip arthroscopy has become a very popular procedure. It is a "new frontier" for the arthroscopist, so all scope docs want to "stake their claim" for a piece of the action. Having just completed interviews for our sports medicine fellowship, I can tell you that this is a "hot topic." However, as I discussed with the fellow applicants, I must offer a word of caution—"not so fast." Like all things in orthopedic surgery, the pendulum swings. All of the current "indications" for hip arthroscopy may prove to not significantly improve outcomes with long-term follow-up. Additionally, and perhaps most importantly, hip arthroscopy is not a niche trick that you can pull out a few times a year. Like every other procedure, getting good at hip arthroscopy requires practice—several times a week. So ... perhaps many of us should leave hip arthroscopy to the experts—like the surgeons who are included in this edition of *Clinics in Sports Medicine.*

This edition is guest edited by Dr Brian D. Busconi, of the University of Massachusetts. I discovered that Brian had a special interest in hip arthroscopy several years ago and have asked him to contribute to several projects where I needed an expert in this area. He has come through every time, and this effort is certainly no exception. As always, he has developed a logical, thorough, and complete treatise on this subject. The articles begin with a review of the brief history of hip arthroscopy, describe the appropriate workup, and then cover the gambit of conditions. Note that to be complete, he has also included hip and groin pathology that cannot be treated arthroscopically—at least yet!

So ... if you decide that you want to specialize in this area, then spend the time to really learn it. This is a great place to start. Thank you!

Mark D. Miller, MD
S. Ward Casscells Professor of Orthopaedic Surgery
University of Virginia
Team Physician, James Madison University
400 Ray C. Hunt Drive, Suite 330
Charlottesville, VA 22908-0159, USA

E-mail address:
mdm3p@virginia.edu

Clin Sports Med 30 (2011) xiii
doi:10.1016/j.csm.2011.01.005
0278-5919/11/$ – see front matter

Preface

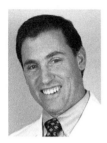

Brian D. Busconi, MD
Guest Editor

Management of sports-related hip injuries is currently one of the fastest growing, challenging, and dynamic fields in sports medicine. Interest in this field has risen due to greater comprehension of the hip's normal function, biomechanics, and pathologic states. Through research and greater success in the effectiveness of surgical procedures, more physicians have a heightened interest in treating sports-related hip injuries. It was my goal to provide to the sports medical practitioner a complete and state-of-the-art overview from some of the world's experts on the treatment of hip injuries, from diagnosis to nonoperative treatment to surgical intervention.

This issue is designed to provide the sports medicine practitioner, surgeon, and allied health professional a detailed and comprehensive summary of the most current knowledge of the athlete's hip. The first article was written by one of my mentors and pioneers of hip arthroscopy, Dr Joseph McCarthy. He shows us where we have been and where we are going in the world of hip arthroscopy. The next three articles by Drs Plante, Patel, and Boyle help us to better differentiate and diagnose hip pain through careful history, physical examination, diagnostic imaging selective injections, and the basic principles of arthroscopic evaluation.

The articles following our preliminary diagnosis of hip pain break down the hip joint into problems involving compartment pathology. We first explore areas of injury to the static structures of the central compartment, the labrum, the articular cartilage, and capsule by Drs Safran, Philippon, and Sampson.

We move from static pathologies to more pathologic dynamic conditions involving the peripheral compartment and how these conditions ultimately affect the central compartment. Drs Safran, Philippon, and Kelly provide us with cutting edge thoughts on these clinical concepts.

The next two articles look at specific injuries involving the peri-trochanteric compartment and soft tissue structures surrounding the hip by Drs Ilizaliturri and Litwin. Our final articles concentrate on specific concerns of the adolescent and mature hip by Drs Kocher and Browne and rehabilitating the athlete with hip pain by physical therapists Wahoff and Ryan.

This issue of *Clinics in Sports Medicine* could not have come to fruition without the great effort of all of the contributing authors, many of them pioneers in the field, and for

Clin Sports Med 30 (2011) xv–xvi
doi:10.1016/j.csm.2011.01.004
0278-5919/11/$ – see front matter © 2011 Elsevier Inc. All rights reserved.

which I am grateful of their time and effort. I would like to thank my four fellows, Drs Wallace, Mc Millan, Plante, and Boyle, for their dedication and late night organizational skills. I would like to thank the consulting editor Dr Miller for allowing me to be the lead editor for this section. Special thanks to Ruth Malwitz of Elsevier, who now is editing her own chapter on motherhood, and Jessica Demetriou of Elsevier, for keeping the project on task. Finally, to my loving wife, Karolyn, and my children, Liam and Aidan, thanks for putting up with me, and I promise more time looking for sea glass this summer. It has been a pleasure to work with such experts in the field of sport injuries In the hip.

Brian D. Busconi, MD
Department of Orthopedics and Physical Rehabilitation
University of Massachusetts Medical School
281 Lincoln Street
Worcester, MA 01605-2192, USA

E-mail address:
brian.busconi@umassmemorial.org

History of Hip Arthroscopy: Challenges and Opportunities

Joseph C. McCarthy, MD[a,b,]*, Jo-Ann Lee, MS[a,b]

KEYWORDS

• Hip arthroscopy • Hip anatomy • Chondral lesion
• Labral injury • Chondral injury

In 1983, a 36-year-old mother of two young children presented with ongoing and recurrent anterior groin pain. This pain persisted despite consultations with five physicians and multiple radiologic imaging studies, all of which were negative. These imaging studies included multiple radiographs, a CAT scan, and an MRI scan. She also underwent extensive blood testing. Despite this evaluation, no specific diagnosis could be made. Because of her particular symptoms and abnormal hip clinical examination, the patient underwent a mini-open anterior hip surgery, during which 25 loose bodies were extracted from her hip joint. These chondral loose bodies were from synovial chondromatosis. This surgical procedure relieved her symptoms and the patient was able to return to full-time employment. This experience prompted a literature review and, because of the paucity of scientific literature, an extensive cadaveric study to ascertain safe arthroscopic access to the joint.

HIP ANATOMY AND ACCESS

The hip joint is uniquely recessed within an extensive soft tissue envelope, making access more difficult than with other joints. In addition, the convex surface of the femoral head and concave surface of the acetabulum are deterrents to arthroscopic intervention. Furthermore, the hip joint inherently has negative pressure, and this vacuum phenomenon resists distraction of the hip. Finally, the ligamentous structures, especially the iliofemoral ligament, are inelastic and also resist separation of femoral head from the socket. Because of these structural factors, arthroscopic procedures for the hip joint lagged far behind those for the knee and the shoulder joints.

Cadaveric investigation examined access portals and avoidance of the neurovascular structures in and around the hip joint. This endeavor resulted in an understanding of

[a] Department of Orthopaedics, Massachusetts General Hospital, 55 Fruit Street, Boston, MA 02114, USA
[b] Kaplan Center for Joint Reconstructive Surgery, Newton Wellesley Hospital, 2014 Washington Street, Newton, MA 02462, USA
* Corresponding author.
E-mail address: jcmccarthy1@partners.org

Clin Sports Med 30 (2011) 217–224
doi:10.1016/j.csm.2010.12.001
0278-5919/11/$ – see front matter © 2011 Elsevier Inc. All rights reserved.

safe access anteriorly and laterally, and resulted in further understanding of the distraction methods necessary to perform this procedure.[1] A study by Burman[2] in 1931 showed access to the joint, although his work in cadavers accessed only the peripheral compartment. Erikson and Sebik[3] later showed the forces necessary to enter the central compartment with distraction. These investigators understood that the forces were reduced in an anesthetized patient experiencing muscle relaxation.

DISTRACTION EQUIPMENT

Initially, the only device used for hip distraction was a fracture table. Although this was more than adequate for hip fractures in elderly patients, the device had considerable limitations for young or muscular patients who required procedures within their biologic hip joint. The resistance to distraction by the muscular and ligamentous structures precluded access in many cases. Glick[4] published that as many as 40% of patients were inaccessible in his early experience. Because of these limitations, hip-specific distractors were eventually developed, including the Arthronix distractor, which allowed hip arthroscopy in the lateral position, and the Innomed hip distractor, which improved mechanical advantage to distract the hip away from the acetabular socket. The device was also was the first distractor to allow both rotation of the foot and flexion and movement of the extremity during the procedure. More recently, Smith and Nephew (Hip Positioning System, Andover, MA, USA) developed a distractor that allows dynamic hip motion, including flexion.

ANATOMIC POSITIONING

Initially hip arthroscopy was performed in the supine position on a fracture table. Both Johnson[5] and later Byrd and colleagues[6] described techniques for accessing the hip joint in the supine position. Conversely, in 1987 Glick and colleagues[7] published the essentials of arthroscopic access from the lateral decubitus position using the Arthronix distractor. The technique continues to be refined.

COMPARTMENT ACCESS
Peripheral Compartment

Initially, access to the joint was through the peripheral compartment only, as shown in Burman's[2] publication in 1931 in *The Journal of Bone and Joint Surgery*. In 1987, Dorfmann and Boyer[8] also published their experience of peripheral compartment access without distraction, and in 2001, Dienst and Kohn[9] published on peripheral compartment access of the hip joint and the appropriate anatomy in this area. More recently, Philippon and colleagues,[10] Enseki and colleagues,[11] and Guanche and Bare[12] described the anatomic structures and surgical procedures possible within the peripheral joint.

Central Compartment

Once distraction methods were refined, the central compartment became accessible. Gross[13] initially showed access in pediatric patients, and Holgersson and colleagues[14] showed biopsy of the joint. Later, Locker and Beguin,[15] Johnson[5] in 1986, Glick[16] in 1991, McCarthy and Busconi[17] in 1995, and others[18–20] all published on diagnosis and treatment of central compartment pathology.

Portals

Once distraction techniques were developed for access to the central and peripheral compartments, safe portal access became paramount. Johnson,[5] Byrd and colleagues,[21] Philippon and colleagues,[10] Dorfmann and colleagues,[22] and Villar[23] all published on techniques of safe hip joint access in the supine position. Conversely, both Glick and colleagues[7] and McCarthy and Busconi[17] published techniques of safe portal placement for patients in the lateral decubitus position. These portals avoided the major neurovascular structures in and around the hip joint, allowed access to all compartments of the hip joint, and enabled surgical interventions.

Instrumentation

Initially, instrumentation for hip procedures was adopted from knee and shoulder joint equipment. These instruments, however, had limitations in length and curvature for hip procedures. Somewhat later, several companies began to develop hip-specific instruments, including telescoping cannulas for the joint, and both hand and motorized tools. These telescoping cannulas maintained portal access throughout the surgical procedure, and larger interchangeable cannulas could be used if loose bodies needed to be removed. In addition to improvements in optical resolution, the hip-specific tools included long alligator-type graspers; straight, curved, and motorized shavers; and burrs for removing bony or chondral pathology. More recently, electrothermal tools were used for both cartilage and synovial pathology within the hip joint. Additional tools continue to be developed.

Imaging

Historically, diagnostic imaging capabilities limited the indications for hip arthroscopy. Although radiographs provide an excellent overview of the bony morphology of the hip joint, they are not able to visualize chondral or synovial pathology. Digital imaging such as CAT scans and later MRI scans improved soft tissue visualization, particularly of the muscles; vascular supply to the femoral head; and ligamentous structures in and around the hip joint. However, multiple authors showed the limitations of the noncontrast MRI scan in diagnosing chondral pathology of the hip joint. The gadolinium arthrogram MRI scan was developed.[24–28] This contrast technique showed marked improvement in diagnosing the labral pathology within the hip joint. In addition to the improved resolution provided by the contrast, oblique and radial imaging allowed better visualization of the anterior half of the hip joint where much of the labral pathology exists. More recently, Leunig and colleagues[29] and Potter and colleagues[30] showed considerable improvement in noncontrast MRI imaging using multiple radial thin-slice high-resolution imaging to further improve the diagnostic capability.

Procedural Treatment

Initially, hip arthroscopy was used for diagnostic purposes only. This technique was performed in hundreds of cases in Japan as part of a pelvic osteotomy, but no surgical procedure was performed. Once adequate distraction techniques were developed and tools created for treatment, therapeutic procedures were instituted. Initially these procedures consisted of biopsy of the synovium, and were performed by Aignan[31] in 1975 and Holgersson and colleagues[13] in 1981, particularly for children with collagen vascular disease. Later, loose bodies were removed, and in 1980 Warren and Brooker[32] published on the removal of bone cement after a dislocated total hip replacement. Both Glick[4] and McCarthy and Lee[33] published on loose body removal.

The Labrum

Although initially labral injuries were not thought possible, improvements in imaging and direct visualization with arthroscopy conclusively proved the existence of this labral pathology. McCarthy and colleagues[19,20] performed a vascular study on the labrum and showed that most labral injuries occur in a white, nonvascularized zone of the labrum, and consequently that surgical intervention is necessary for symptomatic improvement in these patients. Later, Philippon[34] corroborated this study, showing that the vascularized red zone existed only adjacent to the capsular insertion. For this reason, the treatment of labral tears expanded considerably throughout the past 20 years. McCarthy and Lee[33] published a classification of the labral tears, showing that the outcome of an arthroscopic hip procedure was related to not only treatment of a labral tear but also the extent of chondral damage to the acetabulum and femoral head. This finding has been corroborated by multiple subsequent studies performed even 10 years later.[35–38] Glick[16] and Villar[23] also classified labral tears and showed similar findings. Labral repair has become progressively more important as knowledge of the suction seal and its mechanical role continues to evolve. These repair techniques have paralleled further developments in hip-specific instrumentation, including suture. Multiple authors have shown equivalent or improved outcomes of labral repair in appropriate lesions at short-term follow-up.[38–40]

Chondral Lesions

Chondral lesions of the hip joint occur with considerable frequency. In the study by McCarthy and colleagues,[20] they were numerically more frequent than labral lesions. Preoperative diagnosis of chondral lesions using contemporary imaging is difficult. Improvements in chondral imaging, such as dGEMRIC, are gradually improving diagnosis of chondral lesions within the joint. These lesions, which are always white-zone lesions, must be diagnosed and treated at the time of the procedure or symptoms will not resolve. Studies have shown that the existence and size of chondral lesions largely determine patient outcome.[9,17,35,36,41,42]

Extra-articular Lesions

Although arthroscopy of the hip was initially confined to central and peripheral compartment access, more recently extra-articular procedures have been performed with increasing frequency. These areas of access include the iliopsoas tendon. Glick[4] initially published on this for patients with recurrent psoas tendinitis. The tendon release was initially at the lesser trochanter. Wettstein and colleagues[43] on recession at the joint capsule level (personal communication), Ilizaliturri and colleagues[44] published a technique of arthroscopic iliotibial band resection, and Voos and colleagues[45] published on techniques for addressing tears of the gluteus medius tendon. In addition, Byrd has described removal of heterotropic bone in the extra-articular space from an old rectus avulsion fracture.[46] Further developments in extra-articular access and treatment are expected.

Peripheral Compartment

Perhaps the area of most significant interest in recent years has been treatment of peripheral compartment pathologies. Initially, peripheral compartment visualization allowed treatments for loose bodies either individually or as part of synovial chondromatosis. Synovectomy could also be performed for conditions such as pigmented villonodular synovitis, rheumatoid arthritis, and recurrent synovitis. Most recently, interest is evolving in treatment of bony morphologic abnormalities of the femoral head or acetabulum. These cam (femoral head neck junction) or pincer (acetabulum) deformities have been found to limit hip motion or result in the development of hip intra-articular cartilage pathology. Further improvements in radiologic imaging and three-dimensional CT scan imaging have helped promote further understand of these deformities. Ganz, Leunig,[47] Philippon and colleagues,[10,48] and others[49,50] have contributed greatly to the understanding of these conditions. Published work in this area has been limited by short follow-up, but initial results are encouraging.

Brunner and colleagues[51] evaluated 50 patients whose peripheral compartments were decompressed arthroscopically with or without a CT-guided navigation system. Both groups had a 24% rate of inadequate decompression according to radiologic guidelines, but neither showed a clinical difference.

Classification of Lesions

Labral lesions have been categorized both descriptively initially and later functionally as related to the cartilage surfaces of the joint. In addition, the outcome of a hip procedure has been shown to be directly correlated with the extent of arthritic wear. These findings have been corroborated with later follow-up.[17,40] Initially, the Harris Hip Score was used to determine outcome, but because of its limitations in a young active population, other scoring systems were developed. The first validated outcome score in young patients that included an activity scale was the Nonarthritic Hip Score, and this was validated in several languages.[52] Later the hip outcome score was developed and is analogous in purpose.[53]

The Future

Interest in hip arthroscopy and understanding of the biologic joint continues to evolve exponentially. This interest is multinational and underscores the importance of common definitions of pathology and of outcome. For this reason, MAHORN (Multicenter Arthroscopic Hip Outcome Research Network) was developed, which is a multinational study group working to help elucidate and classify uniformly the definition of labral and chondral injuries of the femoral head and the acetabulum, and both ligament and capsular deformities in and about the hip. This type of multinational group endeavor will improve the clarity of lesions and their treatment. In addition, a MAHORN hip outcome tool has been finalized. This 14- or 33-question scoring system has been validated and refined, and will be validated in multiple languages. This type of endeavor will allow further prospective multicenter studies. As an outgrowth of these efforts, the International Society of Hip Arthroscopy was developed with the goal of furthering the work of clinical research via the MAHORN group and increasing the basic science understanding of labral, chondral, and bony abnormalities in and about the hip joint. It is working toward an international registry that will further allow development of prospective studies using the same classification systems, and is spawning the development of further social networking, allowing immediate information exchange among like-minded clinicians around the world.

SUMMARY

Hip arthroscopy is continuing to evolve. Like the knee and shoulder joints, it began with resection of pathologies and later progressed to repair of different tissues. There is an increasing impetus for reconstruction of biologic joints; although this has occurred with other joints, hip arthroscopic procedures are now headed in this direction. Thus, despite considerable initial challenges, multiple opportunities are now available in this fertile field.

REFERENCES

1. Robertson WJ, Kelly BT. The safe zone for hip arthroscopy: a cadaveric assessment of central, peripheral, and lateral compartment portal placement. Arthroscopy 2008;24(9):1019–26.
2. Burman M. Arthroscopy or the direct visualization of joints. J Bone Joint Surg 1931;4:669–95.
3. Eriksson E, Sebik A. Arthroscopy and arthroscopic surgery in a gas versus a fluid medium. Orthop Clin North Am 1982;13(2):293–8.
4. Glick JM. Hip arthroscopy using the lateral approach. Instr Course Lect 1988;37: 223–31.
5. Johnson L. Arthroscopic surgery principles and practice. St Louis (MO): CV Mosby; 1986.
6. Byrd JW, Pappas JN, Pedley MJ. Hip arthroscopy: an anatomic study of portal placement and relationship to the extra-articular structures [see comments]. Arthroscopy 1995;11(4):418–23.
7. Glick JM, Sampson TG, Gordon RB, et al. Hip arthroscopy by the lateral approach. Arthroscopy 1987;3(1):4–12.
8. Dorfmann H, Boyer T. Hip arthroscopy utilizing the supine position. Arthroscopy 1996;12(2):264–7.
9. Dienst M, Kohn D. [Hip arthroscopy. Minimal invasive diagnosis and therapy of the diseased or injured hip joint]. Unfallchirurg 2001;104(1):2–18 [in German].
10. Philippon MJ, Yen YM, Briggs KK, et al. Early outcomes after hip arthroscopy for femoroacetabular impingement in the athletic adolescent patient: a preliminary report. J Pediatr Orthop 2008;28(7):705–10.
11. Enseki KR, Martin RL, Draovitch P, et al. The hip joint: arthroscopic procedures and postoperative rehabilitation. J Orthop Sports Phys Ther 2006;36(7):516–25.
12. Guanche CA, Bare AA. Arthroscopic treatment of femoroacetabular impingement. Arthroscopy 2006;22(1):95–106.
13. Gross R. Arthroscopy in hip disorders in children. Orthop Rev 1977;6:43–9.
14. Holgersson S, Brattstrom H, Mogensen B, et al. Arthroscopy of the hip in juvenile chronic arthritis. J Pediatr Orthop 1981;1(3):273–8.
15. Locker B, Beguin J. L'arthroscopie de hanche. J Med Lyon 1984;1394:25–6.
16. Glick J. Operative arthroscopy. New York: Raven Press; 1991.
17. McCarthy JC, Busconi B. The role of hip arthroscopy in the diagnosis and treatment of hip disease. Orthopedics 1995;18(8):753–6.
18. Farjo LA, Glick JM, Sampson TG. Hip arthroscopy for acetabular labral tears. Arthroscopy 1999;15(2):132–7.
19. McCarthy JC, Noble PC, Schuck MR, et al. The watershed labral lesion: its relationship to early arthritis of the hip. J Arthroplasty 2001;16(8 Suppl 1):81–7.
20. McCarthy JC, Noble PC, Schuck MR, et al. The Otto E. Aufranc award: the role of labral lesions to development of early degenerative hip disease. Clin Orthop 2001;393:25–37.
21. Byrd JW, Pappas JN, Pedley MJ. Hip arthroscopy: an anatomic study of portal placement and relationship to the extra-articular structures. Arthroscopy 1995; 11(4):418–23.
22. Dorfmann H, Boyer T, De Bie B. [Arthroscopy of the hip. Methods and values]. Rev Rhum Ed Fr 1993;60(5):330–4 [in French].
23. Villar RN. Hip arthroscopy. Br J Hosp Med 1992;47(10):763–6.
24. Bencardino JT, Kassarjian A, Palmer WE. Magnetic resonance imaging of the hip: sports-related injuries. Top Magn Reson Imaging 2003;14(2):145–60.

25. Schedel H, Wicht L, Maurer J, et al. Differential diagnosis in variants or abnormal-ities of the hip on MRI. Bildgebung 1994;61(1):20–4.
26. Newman JS, Newberg AH. MRI of the painful hip in athletes. Clin Sports Med 2006;25(4):613–33.
27. Newberg AH, Newman JS. Imaging the painful hip. Clin Orthop Relat Res 2003; 406:19–28.
28. Palmer WE. MR arthrography of the hip. Semin Musculoskelet Radiol 1998;2(4): 349–62.
29. Leunig M, Werlen S, Ungersbock A, et al. Evaluation of the acetabular labrum by MR arthrography. J Bone Joint Surg Br 1997;79(2):230–4.
30. Potter HG, Schachar J. High resolution noncontrast MRI of the hip. J Magn Reson Imaging 2010;31(2):268–78.
31. Aignan M. Arthroscopy of the hip. In: Proceedings of the International Association of Arthroscopy. Rev Int Rheumatol 1976:33.
32. Warren SB, Brooker AF Jr. Excision of heterotopic bone followed by irradiation after total hip arthroplasty. J Bone Joint Surg Am 1992;74(2):201–10.
33. McCarthy JC, Lee JA. Arthroscopic intervention in early hip disease. Clin Orthop Relat Res 2004;429:157–62.
34. Philippon MJ. New frontiers in hip arthroscopy: the role of arthroscopic hip labral repair and capsulorrhaphy in the treatment of hip disorders. Instr Course Lect 2006;55:309–16.
35. McCarthy JC, Jarrett BT, Ojeifo O, et al. What factors influence long-term survivor-ship after hip arthroscopy? Clin Orthop Relat Res 2011;469(2):362–71.
36. Byrd JW, Jones KS. Hip arthroscopy for labral pathology: prospective analysis with 10-year follow-up. Arthroscopy 2009;25(4):365–8.
37. Byrd JW, Jones KS. Hip arthroscopy in athletes: 10-year follow-up. Am J Sports Med 2009;37(11):2140–3.
38. Kelly BT, Weiland DE, Schenker ML, et al. Arthroscopic labral repair in the hip: surgical technique and review of the literature. Arthroscopy 2005;21(12): 1496–504.
39. Philippon MJ, Schroder e Souza BG, Briggs KK. Labrum: resection, repair and reconstruction sports medicine and arthroscopy review. Sports Med Arthrosc 2010;18(2):76–82.
40. Safran MR. The acetabular labrum: anatomic and functional characteristics and rationale for surgical intervention. J Am Acad Orthop Surg 2010;18(6): 338–45.
41. McCarthy JC, Lee JA. Acetabular dysplasia: a paradigm of arthroscopic exami-nation of chondral injuries. Clin Orthop 2002;405:122–8.
42. Margheritini F, Villar RN. The efficacy of arthroscopy in the treatment of hip oste-oarthritis. Chir Organi Mov 1999;84(3):257–61.
43. Wettstein M, Jung J, Dienst M. Arthroscopic psoas tenotomy. Arthroscopy 2006; 22:907.
44. Ilizaliturri VM Jr, Martinez-Escalante FA, Chaidez PA, et al. Endoscopic iliotibial band release for external snapping hip syndrome. Arthroscopy 2006;22(5):505–10.
45. Voos JE, Shindle MK, Pruett A, et al. Endoscopic repair of gluteus medius tendon tears of the hip. Am J Sports Med 2009;37(4):743–7.
46. Byrd JC. Advanced arthroscopy. In: Arthroscopy of the hip and application: supine position. p. 318. Chapter 27.
47. Leunig M, Beaule PE, Ganz R. The concept of femoroacetabular impingement: current status and future perspectives. Clin Orthop Relat Res 2009;467(3): 616–22.

48. Philippon MJ, Briggs KK, Hay CJ, et al. Arthroscopic labral reconstruction in the hip using iliotibial band autograft: technique and early outcomes. Arthroscopy 2010;26(6):750–6.
49. Reichenbach S, Juni P, Werlen S, et al. Prevalence of cam-type deformity on hip magnetic resonance imaging in young males: a cross-sectional study. Arthritis Care Res (Hoboken) 2010;62(9):1319–27.
50. Shetty VD, Villar RN. Hip arthroscopy: current concepts and review of literature. Br J Sports Med 2007;41(2):64–8 [discussion: 68].
51. Brunner A, Horisberger M, Herzog RF. Evaluation of a computed tomography-based navigation system prototype for hip arthroscopy in the treatment of femoroacetabular cam impingement. Arthroscopy 2009;25(4):382–91.
52. Christensen CP, Althausen PL, Mittleman MA, et al. The nonarthritic hip score: reliable and validated. Clin Orthop Relat Res 2003;406:75–83.
53. Martin RL, Philippon MJ. Evidence of reliability and responsiveness for the hip outcome score. Arthroscopy 2008;24(6):676–82.

Clinical Diagnosis of Hip Pain

Matthew Plante, MD[a],*, Roxanne Wallace, MD[b],
Brian D. Busconi, MD[c]

KEYWORDS

- Hip pain • Intra-articular hip pathology
- Extra-articular hip pathology • Clinical history of hip pain

This article reviews the evaluation of the hip including the clinical history and physical examination. Of all the major joints, the hip remains the most difficult to evaluate for most orthopedic clinicians. Before the advent of MRI and hip arthroscopy, osteoarthritis was the major diagnosis associated with this joint. A recent study estimated that more than 25% of the population will develop symptomatic hip arthritis before the age of 85.[1] As our understanding of hip pathology evolves, and arthroscopic and other minimally invasive operative techniques continue to improve, the focus is shifting toward earlier identification of hip pathology. Risk factors for the development of arthritis are now well established and include femoral acetabular impingement (FAI), labral tearing, developmental dysplasia, and slipped capital femoral epiphysis (SCFE).[2–6] Emerging treatment options may address these conditions in the early stages and prevent or slow the progression of hip degeneration.

HISTORY

The first step in evaluating the hip is to obtain a thorough history from the patient. The presence or absence of trauma, as well as the duration and severity of symptoms, should be determined. The examiner should inquire about prior hip consultations, past surgeries, and old injuries. Exacerbating and alleviating factors should be identified. Specific activities of daily living that are limited should be documented. Information regarding prior treatments including activity modifications, oral medications, physical therapy, injections, and assistive devices should be obtained.

The first step is to delineate intra-articular versus extra-articular disorders. This is accomplished by determining the exact location of the pain (**Fig. 1**). Typically, intra-

[a] Foundry Orthopedics & Sports Medicine, 285 Promenade Street, Providence, RI 02908, USA
[b] Department of Sports Medicine, University of Massachusetts Memorial Medical Center, 281 Lincoln Street, Worcester, MA 01605, USA
[c] Department of Orthopedics and Physical Rehabilitation, University of Massachusetts Medical School, 281 Lincoln Street, Worcester, MA 01605-2192, USA
* Corresponding author.
E-mail address: mplante1414@hotmail.com

Clin Sports Med 30 (2011) 225–238
doi:10.1016/j.csm.2010.12.003
0278-5919/11/$ – see front matter © 2011 Elsevier Inc. All rights reserved.

sportsmed.theclinics.com

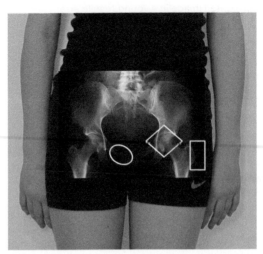

Fig. 1. Intra-articular pathology presents as groin pain, diamond shape. Extra-articular pathology such as lower abdomen or at the adductor tubercle can indicate athletic pubalgia, oval shape. Pain located around the greater trochanter and associated with snapping can be snapping hip syndrome/trochanteric bursitis, rectangle shape.

articular pathology presents as groin pain that may radiate to the knee. Pain located in the thigh or buttocks, or pain that radiates distally below the knee, is likely to originate from the lumbar spine or buttock and proximal thigh musculature.[7] Pain located in the lower abdomen and/or at the adductor tubercle can indicate athletic pubalgia. Pain located around the greater trochanter and associated with snapping can be snapping hip syndrome. Identification of associated symptoms such as weakness or numbness, back pain, and exacerbation with coughing or sneezing, may indicate thoracolumbar pathology.[8]

Past medical and surgical history, as well as any developmental problems should be explored. Patients should specifically be asked about systemic illnesses such as malignancy, coagulopathies, and inflammatory disorders. Various coagulation and metabolic disorders have been shown to impede vascular supply to the femoral head.[9] Social history should be reviewed to determine current or prior use of alcohol, steroids, and tobacco, which might place the patient at risk for osteonecrosis.[7]

Recreational history and athletic participation should be probed, as certain sports including soccer, rugby, martial arts, and long-distance running are associated with an increased incidence of degenerative hip disease when compared with the general population.[10] Hip pain in elite athletes and patients sustaining low-energy trauma is often caused by anterior labral tears and acetabular chondral defects.[11] Patients with clicking or locking are likely to have a mechanical cause, such as labral tearing or loose bodies. Traumatic or inflammatory conditions more frequently present with anterior groin pain and decreased range of motion.

To help quantify the severity of symptoms, various hip-scoring systems have been developed.[12] Some quantify hip function into numeric value, whereas others categorize using descriptive terms such as excellent, good, fair, and poor.[13] The most frequently used functional scores include the Harris Hip Score, the Charnley Hip Score, the Hospital for Special Surgery Score, and the Merle d'Aubigné. Visual analog pain score is frequently used because of its simplicity and ease of use.

Although frequently cited in surgical outcomes literature, different scoring systems may produce varying assessments of the same individual.

PHYSICAL EXAMINATION

Because hip pain may be a result of intra-articular hip pathology as well as a myriad of extra-articular and referred sources of pain, it is crucial to perform a consistent, comprehensive physical examination to best identify the underlying diagnosis. An appropriate physical examination should begin with documentation of vital signs including patient temperature. Although rare, hip pyathrosis should be considered in any febrile patient with hip pain. Other conditions that may produce fever and pain radiating to the hip include pelvic inflammatory disease, urinary tract infection, psoas abscess, and prostatitis.[7] The position in which the patient keeps the hip while at rest may provide useful information regarding the underlying pathology. Patients with synovitis or a hip effusion will often keep the hip in a flexed, abducted, and externally rotated position, as this position places the hip capsule at its largest potential volume.

Upright Exam

Examining the upright patient can provide useful information regarding the diagnosis. This portion of the evaluation should include evaluation of gait, pelvic obliquity, and single leg stance. Assessment of gait should be performed in an area large enough to accommodate several patient strides. An antalgic gait will have a shortened stance phase to limit the duration of weight bearing on the affected side. Exaggeration of normal pelvic rotation may also be observed with certain pathologic conditions. A Trendelenburg gait is characterized by abductor weakness. Clinically, the gluteus medius and minimus are not strong enough to keep the pelvis level, and as a result, the pelvis will drop on the contralateral side during the stance phase of gait. As this weakness progresses, a compensatory shift of weight toward the affected side may occur. Known as an abductor lurch, this gait pattern places the center of gravity closer to the hip and thus decreases the force required from the abductors. These gait patterns may be an indicator of underlying intra-articular pathology but are also seen in patients with certain extra-articular problems.[7]

Pelvic obliquity may reflect either an underlying scoliosis or leg length discrepancy. Normally, when a patient stands, the height of the iliac crests should be symmetric. Pelvic obliquity is present if an imaginary line drawn between the iliac crests is not level with the floor. A true leg length discrepancy is present if the distance from the femoral head to the plantar aspect of the foot is not symmetric when measured on long leg radiographs. This may occur as the result of significant angular deformity of the hip, congenital hypoplasia, or a femoral or tibial growth plate injury. On physical examination, leg length is measured using a tape measure to determine the distance between the anterior superior iliac spine (ASIS) and the distal aspect of the ipsilateral medial malleolus. Leg length discrepancy has been postulated to contribute to an array of associated orthopedic conditions.[14–16]

If the leg lengths are equal in the presence of pelvic obliquity, a functional leg length discrepancy is present. This is assessed clinically by measuring the distance from the umbilicus to bilateral medial malleoli. Contractures of the hip have been implicated as a cause of functional leg length discrepancy[17,18] Compensation for these contractures produces a pelvic obliquity.

A single leg stance, or Trendelenburg test, is helpful in identifying a patient with weakened abductor muscles (**Fig. 2**). This test is performed by having the patient stand on one leg with the contralateral knee and hip flexed. A patient with intact

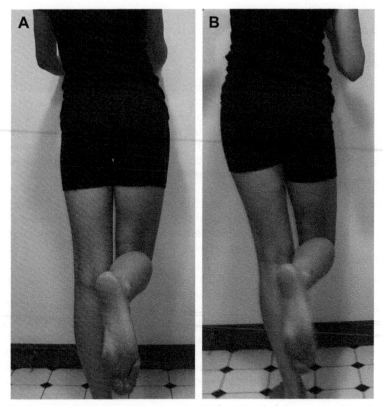

Fig. 2. The Trendelenburg test (*A*) is normal with functional abductors resulting in a level pelvis. (*B*) Weak abductors allow the pelvis to fall into obliquity.

abductors will lift the pelvis level with the stance limb. Abductor weakness is present if the pelvis drops contralateral to the stance leg or the patient shifts his or her entire body over the stance leg to compensate for the deficient abductors.

Having the standing patient identify the site of greatest discomfort can provide clues to the underlying diagnosis. A frequently reported sign in patients with intra-articular hip pathology is the "C-Sign" (**Fig. 3**).[8] When asked to localize the pain, the patient will hold his or her hand in the shape of a C with the thumb positioned superior to the greater trochanter and the index finger over the groin.

Palpation

Identifying localized tenderness may help determine the patient's diagnosis. Palpating bony prominences around the hip is an essential part of the physical examination. The ASIS is the origin of the sartorius, a common location of apophyseal avulsion fractures in adolescent athletes. Just medial to the ASIS, the lateral femoral cutaneous nerve crosses under the inguinal ligament. Compression of the nerve at this site, known as meralgia parasthetica, may produce dysesthesias over the proximal anterolateral aspect of the thigh. Reproduction of symptoms with deep palpation just medial to the ASIS is diagnostic for this condition. Tenderness and swelling at the iliac crest following direct trauma is caused by hematoma formation and is commonly known as a "hip pointer." The anterior inferior iliac spine (AIIS) is the origin of the rectus

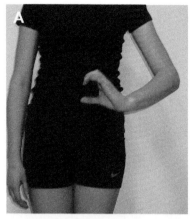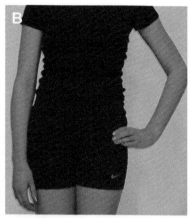

Fig. 3. The "C" sign (*A*) and placed over the hip (*B*).

femoris. Tenderness at this location in a skeletally immature athlete suggests an apophyseal avulsion injury.

Tenderness at the pubic symphysis or ramus may occur as the result of recurrent stress created by powerful adductors. This condition, termed pubic syphysitis or osteitis pubis, is most frequently seen in soccer and hockey players.[19] Tenderness over the greater trochanter is seen with trochanteric bursitis. Tenderness posterior to the greater trochanter is suggestive of piriformis tendonitis, whereas tenderness just superior to the greater trochanter may be because of gluteus medius tendonitis.

The ischial tuberosity may be palpated with the patient either prone or in the supine position with the hip flexed. Acute tenderness at this site is found in hamstring avulsion injuries. Tenderness in the absence of acute injury may be attributable to inflammation of the overlying bursa. Ischiogluteal bursitis, or *weaver's bottom*, is most commonly found in seated athletes such as rowers, bikers, and equestrian athletes.[20]

Range of Motion

It is important to evaluate hip range of motion with the patient in both the seated and supine positions (**Fig. 4**). The seated position allows for a more accurate assessment of hip rotation, as the pelvis is better stabilized in this position. Always remember to assess both the affected and contralateral sides for comparison. Diminished internal rotation suggests intra-articular pathology. Excessive femoral anteversion will present with increased internal rotation and decreased external rotation. Clinically, femoral anteversion is assessed with the patient in the prone position. The knee is then flexed to 90°, and using the leg as a lever, the hip is internally rotated until the lateral aspect of the greater trochanter is felt to be most prominent. Femoral anteversion is measured by the angle between the tibia and an imaginary vertical line.

Hip flexion and extension are best assessed with the patient supine on the examining table. It is important to distinguish motion from the hip joint itself from complementary or compensatory motion occurring in the pelvis and lumbar spine.[21] From this position, the knee is flexed and brought toward the patient's chest. To assess hip extension, both hips are first maximally flexed at the same time. The side being tested for extension is then brought back down to the table while the contralateral side is held tightly flexed. Neutral extension is achieved if the posterior aspect of the extending thigh makes contact with the examination table. A flexion contracture

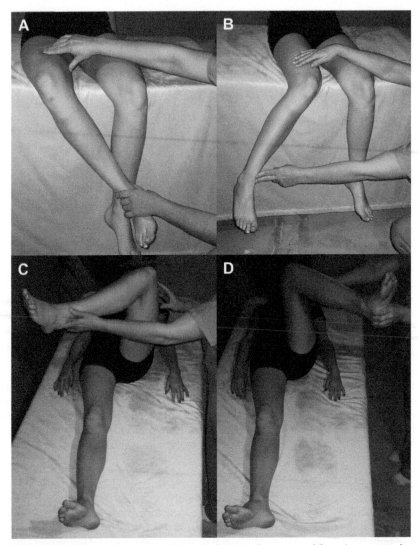

Fig. 4. (A) Seated external rotation; (B) seated internal rotation; (C) supine external rotation; (D) supine internal rotation.

is present if the thigh cannot touch the table (Thompson test) (**Fig. 5**). Abduction and adduction are measured in the supine position, with the hip either flexed or extended (**Fig. 6**). Care must be taken to stabilize the pelvis with one hand to get accurate measurements.

Provocative Tests

Intra-articular pathology

The dynamic external rotatory impingement test (DEXRIT) and the dynamic internal rotatory impingement test (DIRI) are both performed with the patient lying supine with the contralateral leg maximally flexed to eliminate lumbar lordosis. The affected hip is then brought to 90° of flexion. In the DIRI, the hip is passively ranged through a wide

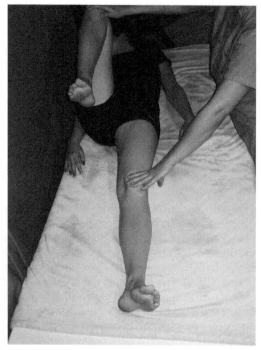

Fig. 5. The Thompson test.

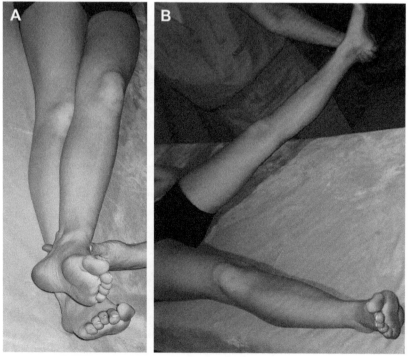

Fig. 6. (*A, B*) Adduction and abduction.

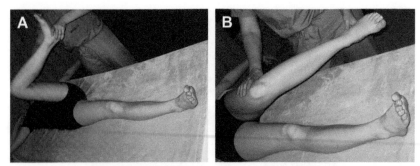

Fig. 7. DIRI, dynamic internal rotation impingement test: (*A*) beginning position, (*B*) end position.

arc of adduction and internal rotation (**Fig. 7**). In the DEXRIT, the hip is passively ranged through a wide arc of abduction and external rotation (**Fig. 8**). For both maneuvers, a positive test will recreate the patient's pain. Both tests may be performed during arthroscopy to provide direct visualization of femoral neck and acetabular congruence.

The flexion/adduction/internal rotation (FADDIR) test may be performed in either the supine or lateral positions (**Fig. 9**). The examined hip is passively brought into flexion, adduction, and internal rotation. Reproduction of the patient's pain indicates a positive test. The degree of flexion and internal rotation achieved at the onset of pain should be documented. Although very sensitive for intra-articular hip pathology, this test has been shown to yield a high percentage of false positive results.[22]

The groin pain provoked by the dynamic test described by McCarthy[23] indicates intra-articular pathology as well. It is performed by starting with maximum flexion, adduction, and internal rotation moving to full extension, then immediately moving into maximum flexion, abduction, and external rotation moving to full extension.

Having the patient perform a straight leg raise against resistance, known as the Stinchfield test, is an effective screening tool for intra-articular hip pathology. The patient is asked to perform an active straight leg raise to 45°, and then the examiner directs a downward force just superior to the patient's knee. A positive test produces either pain or weakness. This maneuver is designed to simulate normal walking and creates a force double the patient's body weight across the hip joint.[21] With active resistance, the psoas places pressure on the labrum, and thus helps detect intra-articular pathology.

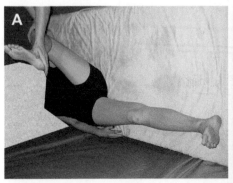
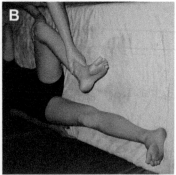

Fig. 8. DEXRIT, dynamic external rotation impingement test: (*A*) starting position, (*B*) end position.

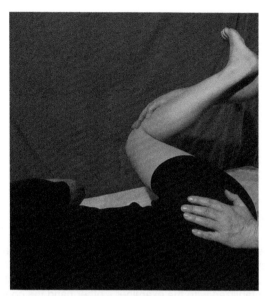

Fig. 9. FADDIR, flexion adduction and internal rotation test. Shown in the lateral position.

Extra-articular pathologies, including hip flexor tendonitis, a hip flexor avulsion fracture, or a psoas abscess, will also produce a positive result.

The foveal distraction test is performed with the patient in the supine position. The leg is abducted 30° and axial traction is placed on the leg. This maneuver reduces intra-articular pressure, and relief of pain is indicative of an intra-articular source of hip pain.

The heel strike test is a useful test to evaluate for a femoral neck stress fracture. With the examined leg lying straight on the table, the heel is struck firmly. This maneuver simulates the onset of the stance phase of gait, when stresses across the femoral neck are greatest. Pain in the groin with heel strike is suggestive of possible stress fracture.[24] The hop test is another effective test to diagnose a stress fracture. The patient performs a single leg hop on the affected leg. Pain in the groin, hip, or anterior thigh is considered a positive test.

Extra-articular pathology
Sacroiliac joint The flexion/abduction/external rotation test (FABER), also know as the Patrick test, is helpful to detect sacroiliac pain (**Fig. 10**). The patient is placed supine and the examined extremity is place in the figure-4 position with the knee flexed and the ipsilateral ankle resting on the contralateral thigh. The examiner directs a downward force of the flexed knee with one hand while stabilizing the pelvis at the contralateral ASIS with the other hand. This test stresses the sacroiliac joint and should not normally produce pain. If this maneuver produces posterior hip pain, sacroiliac joint pathology should be suspected. The FABER test will often elicit pain with true intra-articular hip pathology; however, the pain will typically be localized to the anterior groin.[21,23]

Gaenslen's test is another test that places stress on the sacroiliac (SI) joint. The patient is positioned supine with the examined hip shifted toward the side of the table. Both knees are flexed up toward the patient's chest. The examiner stabilizes the pelvis with one hand while extending the examined thigh over the edge of the table. This maneuver stresses the sacroiliac joint and is positive if the patient experiences pain on the provoked side.[25]

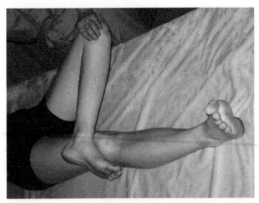

Fig. 10. FABER test, flexion abduction and external rotation.

The posterior pelvic pain provocation test is another means of assessing SI joint pathology. The test is performed with the patient supine and the hip to be tested flexed to an angle of 90°. An axial load is then applied along the longitudinal axis of the femur while the pelvis is stabilized with the examiner's other hand the contralateral ASIS. A positive test will reproduce the patient's pain deep in the gluteal region.[25]

Pubic symphysis The pubic symphysis stress test is useful for identifying pathology at that site. The test is performed in the supine position. One of the examiner's hands is placed at the superior border at one side of the pubis, and the other is placed at the inferior border of the pubis on the contralateral side. The two hands are then pressed together, creating a shearing force at the pubic symphysis.[21] A positive test will reproduce the patient's pain at this location.

The lateral pelvic compression test may be performed in the supine or lateral positions. In the lateral position, the examiner directs a downward force on the iliac crest, compressing the pelvis against the examining table. In the supine position, the examiner uses both hands to compress the iliac crests together. These maneuvers produce a compression force at the pubic symphysis, which, in a positive test, will cause pain at that site.

Contractures A number of tests are useful for diagnosing extra-articular hip pathology. Ober's test is useful for diagnosing a contracture of the iliotibial band. A tight iliotibial band is associated with trochanteric bursitis and external snapping hip syndrome,[26] as well as knee pathology, such as iliotibial band friction syndrome and patellofemoral dysfunction.[27] Ober's test is performed in the lateral decubitus position with the affected side facing up. The knee is flexed 90° and the hip is brought into maximal extension (**Fig. 11**). While stabilizing the pelvis, knee flexion and hip extension is maintained while the leg is adducted. Inability to adduct the hip past the midline of the body indicates the presence of an iliotibial band contracture.

Hamstring tightness may be diagnosed by the presence of a tripod sign. The patient sits on the edge of the examining table. The examiner then passively extends the patient's knee and watches for any compensatory motion at the hips. Normally, the patient should obtain full passive knee extension while remaining in the seated, upright position. The presence of hamstring tightness will result in compensatory extension of the ipsilateral hip, seen clinically as the leaning back.

The Ely test is helpful in diagnosing contractures of the rectus femoris muscle. The test is performed with the patient in the prone position and both knees extended. The

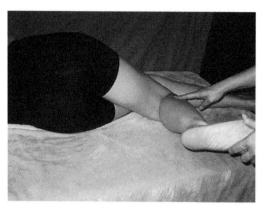

Fig. 11. Ober's test: maximal extension and adduction in the lateral position tests for iliotibial band tightness.

knee on the examined side is then passively flexed. Normally, the knee should flex fully without any compensatory movement from the hip or pelvis. Because the rectus femoris crosses both the knee and hip, in the case of a contracture, full passive flexion will cause an involuntary, compensatory flexion of the hip.

The Phelps test is helpful to diagnose contractures of the gracilis muscle. With the patient in the prone position, both knees are fully extended. Both hips are then maximally abducted. The knees are then flexed to relax the gracilis muscles. If the hips are able to abduct further with the knees flexed, then a gracilis contracture is present. This phenomenon occurs because the gracilis crosses both the hip and knee joints.

Snapping hip The diagnosis of snapping hip syndrome is guided by history and physical examination. Symptom onset is generally insidious. Localization of the pain can help distinguish external from internal causes. External snapping hip (coxa sultans externa) produces tenderness over the greater trochanter, and the pain can be reproduced with repetitive flexion and extension. Ober's test is helpful in establishing the diagnosis of a contracted iliotibial band. The bicycle test is also helpful in diagnosing external snapping hip syndrome. The test is performed with the patient in the lateral position with the tested side up. A bicycle pedaling motion is simulated, and a positive test will reproduce snapping of the iliotibial band.

Internal causes of snapping hip produce pain along the inguinal crease and medial thigh. The snapping occurs when the iliopsoas is suddenly forced under tension over the iliopectineal eminence or the femoral head. The snap can be made more obvious if the hip is ranged from a flexed, abducted, and externally rotated position to an adducted, internally rotated, and extended position. This motion moves the iliopsoas tendon from a position lateral to the femoral head to a position medial to the femoral head and is associated with a very loud clunk. Gentle pressure over the femoral head prohibits the snap from occurring.

Nerve root compression The femoral nerve traction test is performed with the patient in the prone position with a pillow placed under the abdomen. The knee is flexed to 90° and the hip is passively extended. A positive test will produce pain in the anterior or lateral thigh. This finding indicates L2-L4 nerve root impingement.[28]

Sports hernia The resisted sit-up test is helpful in diagnosing a sports hernia. With the patient in the supine position, legs extended, the examiner places a hand on the patient's chest and provides resistance (**Fig. 12**). A positive test produces pain at

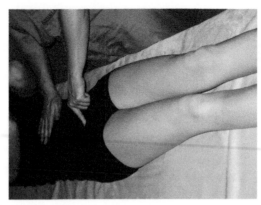

Fig. 12. Resisted sit up: legs extended.

the rectus abdominus insertion or in the groin. The origin of the adductor longus can also be involved in this pathology. The resisted sit-up test is repeated this time with both knees flexed to 90° with the feet remaining flat on the examining table: the examiner uses one hand to brace the patient's feet while a sit-up is initiated, and uses the other hand to provide resistance. This will provoke pain at the adductor longus tendon origin (**Fig. 13**). There will also be tenderness to palpation of the proximal tendon of the adductor longus and pain at this site is provoked by resisted adduction of the hip.

Referred pain When performing a thorough musculoskeletal examination of the hip region, it is important to consider potential sources of referred pain. The groin should be evaluated for femoral or inguinal hernias. An abdominal examination should be performed to rule out a gastrointestinal cause of pain. Other known sources of referred pain include renal problems, such as nephrolithiasis, and gynecologic issues, such as ovarian cysts and pelvic inflammatory disease. Vascular problems such femoral aneurysms and pseudoaneurysms often present as hip pain and are diagnosed as a palpable, pulsatile mass.[7]

DIAGNOSTIC STUDIES

Laboratory studies have a limited role in the evaluation of hip pathology, and no studies are routinely ordered in this setting. If there is concern for a possible infectious

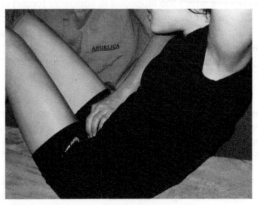

Fig. 13. Resisted sit up: legs flexed.

etiology, a complete blood count (CBC), erythrocyte sedimentation rate (ESR), and C-reactive protein (CRP) may be helpful to establish a diagnosis. In certain areas, Lyme infection should be added. Occasional gout can produce hip pain and can be diagnosed by a joint aspiration tested for crystals. For patients with potential rheumatologic causes of hip pain, rheumatoid factor (RF) and human leukocyte antigen B27 (HLA-B27) should be obtained.[7]

SUMMARY

It is vitally important to elucidate intra-articular versus extra-articular pathology of hip pain in every step of the patient encounter: history, physical examination, and imaging. The role of imaging studies will be discussed in another article.

REFERENCES

1. Murphy LB, Helmick CG, Schwartz TA, et al. One in four people may develop symptomatic hip osteoarthritis in his or her lifetime. Osteoarthritis Cartilage 2010;18:1372–9.
2. Ganz R, Parvizi J, Beck M, et al. Femoroacetabular impingement: a cause for osteoarthritis of the hip. Clin Orthop Relat Res 2003;417:112–20.
3. Leunig M, Ganz R. Femoroacetabular impingement. A common cause of hip complaints leading to arthrosis. Unfallchirurg 2005;108(1):9–10, 12–7 [in German].
4. Jessel RH, Zurakowski D, Zilkens C, et al. Radiographic and patient factors associated with pre-radiographic osteoarthritis in hip dysplasia. J Bone Joint Surg Am 2009;91(5):1120–9.
5. Klaue K, Durnin CW, Ganz R. The acetabular rim syndrome. A clinical presentation of dysplasia of the hip. J Bone Joint Surg Br 1991;73(3):423–9.
6. Leunig M, Fraitzl CR, Ganz R. Early damage to the acetabular cartilage in slipped capital femoral epiphysis. Therapeutic consequences. Orthopade 2002;31(9): 894–9 [in German].
7. DeAngelis NA, Busconi BD. Assessment and differential diagnosis of the painful hip. Clin Orthop Relat Res 2003;406:11–8.
8. Martin HD, Shears SA, Palmer IJ. Evaluation of the hip. Sports Med Arthrosc 2010;18(2):63–75.
9. Petrigliano FA, Lieberman JR. Osteonecrosis of the hip: novel approaches to evaluation and treatment. Clin Orthop Relat Res 2007;465:53–62.
10. Kujala UM, Kaprio J, Sarna S. Osteoarthritis of weight-bearing joints of lower limbs in former elite male athletes. BMJ 1994;308(6923):231–4.
11. Fitzgerald RH Jr. Acetabular labrum tears. Diagnosis and treatment. Clin Orthop Relat Res 1995;311:60–8.
12. Andersson G. Hip assessment: a comparison of nine different methods. J Bone Joint Surg Br 1972;54(4):621–5.
13. Bach CM, Feizelmeier H, Kaufmann G, et al. Categorization diminishes the reliability of hip scores. Clin Orthop Relat Res 2003;411:166–73.
14. Harvey WF, Yang M, Cooke TD, et al. Association of leg-length inequality with knee osteoarthritis: a cohort study. Ann Intern Med 2010;152(5):287–95.
15. Segal NA, Harvey W, Felson DT, et al. Leg-length inequality is not associated with greater trochanteric pain syndrome. Arthritis Res Ther 2008;10(3):R62.
16. Soukka A, Alaranta H, Tallroth K, et al. Leg-length inequality in people of working age. The association between mild inequality and low-back pain is questionable. Spine (Phila Pa 1976) 1991;16(4):429–31.

17. Longjohn D, Dorr LD. Soft tissue balance of the hip. J Arthroplasty 1998;13(1): 97–100.
18. Ranawat CS, Rodriguez JA. Functional leg-length inequality following total hip arthroplasty. J Arthroplasty 1997;12(4):359–64.
19. LeBlanc KE, LeBlanc KA. Groin pain in athletes. Hernia 2003;7(2):68–71.
20. Cho KH, Lee SM, Lee YH, et al. Non-infectious ischiogluteal bursitis: MRI findings. Korean J Radiol 2004;5(4):280–6.
21. Reider B. The orthopedic physical examination. 2nd edition. Philadelphia: Elsevior, Inc; 2005.
22. Martin RL, Irrgang JJ, Sekiya JK. The diagnostic accuracy of a clinical examination in determining intra-articular hip pain for potential hip arthroscopy candidates. Arthroscopy 2008;24(9):1013–8.
23. Martin HD, Kelly BT, Leunig M, et al. The pattern and technique in the clinical evaluation of the adult hip: the common physical examination tests of hip specialists. Arthroscopy 2010;26(2):161–72.
24. Ni C. Influence of calcar femoral on stress distribution of the upper femur and its clinical application. Zhonghua Wai Ke Za Zhi 1989;27(6):333–6, 381 [in Chinese].
25. Vleeming A, Albert HB, Ostgaard HC, et al. European guidelines for the diagnosis and treatment of pelvic girdle pain. Eur Spine J 2008;17(6):794–819.
26. Tibor LM, Sekiya JK. Differential diagnosis of pain around the hip joint. Arthroscopy 2008;24(12):1407–21.
27. Puniello MS. Iliotibial band tightness and medial patellar glide in patients with patellofemoral dysfunction. J Orthop Sports Phys Ther 1993;17(3):144–8.
28. Dyck P. The femoral nerve traction test with lumbar disc protrusions. Surg Neurol 1976;3:163–6.

Radiology

Ketan Patel, MD[a,b,*], Roxanne Wallace, MD[c],
Brian D. Busconi, MD[d]

KEYWORDS

- Acetabular labrum tear • Femoroacetabular Impingement (FAI)
- Athletic pubalgia • Bursitis • Stress fracture • Avulsion injuries
- Hip abductor injury

Hip and groin pain are a common complaint among athletes of all ages, and may result from an acute injury or from chronic, repetitive trauma.[1] The hip joint is a functionally and structurally complex joint, consisting of the acetabulum, femoral articulation, supporting soft tissue, muscle, and cartilage structures. Hip injuries can be intraarticular, extraarticular, or both. Clinical findings with such injuries are highly variable. Labral abnormalities may occur in asymptomatic patients as well as in those with incapacitating symptoms and signs.[2] Athletic hip injury leading to disabling intraarticular hip pain most commonly involves labral tear.[3] The extraarticular causes are usually the result of overuse activity, leading to inflammation, tendonitis, or bursitis. In clinical practice, the term athletic pubalgia is used to describe exertional pubic or groin pain. There are many causes of pubalgia, including labral tear of the hip, sacroiliitis, lower lumbar disc disease, adductor dysfunction, osteitis pubis, and athletic pubalgia (also termed sportsman's hernia).[4]

LABRAL CONDITIONS

In young athletes the mechanism of injury is usually trauma, ranging from twisting injury to hip dislocation. Acute traumatic labral tear are more common in sports, requiring extreme hip rotation and flexion. In middle-aged patients (<50 years of age) femoroacetabular impingement (FAI) is a frequent contributing factor. In older patients degenerative tears associated with osteoarthritis of the hip are most commonly seen. Patients with previous hip dislocations and hip dysplasia are at increased risk.

The author has nothing to disclose.
[a] Shields Healthcare Group, 265 Westgate Drive, Brockton, MA 02301, USA
[b] UMASS Medical Center, Department of Radiology, University Campus, 55 Lake Avenue North, Worcester, MA 01655, USA
[c] Department of Sports Medicine, University of Massachusetts Memorial Medical Center, 281 Lincoln Street, Worcester, MA 01605, USA
[d] Department of Orthopedics and Physical Rehabilitation, University of Massachusetts Medical School, 281 Lincoln Street, Worcester, MA 01605-2192, USA
* Corresponding author. Shields Healthcare Group, 265 Westgate Drive, Brockton, MA 02301.
E-mail address: patelketan@me.com

LABRAL VARIANT

The acetabular labrum (**Fig. 1**) is a fibrocartilaginous rim that deepens the socket of the hip joint, although its role in hip stability remains unclear.[5] The labrum is present in approximately two-thirds to three-fourths of the circumference of the acetabulum and is absent along the inferior aspect. The transverse acetabular ligament extends from the anterior to the posterior aspect at the inferior acetabular fossa.

Several labral variations and clinically insignificant findings have been described in asymptomatic patients.[6–8] The posterior inferior sublabral sulcus (**Fig. 2A**) should not be misinterpreted as posterior labral tear on axial images.[9] This condition is seen on 1 or 2 axial oblique images superior to the transition between the transverse ligament and the posterior inferior labrum. An anterosuperior cleft (see **Fig. 2B**) may be seen as a normal variant in the presence of a normal lateral acetabular labrum. On anterior coronal or sagittal images, this cleft is seen as a partial undercutting of the labrum on a single image. The extension of the fluid into this cleft occurs from the femoral side and is more commonly seen in labral hypertrophy associated with mild developmental dysplasia of the hip. A transverse ligament labral junction sulcus (see **Fig. 2C**) is a normal sulcus or recess that may be seen between the transverse ligament and the labrum either anteriorly or posteriorly. The perilabral sulcus (see **Fig. 2D**) represents a normal space between the acetabular labrum and capsule visualized on coronal images. With regard to labrum shape, more reports document that a triangular appearance is most common (70%–80%), although the labrum may be round, flat, irregular, or even absent (1%–14%) in asymptomatic persons. An enlarged or hypertrophic labrum may occur in patients with mild developmental dysplasia of the hip (**Fig. 3**).

The stellate lesion or crease (**Fig. 4**) is a bare area deficient in hyaline cartilage above the anterosuperior margin of the acetabular fossa within the articular area of the acetabulum. This lesion should not be confused with an osteochondral lesion. The tubular acetabular intraosseous contrast tracking (**Fig. 5**) is a common magnetic resonance (MR) arthrographic finding that seems to have little or no clinical significance. Although the exact pathophysiologic mechanism is unknown, it is thought to represent dilatation of nutrient foramina along the anterior and posterior margin of the acetabular fossa.[10] The pectinofoveal fold (**Fig. 6**) is almost always visualized at MR arthrography.

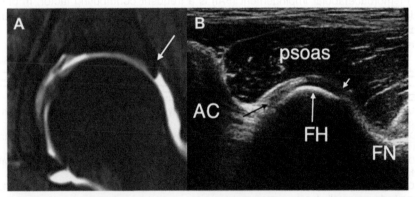

Fig. 1. (*A*) Coronal T1 fat-saturated (FS)-weighted image shows triangular shaped superior labrum (*arrow*). (*B*) Oblique sagittal ultrasound image shows anterior labrum (*black arrow*), femoral head (FH) cortex (*large white arrow*), anterior joint capsule (*small white arrow*), femoral neck (FN), iliopsoas muscle (psoas), acetabulum (AC).

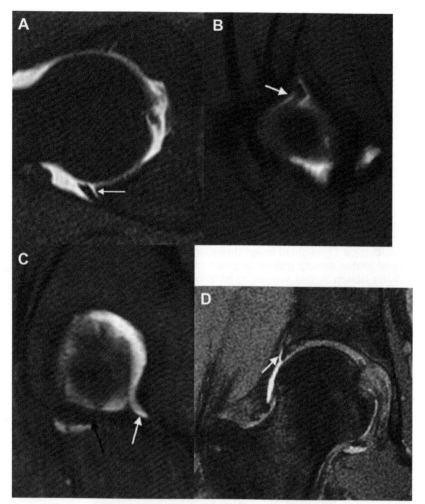

Fig. 2. (*A*) The posterior inferior sublabral sulcus or groove (*arrow*) does not extend completely underneath the labrum. (*B*) The anterosuperior cleft (*arrow*) partially undercuts the labrum on a single coronal image, which does not extend completely through the labrum. (*C*) Normal transverse ligament labral sulcus (*white arrow*) and transverse acetabular ligament (*black arrow*), which extends from the anterior to the posterior aspect at the inferior acetabular fossa. (*D*) The perilabral sulcus (*arrow*), a normal space between the capsule, lateral acetabular rim, and labrum.

This fold may resemble a hip plica and can have various appearances and attachment sites. The pectinofoveal fold has had only limited study in the clinical and anatomic literature.[11] A prospective study is needed to determine whether the pectinofoveal fold can be a cause of impingement that results in hip pain.

LABRUM TEAR

MR arthrography shows excellent accuracy in the detection and staging of acetabular labral lesions compared with conventional MR imaging (MRI).[12] The hip joint is situated deep within the body and has small structures that can have significant

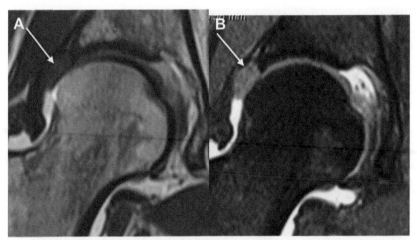

Fig. 3. (*A*) Coronal T1-weighted image shows large hypertrophic superior labrum (*arrow*). (*B*) Coronal proton density (PD) FS-weighted image shows increased signal intensity of hypertrophic labrum (*arrow*), suggesting intralabral degeneration.

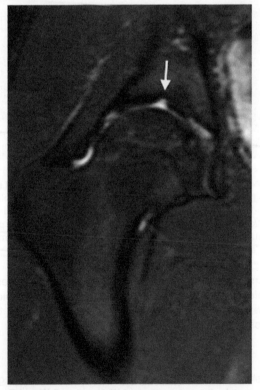

Fig. 4. The stellate crease (*arrow*) represents a bare area deficient in hyaline cartilage and not degeneration.

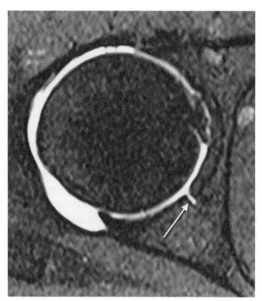

Fig. 5. Axial T1 FS-weighted images shows tubular acetabular intraosseous contrast tracking (*arrow*) along the posterior margin of the acetabular fossa, which likely represents dilatation of the nutrient foramina.

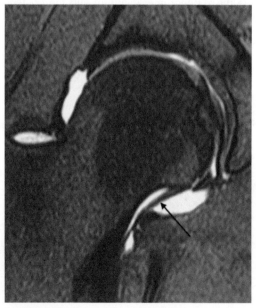

Fig. 6. Coronal T1 FS-weighted images shows the pectinofoveal fold (*arrow*) arising from the medial aspect of the femoral neck, extending inferiorly to attach on to the proximal femur. The relationship of this fold to internal impingement is not known.

consequences clinically. Small field-of-view high-resolution imaging is required to delineate normal anatomy and pathologic processes. MRI protocol varies from 1 institute to other. Axial oblique images parallel to the femoral neck are used to assess FAI (**Fig. 7**). Knuesel and colleagues[13] attempted to improve the cartilage lesion visibility on postarthrographic MR images by comparing a three-dimensional (3D) water-excitation technique with standard T1-weighted spin-echo images. 3D water-excitation true fast imaging with steady-state precession (FISP) or spoiled gradient echo images can be obtained with a 1.5- or 3-T MR system. 3D imaging data can be reconstructed in axial, coronal, sagittal, oblique axial, and radial planes (**Fig. 8**).

There is no uniformly accepted classification system for pathologic lesions of the acetabular labrum. In the arthroscopic classification, injuries are described as either labral detachment from bone or intrasubstance splits. Philippon[14] has defined 5 types of labral pathology: a primary labral tear, primary capsular laxity with minor labral pathology, capsular laxity with pronounced labral involvement, FAI with an associated labral tear, and articular cartilage degeneration with an associated labral tear. Czerny and coworkers[15] established a classification system dependent on the labral appearance as seen on the MR images: labrum morphology, effacement of perilabral sulcus, intralabral signal, contrast extension into the labrum, and detachment.

Most labral tear occurs in the anterior superior labrum or posterior superior (more common in the younger population) and run along the base of the labrum or along the long axis (longitudinal tear). The diagnosis of labral tear is established when gadolinium is seen traversing or undercutting the labrum (**Fig. 9**). A spectrum of labral lesions, including fibrillation and radial and longitudinal morphology, may be seen, as well as chondrolabral separation (**Fig. 10**). Displacement of a portion of labrum (**Fig. 11**) or the presence of a paralabral cyst can increase diagnostic confidence. The oblique axial and sagittal planes are the most useful in identifying anterior superior labrum tear (**Fig. 12**). Most labral tears involve the anterior/superior labrum but the tear can extend to involve the superior/lateral labrum and the posterior superior labrum (**Fig. 13**). The isolated tears in other portions of the labrum can occur but are less common. In the presence of a complete labral tear, synovial fluid or gadolinium or

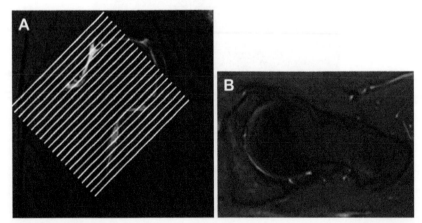

Fig. 7. (*A*) A coronal image is used to prescribe (*B*) oblique axial images, which are oriented parallel to the femoral neck. Femoral head-neck offset is quantified from oblique axial images.

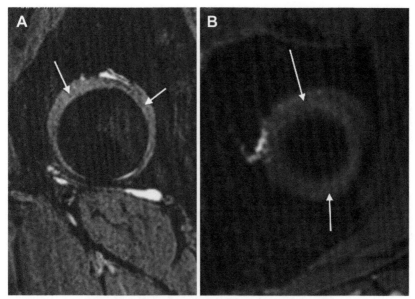

Fig. 8. (*A*) 3D true FISP images originally obtained in the sagittal plane. (*B*) Images are reconstructed in the axial plane from sagittal imaging data. Articular cartilage shows intermediate signal intensity (*arrows*).

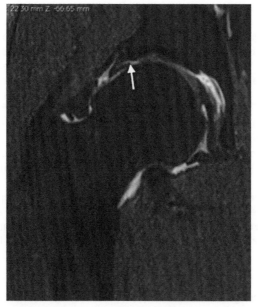

Fig. 9. Coronal T1 FS image shows a longitudinal cleavage tear (*arrow*) of the hypertrophic anterior superior labrum.

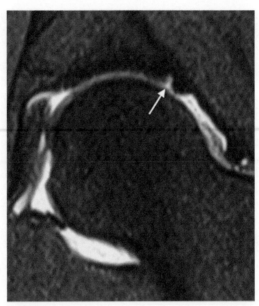

Fig. 10. Coronal T1 FS-weighted image shows chondrolabral tear (*arrow*) perpendicular to the long axis of the labrum.

both can traverse the entire thickness of the labrum and form a paralabral cyst of variable size (**Fig. 14**). Complete absence of the labrum, often with replacement by a large bone acetabular spur, suggests longstanding chronic labral tearing with eventual resorption of the torn and degenerated labrum (**Fig. 15**).

Although uncommon, tears of the ligamentum teres are a known cause for hip pain. The role of this injury in instability of the hip is unclear. MR arthrography can show disruption of the fibers of the ligamentum teres and is best identified on coronal and axial images (**Fig. 16**). Another injury that can occur with a sudden twisting motion of the hip is a tear of the joint capsule. Clinically, this can mimic a labral tear. At MRI, the defect in the capsule can be clearly shown with gadolinium traversing the defect (**Fig. 17**).

Delamination articular cartilage injuries are commonly seen in patients with FAI. Delamination occurs when full-thickness cartilage (**Figs. 18** and **19**) separates from the underlying subchondral bone plate and forms an unstable cartilage flap. MR arthrography has low sensitivity (20%) for delamination injury but high specificity (100%).[16]

Labrum tears are frequently associated with developmental dysplasia, FAI, Legg-Calvé-Perthes disease, slipped capital femoral epiphysis (SCFE), and degenerative hip disease. Traumatic tears may occur along the inner free margin with a radial flap, the most common type, or they may be unstable and displaced longitudinal tears.

FAI

FAI is a recently recognized cause of hip pain in all age groups.[17] FAI was previously called acetabular rim syndrome or cervicoacetabular impingement. Several predisposing conditions have been described that, because of the resultant deformity of

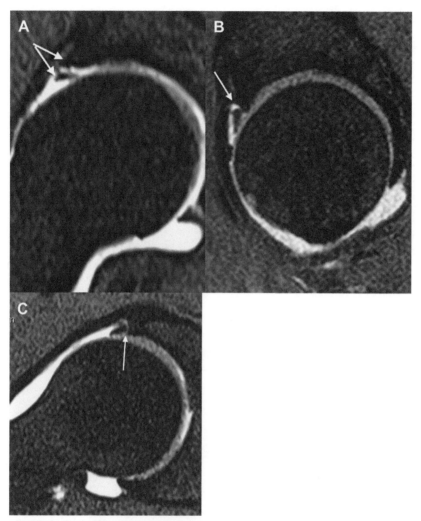

Fig. 11. (*A*) Coronal T1 FS-weighted image shows longitudinal bucket-handle type tear with labral fragments (*arrows*). (*B*) Sagittal 3D true FISP image and (*C*) oblique axial T1 FS-weighted image show detachment (*arrow*) of the anterior labrum.

the femur or the acetabulum or both, result in abnormal contact between these 2 structures during flexion and internal rotation. It is a major cause of early osteoarthritis of the hip, especially in young and active patients.[17,18] Classically, 2 types of FAI have been described depending on clinical and radiographic findings. The cam-type is the femoral cause and is often seen in young athletic males. The predominant abnormality is caused by an aspherical portion of the femoral head-neck junction with decreased offset (OS).[19] The pincer-type is the acetabular cause and is more common in middle-aged and older women. The predominant abnormality has an acetabular cause and is characterized by focal or general overcoverage of the femoral head. Most patients (86%) have a combination of both forms of impingement, which is called mixed pincer

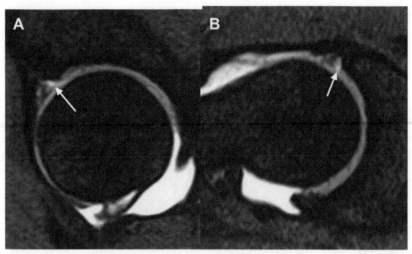

Fig. 12. (*A*) Sagittal T1 FS-weighted image and (*B*) oblique axial T1 FS-weighted image show an anterior superior labral tear (*arrow*).

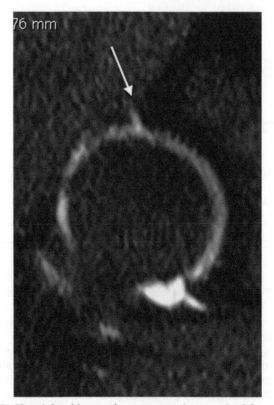

Fig. 13. Coronal T1 FS-weighted image shows a posterior superior labrum tear (*arrow*).

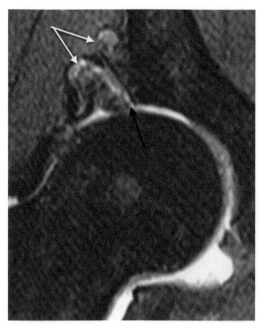

Fig. 14. Coronal T1 FS-weighted image shows a complete labral tear (*black arrow*) and paralabral cyst (*white arrows*).

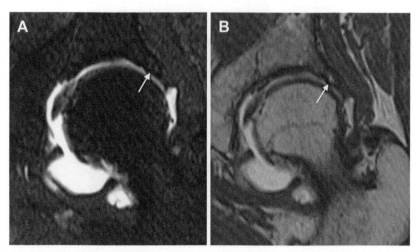

Fig. 15. (*A*) Coronal T1 FS-weighted image and (*B*) coronal T1-weighted image show degenerative changes, complete absence of labrum, and large acetabular bone spur (*arrow*).

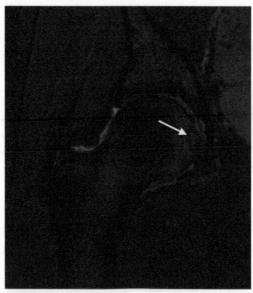

Fig. 16. Coronal PD FS-weighted image shows a tear of the ligamentum teres (*arrow*) and bone contusion after hip sprain.

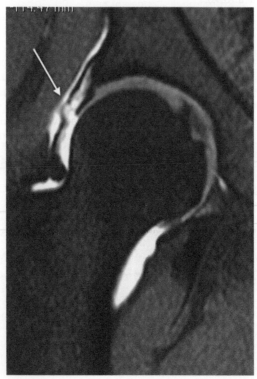

Fig. 17. Coronal T1 FS-weighted image shows a proximal iliofemoral ligament tear (*arrow*) and extraarticular contrast leak.

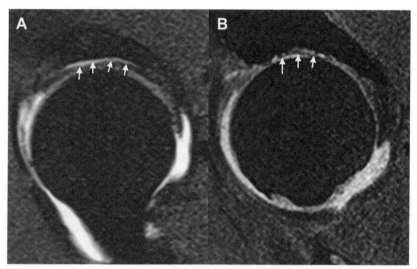

Fig. 18. (*A*) Sagittal T1 FS-weighted image shows articular cartilage delamination (*arrows*). (*B*) Sagittal 3D true FISP image shows articular cartilage fragmentation and peel-off (*arrows*).

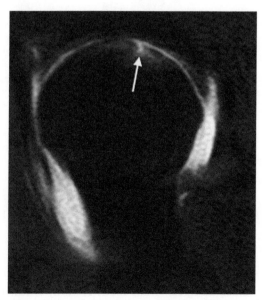

Fig. 19. Direct MR arthrography of right hip in a 24-year-old runner shows femoral head osteochondral injury with delamination of articular cartilage (*arrow*).

and cam impingement, with only a minority (14%) having the pure FAI form of either cam or pincer impingement.[20]

CAM IMPINGEMENT

Femoral causes of cam impingement include insufficient femoral head-neck OS, subtle displacement of the femoral epiphysis, SCFE, and postsurgical or traumatic deformities. As the hip is placed in flexion and internal rotation, because of the loss of normal concavity in this region, the femur abnormally touches the acetabular rim. This abnormal contact results in damage to the cartilage, predominately the anterior/superior acetabular cartilage and labrum.

The abnormal morphology of the femoral head-neck junction can be seen on anteroposterior (AP), frog lateral, or true lateral radiograph. On the AP view of the hip, the normal concavity along the lateral aspect of the femoral head-neck junction becomes flattened or slightly convex (**Fig. 20**). This condition has been referred to as the pistol grip deformity. The anterior femoral head-neck OS is defined as the difference in radius between the anterior femoral head and the anterior femoral neck on a cross-table axial view of the proximal femur (**Fig. 21**). The same morphologic abnormalities can be seen on oblique axial MR images. The α angle is measured from an oblique image through the center of the femoral neck. A line is drawn along the long axis of the femoral neck, bisecting a circle that outlines the femoral head. A second line is then drawn from the center of the circle to the point at which the anterior femoral cortex protrudes beyond the confines of the circle anteriorly (**Fig. 22**). The angle formed by these 2 lines is the α angle. A normal α angle is less than 45°. An angle

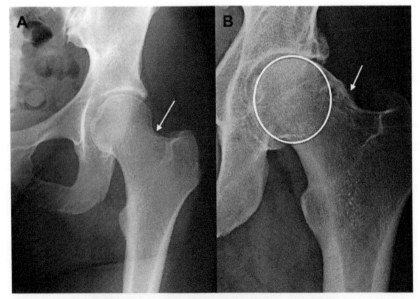

Fig. 20. (*A*) Normal frontal radiograph of hip shows concavity of femoral head and neck (*arrow*). (*B*) Pistol grip deformity with abnormal extension of epiphyseal scar in a patient with cam impingement.

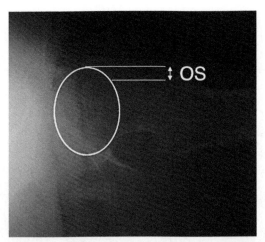

Fig. 21. Anterior OS, which is defined as the difference in radius between the anterior femoral head and the anterior femoral neck on a cross-table axial view of the proximal femur. Less than 10 mm OS is a strong indicator for cam impingement. (Asymptomatic hips, OS is 11.6 ± 0.7 mm; cam impingement has a decreased OS of 7.2 ± 0.7 mm.)

between 45° and 55° is considered borderline. An angle more than 55° is considered abnormal.[21]

A triad of MR arthrographic findings has been described in patients with cam-type FAI.[19] This triad consists of an abnormal α angle, an anterior/superior acetabular cartilage lesion, and an anterior/superior labral tear (**Fig. 23**).

PINCER IMPINGEMENT

In pure pincer-type impingement, the predominant abnormality is with the morphology of the acetabulum. The proximal femur has a normal contour. The acetabular overcoverage can be generalized or focal. General acetabular overcoverage is related to an increased depth of the acetabular fossa: coxa profunda or protrusio acetabuli.[22] At this stage no clear information exists that the 2 entities are a continuation of each

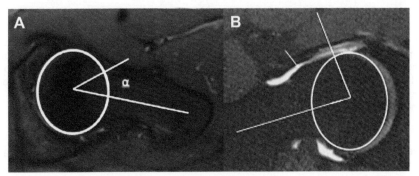

Fig. 22. (A) Oblique T1 FS-weighted image shows lines used for measuring α angle (normal <45°). (B) Oblique T1 FS-weighed images shows an abnormal α angle (78°) because of osseous bump and decreased femoral head-neck OS.

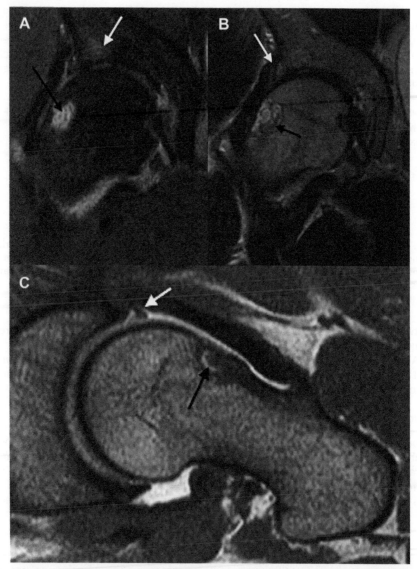

Fig. 23. (A) Coronal PD FS-weighted image shows anterior acetabular cartilage loss, subchondral edema (*white arrow*), osseous bump, and fibrocystic changes of the femoral head (*black arrow*). (B) Coronal T1-weighted image shows absent labrum (*black arrow*) and acetabular bone spur (*white arrow*). (C) Oblique axial T1-weighted image shows a displaced anterior labrum tear (*white arrow*), osseous bump, and fibrocystic changes of femoral neck (*black arrow*).

other. Focal overcoverage can occur in the anterior or the posterior part of the acetabulum. The anterosuperior overcoverage is called acetabular retroversion and causes anterior FAI that can be reproduced clinically with painful flexion and internal rotation. The posterior wall can be too prominent or deficient. A deficient posterior wall is often related to acetabular retroversion or dysplasia. The too-prominent posterior wall can often be seen in hips with coxa profunda or protrusio acetabuli. This situation can cause posterior impingement, with reproducible pain in hip extension and external rotation.

The evaluation of acetabular morphologic abnormality can be challenging on imaging because of the complex orientation and anatomy of the acetabulum. The AP view of the pelvis is the single most important view for defining acetabular morphology. However, care must be taken because slight craniocaudal angulations on an AP view of the pelvis or radiograph centered over the hip can cause pseudoappearance or obscure true retroversion.[22]

The generalized acetabular overcoverage is assessed as the relationship of the acetabular fossa to the ilioischial line. In a normal hip, the acetabular fossa line is lateral to the ilioischial line (**Fig. 24**A). A coxa profunda is defined with the floor of

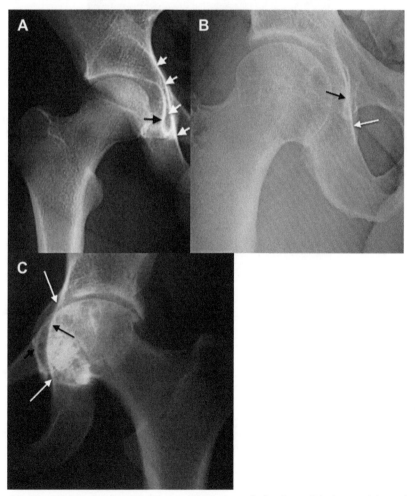

Fig. 24. AP radiograph of pelvis (A) normal hip: acetabular fossa (*black arrow*) lateral to ilioischial line (*multiple white arrows*). (B) Coxa profunda: acetabular fossa (*black arrow*) overlapping ilioischial line (*white arrow*). (C) Protrusio acetabuli: acetabular fossa (*small black arrow*) and femoral head (*large black arrow*) crossing ilioischial line (*white arrow*).

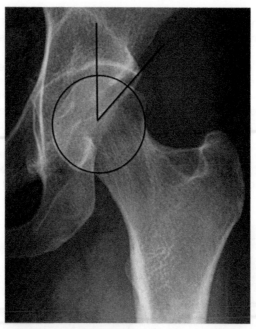

Fig. 25. Lateral-center-edge angle is formed by a vertical line and a line connecting the femoral head center with the lateral acetabular rim. Normal angle varies from 25°(< hip dysplasia) to 39° (> acetabular overcoverage).

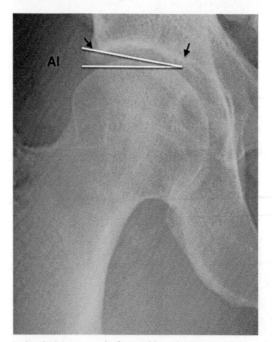

Fig. 26. Acetabular index (AI) is an angle formed by a horizontal line and a line connecting the medial point of the sclerotic zone (*small black arrow*) with the lateral center of the acetabulum. Normal acetabular index is positive while in coxa profunda and protrusio acetabuli AI is o or negative.

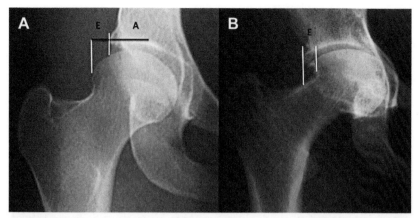

Fig. 27. Femoral head extrusion index [E/A+E]. Normal extrusion index (*A*) is about 25%. In coxa profunda and protrusio acetabuli (*B*) more femoral head is covered and the index is 0 or negative.

acetabular fossa touching or overlapping the ilioischial line (see **Fig. 24**B). Protrusio acetabuli occurs when the femoral head is overlapping the ilioischial line medially (see **Fig. 24**C). The excessive acetabular coverage can be quantified with the lateral-center-edge angle (**Fig. 25**) or the acetabular index (**Fig. 26**).[22] A normal lateral-center-edge angle varies between 25° and 39°. A value less than 25° defines a dysplasia and a value more than 39° indicates acetabular overcoverage. The acetabular index (also known as the acetabular roof angle) is normally positive. The acetabular index is 0° or negative in cases of coxa profunda or protrusio acetabuli. Another parameter for quantification of femoral coverage is the femoral head extrusion index (**Fig. 27**), which defines the percentage of femoral head that is uncovered when a horizontal line is drawn parallel to the interteardrop line. A normal extrusion index is less

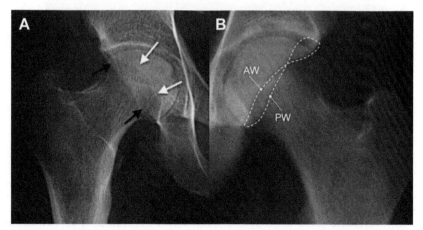

Fig. 28. AP radiograph of pelvis (*A*) normal hip anterior wall (*white arrows*) lies more medial to the posterior wall (*black arrows*). (*B*) Acetabular retroversion is defined when anterior wall (AW) crosses the posterior wall (PW) in the cranial aspect (**Fig. 8** configuration).

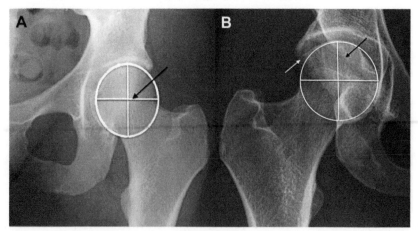

Fig. 29. AP radiograph of pelvis (*A*) normal posterior rim (*black arrow*) descends approximately through the center point of the femoral head. (*B*) Too-prominent posterior wall (*white arrow*) project lateral to the femoral head center.

than 25%. The femoral head extrusion index is decreased in coxa profunda and protrusio acetabuli and increased in developmental dysplasia.

The anterior rim of acetabulum should always project medial to the posterior rim of the acetabulum. In patients with acetabular retroversion, the anterior rim of the acetabulum projects lateral to the posterior rim of the acetabulum. This condition typically involves the superior half of the acetabulum. The edge of the anterior and

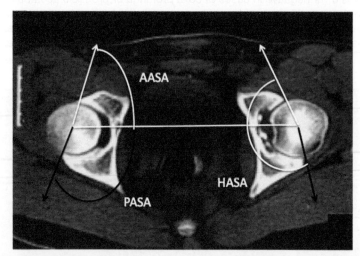

Fig. 30. Horizontal line is drawn through the center of both femoral heads. Anterior coverage is determined by use of the anterior acetabular sector angle (AASA), posterior coverage by posterior acetabular sector angle (PASA), and global acetabular coverage by horizontal acetabular sector angle (HASA). Mean normal AASA value of 63° in males and 64° in females, PASA 105° for both. (*Data from* Anda S, Terjesen T, Kvistad KA, et al. Acetabular angles and femoral anteversion in dysplastic hips in adults: CT investigation. J Comput Assist Tomogr 1991;15:116.)

posterior rim of the acetabulum crosses over on the AP view of the pelvis, the so-called crossover sign (**Fig. 28**). The posterior wall sign was introduced as an indicator for a prominent posterior wall. In a normal hip, the outline of the posterior rim descends approximately through the center point of the femoral head (**Fig. 29**). A deficient posterior wall has the posterior rim medial to the femoral head center and lateral to the femoral head center in a too-prominent posterior wall. The cross-sectional imaging (computed tomography [CT] scan or MRI) can be used for evaluation of acetabular anteversion and lateral-center-edge angle (**Figs. 30** and **31**).[23]

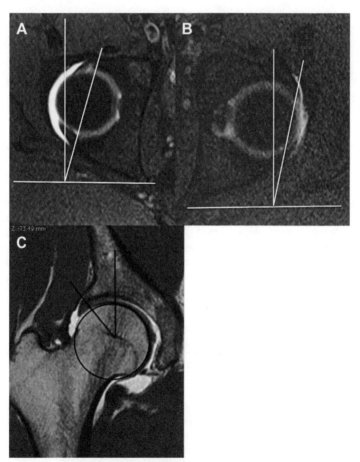

Fig. 31. (*A*) Most superior axial image at the level of the femoral head is used. A horizontal line is drawn connecting the posterior aspect of the ischial. A perpendicular line to this line is constructed. A line is drawn connecting the anterior and posterior acetabular rim. The acetabular anteversion angle is measured between the acetabular rim and the perpendicular line (normal anteversion angle is about 15°). The anterior acetabular rim is medial to the posterior rim. (*B*) Acetabular retroversion: the anterior acetabular rim is lateral to the posterior rim and angle of −10°. (*C*) Lateral-center-edge angle is formed by a vertical line and a line connecting the femoral head center with the lateral acetabular rim (normal angle: 25°–39°).

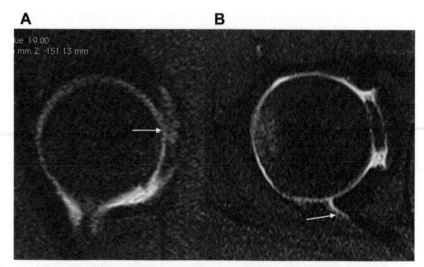

Fig. 32. (*A*) Sagittal (*B*) axial T1 FS image shows posterior labrum tear (*arrow*).

In pincer-type impingement, the cartilage lesions are often seen along the posterior aspect of the acetabulum (**Fig. 32**) as a result of a countercoup type of injury because the femur abnormally touches the acetabular rim. The associated labral degeneration and tears are most common in the anterosuperior labrum.

The exact association of fibrocystic changes (**Fig. 33**) of the femoral neck and FAI is not entirely clear. It is possible that these cysts are more common in patients with pincer-type impingement than cam.[24] An association between an os acetabuli (**Figs. 34** and **35**) and hip impingement has been suggested. Some believe this condition is heterotopic bone formation on the acetabulum rim related to abnormal contact with the femur. The mineralization may be in the soft tissue or in the labrum.

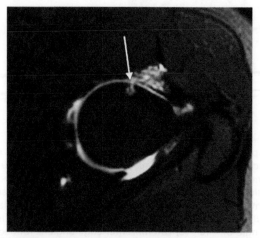

Fig. 33. Axial T1 FS-weighted images shows fibrocystic changes (*arrow*) at the anterior femoral head-neck junction.

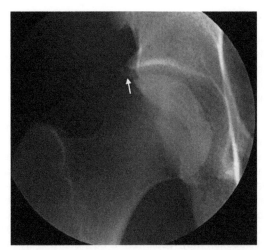

Fig 34. Frontal radiograph shows mineralization along the lateral margin of the acetabulum (*arrow*) and acetabular retroversion.

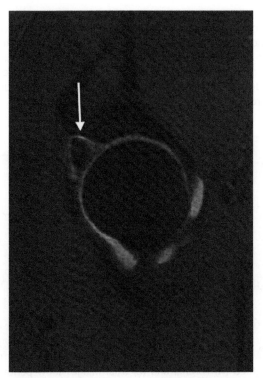

Fig. 35. Sagittal T1 FS-weighted image shows os acetabuli (*arrow*).

HIP SPRAIN AND DISLOCATION

Traumatic hip subluxation is a lesser injury than hip dislocation but may lead to significant clinical manifestation. The most common pattern is posterior, and the injury has been often described in athletes, especially players of American football. The most common mechanism of injury is a fall on a flexed and adducted hip. Radiographs are usually normal or may show small posterior acetabular rim fracture, similar to but often smaller than that accompanying posterior dislocation. MR images may show pericapsular soft tissue edema and traumatic disruption of the iliofemoral ligament near its femoral attachment (**Fig. 36**). The ligamentum teres as well as an ischiofemoral ligament tear from the posterior acetabular rim have been emphasized.

Dislocation of the femoral head with or without an acetabular fracture is an injury that usually follows considerable trauma and that may be associated with significant injury elsewhere in the body. Hip dislocation represents approximately 5% of all dislocations. Hip dislocations are generally classified as anterior, posterior, and central. Posterior dislocation of the hip is most common (approximately 80%–85% of all hip dislocation). This dislocation may result from a dashboard injury in which the flexed knee strikes the dashboard during a head-on automobile collision.[25,26] The frequent occurrence of posterior acetabular rim fractures after posterior dislocation of the hip requires careful analysis of routine radiographs and the use of oblique and lateral projections. Shear or compression fractures of the anterior and inferior portions of the femoral head are seen (**Fig. 37**).

STRESS INJURIES

Stress fractures, encompassing both fatigue and insufficiency fractures, are common injuries. Stress fractures account for as many as 10% of all injuries seen in sports medicine clinics.[27] As described by Wolff,[28] bone is a dynamic tissue in which normal stresses stimulate remodeling, allowing adaptation to a changing mechanical environment. Bone remodeling is stimulated by fatigue damage, and fatigue damage occurs in the form of microfracture.[29]

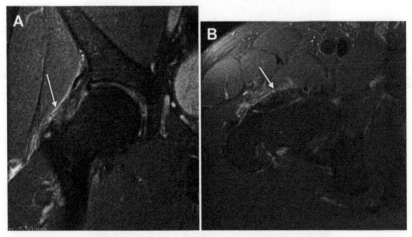

Fig. 36. PD FS-weighted (*A*) coronal and (*B*) axial images show pericapsular edema and partial-thickness iliofemoral ligament tear (*arrows*) after a right hip sprain.

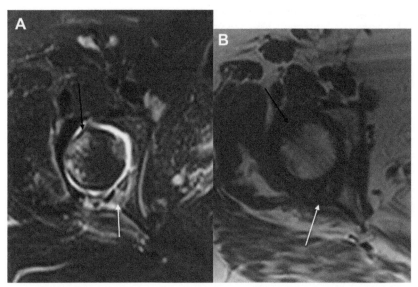

Fig. 37. (*A*) Axial short-tau inversion recovery (STIR)- and (*B*) axial T1-weighted images show posterior acetabular rim fracture (*white arrow*) and compression injury of anterior femoral head (*black arrow*).

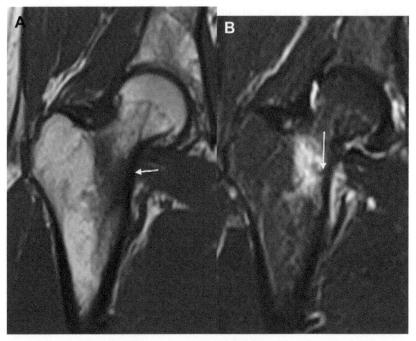

Fig. 38. (*A*) Coronal T1-weighted image shows medial femoral neck cortical thickening and edema (*arrow*). (*B*) Coronal STIR-weighted image shows incomplete fracture line (*arrow*).

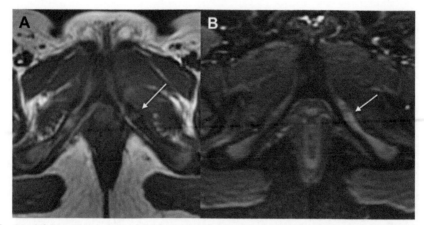

Fig. 39. (*A*) T1-weighted and (*B*) STIR-weighted images show left inferior pubic ramus stress fracture (*arrow*).

The fatigue fractures are more common in runners who have recently started a new and intensive physical activity or who have had a recent change in training regimen.[30] Fatigue fractures are also common in military trainees.[31] Women have a higher incidence of stress fractures in both athletes and military population.[1] The femoral neck is typically involved (**Fig. 38**). The most common other pelvic bones involved are the pubic rami (**Fig. 39**) and sacrum (**Fig. 40**).[32] Insufficiency fractures occur when normal stress is applied to abnormal bone. Risk factors for insufficiency fractures include osteoporosis, irradiation for pelvic malignancy, steroid therapy, hyperparathyroidism,

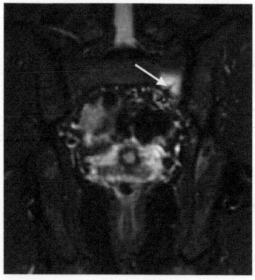

Fig. 40. Coronal STIR-weighted image shows incomplete stress fracture of left sacral ala (*arrow*).

rheumatoid arthritis, osteomalacia, Paget disease, rickets, diabetes mellitus, or osteogenesis imperfecta.[33]

Radiographs are usually the initial imaging performed because of their wide availability and low cost. Plain radiographs are known to be insensitive for stress fracture, with sensitivity approaching 0% for posterior pelvis and sacrum.[32,34] CT scans play a minor role because of high cost, radiation dose, and lack of sensitivity in the early stages of stress injury. The signs of stress-related injury on CT are similar to those seen in radiographs, including periosteal or endosteal elevation, or a fracture line.

Bone scintigraphy is exquisitely sensitive for stress injuries or fracture, which is typically performed with technetium 99m phosphonate analogues. Abnormal bone scan may be seen as early as 6 to 72 hours. Bone scans are not specific for stress fracture, and increased uptake can be seen with infection, tumor, or early stage of avascular necrosis. MRI is reported to be as sensitive as scintigraphy for stress fracture, approaching 100%. MRI also provides high specificity with higher soft tissue and bone marrow contrast.[35]

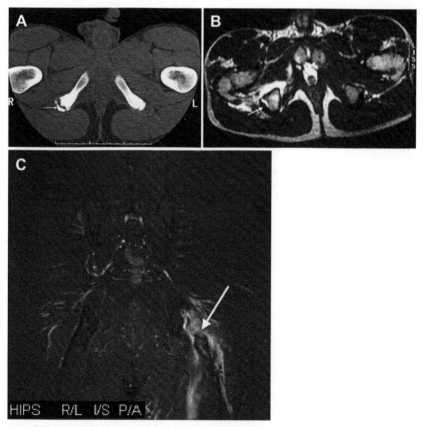

Fig. 41. (*A*) Axial CT scan and (*B*) axial T2-weighted images show avulsion of the right ischial apophysis (*arrow*). (*C*) Coronal STIR image of a 27-year-old football player shows a complete left hamstring origin tear with edema interposed between tendon and ischial tuberosity (*arrow*).

AVULSION INJURIES

Avulsion injuries of the pelvis occur most often in the adolescent athlete, usually result-ing in displacement of an unfused apophysis at the site of tendon attachment. This injury is analogous to a musculotendinous injury in the skeletally mature individual. Apophyseal avulsion injuries are usually detected on radiographs but on occasion may require more advanced imaging such as a CT scan or MRI to identify subtle lesions and delineate the extent of injury. Radiographs are usually adequate to estab-lish the diagnosis of an apophyseal avulsion injury. Comparison with the contralateral

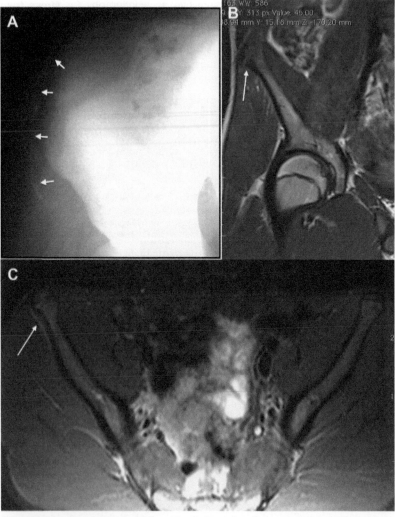

Fig. 42. (A) Magnified frontal radiograph of the pelvis shows anterior superior iliac crest avulsion (*arrows*). (B) Coronal T1-weighted image (*arrow*) and (C) PD FS-weighted image show anterior superior iliac crest avulsion with bone-marrow edema and adjacent soft-tissue edema (*arrow*).

side may be helpful in confirming subtle displacement of apophysis. In the acute setting, if radiographs are indeterminate, MRI can be helpful in identifying minimally displaced or even nondisplaced apophyseal injuries.

Ischial tuberosity is the site of origin of the semimembranosus, semitendinosus, and long head of the biceps femoris tendon. The ischial tuberosity is the most common location for avulsion injury in the pelvis and usually results from a forceful contraction of the hamstring muscles. MRI shows the extent of soft tissue injury, including strain, partial thickness tear, or full-thickness tear of the proximal fibers of the hamstring tendons (**Fig. 41**). The sciatic nerve sits in close proximity to the ischial tuberosity and is best evaluated on axial T1- and T2-weighted images. Stretching injuries of the sciatic nerve have been reported in association with hamstring avulsion injuries.

The anterior superior iliac spine is the site of origin of the sartorius and tensor fascia lata muscle. Avulsion injuries at this level (**Fig. 42**) typically occur in sprinters during forceful extension of the hip with the knee in flexion. The patient complains of point tenderness and swelling directly overlying the site of avulsion. Radiographs of the pelvis usually show cortical avulsion. MRI better defines the extent of adjacent soft tissue injury and retraction of the sartorius tendon.

The anterior inferior iliac spine is the site of origin of the rectus femoris tendon. The anterior inferior iliac spine avulsions usually occur during forceful extension of the hip, resulting in pain and point tenderness directly overlying the site of injury. AP and oblique views of the pelvis better show a nondisplaced or minimally displaced fracture fragment. Chronic injuries may show extensive heterotopic bone formation within the adjacent soft tissues (**Fig. 43**). MRI shows injury of the direct or indirect head of the rectus femoris tendon (**Fig. 44**).

The iliopsoas tendon inserts onto the lesser trochanter along the medial aspect of the proximal femur. Avulsion of the lesser trochanter is an uncommon sports-related injury that occurs most often in adolescent soccer players before closure of the apophyseal growth plate (**Fig. 45**). The apophysis fuses by 16 to 18 years. In adult

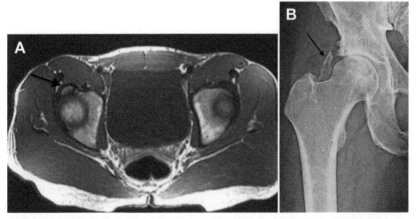

Fig. 43. (*A*) Axial T1-weighted image shows chronic anterior inferior iliac spine avulsion (*arrow*) at the direct head of the rectus femoris origin (*arrow*). (*B*) AP radiograph of the right hip in a different patient shows heterotopic bone (*arrow*) within the proximal rectus femoris 6 months after arthroscopic surgery.

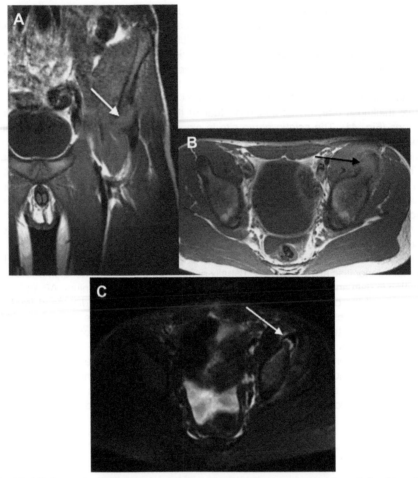

Fig. 44. (A) Coronal and (B) axial T1-weighted images show acute avulsion of direct head of rectus femoris (*arrow*) from anterior inferior iliac spine (AIIS). (C) Axial STIR-weighted image of another patient with acute avulsion injury (*arrow*) of AIIS.

patients, the violent muscular contraction results in a strain or tear of the iliopsoas at the level of the distal musculotendinous junction (**Fig. 46**).

The pubic symphysis and inferior pubic ramus is the site of origin of the adductor longus, adductor brevis, and gracilis muscles, and is also the site of distal attachment of the rectus abdominis muscle.[36] Avulsion injuries at this location are most commonly associated with chronic repetitive stress resulting from excessive twisting and turning movements of the abdomen and pelvis that occur in players of soccer, ice hockey, and tennis. Avulsion injuries of the adductors do not usually result in a displaced bone fragment but rather present as an isolated soft tissue injury. Radiographs are usually normal. MRI shows the extent of adductor origin injury from mild strain to a partial- or full-thickness tear (**Fig. 47**). MRI also commonly shows bone marrow edema adjacent to the site of adductor attachment injury, but fractures of the pubic ramus do not typically occur.

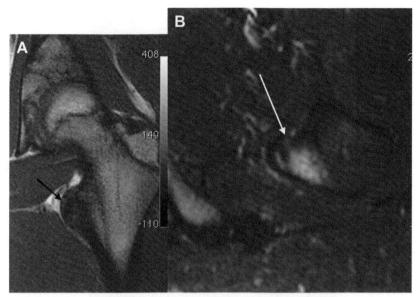

Fig. 45. (A) Coronal T1-weighted image and (B) STIR-weighted image show lesser trochanter avulsion injury with bone-marrow edema (*arrow*).

ATHLETIC PUBALGIA

Groin injuries are common with sports activities such as twisting at the waist, sudden and sharp changes in direction, and side-to-side ambulation. Many athletes with a diagnosis of sports hernia or athletic pubalgia have a spectrum of related pathologic conditions resulting from musculotendinous injuries and subsequent instability of the

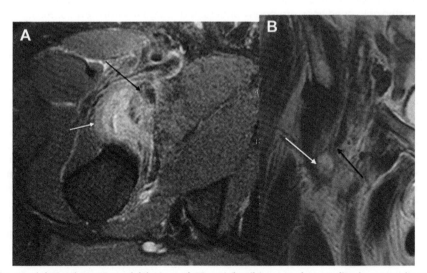

Fig. 46. (A) Axial PD FS- and (B) coronal T2-weighted images show a distal myotendinous junction iliopsoas tendon tear (*black arrow*) and posttraumatic bursitis (*white arrow*).

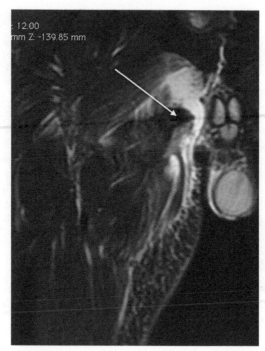

Fig. 47. Coronal T2 FS-weighted image shows avulsed adductor longus tendon (*arrow*) and associated soft-tissue edema.

pubic symphysis without inguinal hernia at physical examination. The mechanisms and pathologic conditions are poorly understood. Large field-of-view screening MRI of the bony pelvis are suboptimal for evaluation of subtle aponeurotic abnormalities at pubic symphysis. Small field-of-view high-resolution MRI of the pubic symphysis should be obtained (**Fig. 48**).

The term sportsman's hernia was first used to describe inguinal pain experienced by athletes without evidence of a hernia at physical examination. The exact location of this weakness or tear was disputed; some investigators favored the external oblique muscle aponeurosis and conjoined tendon,[37,38] whereas others believed it was in the transversalis fascia.[39] The term athletic pubalgia is proposed rather than sports hernia to refer to a group of musculoskeletal processes that occur in and around the pubic symphysis and that share a similar mechanism of injury and common clinical manifestations.[40] The chronic repetitive injury to common aponeurosis of the rectus abdominis and adductor longus tendons along the anterior aspect of the pubic symphysis may lead to eventual avulsion of the tendon or tear in the aponeurosis. The most commonly observed injury is along the lateral border of the rectus abdominis, just cephalad to its pubic attachment, or at the origin of the adductor longus (**Fig. 49**). Hernia-like symptoms may be related to the proximity of the injury site to the medial margin of the superficial ring of the inguinal canal or to lesion extension through the superficial ring and resultant weakening of the posterior wall of the inguinal canal.

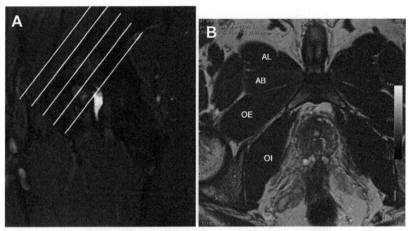

Fig. 48. (*A*) Sagittal image obtained through the arcuate and iliopectineal line is used to prescribe (*B*) small field-of-view oblique axial images of pubic symphysis. AL, adductor longus; AB, adductor brevis; OE, obturator externus; OI, obturator internus.

Other pathologic processes are associated with groin pain such as adductor longus tendinosis, osteitis pubis, inguinal ligament sprain (**Fig. 50**), hockey goalie–baseball pitcher syndrome, pubic stress fracture (**Fig. 51**), septic arthritis, acetabular labral tear, inguinal hernia, nerve entrapment syndrome, and apophysitis.

Hockey goalie–baseball pitcher syndrome results from an epimysial or myofascial herniation of the adductor longus muscle belly several centimeters away from the site of its pubic attachment.[40] Patients with this condition often experience an acute onset of pain, which may be persistent or may intermittently intensify after stretching. There are no well-established MRI findings, and the imaging appearance often is

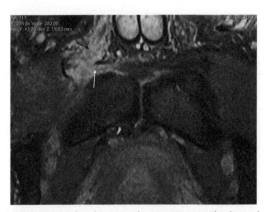

Fig. 49. Oblique axial PD FS-weighted image shows a tear in the lateral aspect of the right rectus abdominis-adductor longus aponeurosis (*white arrow*) with edema-like signal along the superficial inguinal ring (*black arrow*).

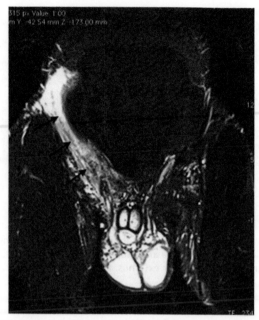

Fig. 50. Coronal STIR-weighted image of professional hockey player shows diffuse soft-tissue edema (*arrows*) of the right inguinal ligament extending along the oblique and transverse abdominis muscle aponeurosis, suggesting an extensive tear. He also suffered an acute rectus abdominis-adductor aponeurosis tear (not shown): an acute injury to all structures of previously disputed sportsman's hernia etiology.

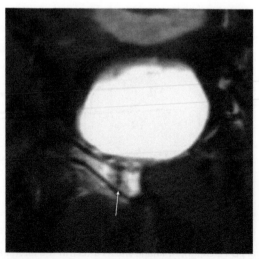

Fig. 51. A 28-year-old runner with groin pain. Coronal STIR-weighted image shows right pubis stress fracture (*arrow*).

normal. MRI may show a proximal myofascial focal bulge, suggesting hernia and edema of the adductor longus muscle belly (**Fig. 52**).

Osteitis pubis is common in soccer players, long-distance runners, and hockey players. It is thought to result from instability of the pubic symphysis because of chronic repetitive shear and distraction injuries and unbalanced tensile stress from

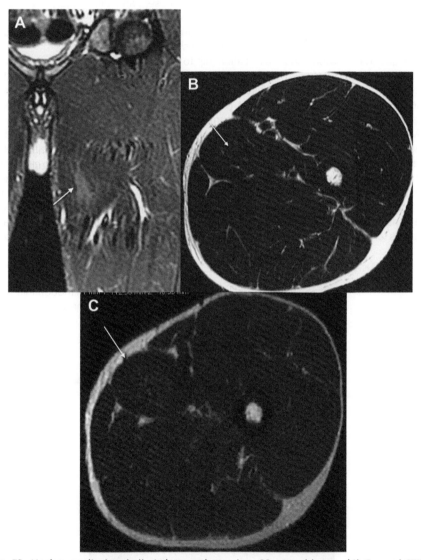

Fig. 52. Hockey-goalie–baseball-pitcher syndrome in a 32-year-old man. (*A*) Coronal STIR-weighted image shows edema-like signal of the left adductor longus muscle (*arrow*) several centimeters from the pubic symphysis. (*B*) Axial T2-weighted image shows mild bulging of fascia and edema-like signal (*arrow*). (*C*) Focal myofascial bulging was more prominent with hip flexion (*arrow*), suggesting myofascial herniation.

the muscle attachment of the pubic symphysis. MR images show diffuse marrow edema extending from the subchondral plate and often involving pubic bone, periostitis, articular surface irregularity, erosions, anterior and posterior osteophytes, and subchondral cysts (**Fig. 53**).

HIP ABDUCTOR INJURIES AND TROCHANTERIC BURSITIS

Gluteus medius and gluteus minimus muscle strains, also referred to as a charley horse or the greater trochanter pain syndrome, represent an indirect injury secondary to overuse, repetitive microtrauma, excessive force, or muscle fiber stretch. Greater trochanteric pain syndrome refers to a broad spectrum of pathologic conditions, often relieved by injections of steroids and analgesics.[41]

The abductor tendons and their relationship to the greater trochanter are analogous to the relationship between the rotator cuff tendons and greater tuberosity in the shoulder. The gluteus minimus inserts on the anterior facet and the gluteus medius inserts on the superoposterior facet (**Fig. 54**). The posterior facet has no tendon attachment and is covered by the trochanteric bursa.

MRI can play a pivotal role in differentiating trochanteric bursitis from abductor tendon avulsion. Radiographs are usually normal. However, on occasion calcific tendinitis or bursitis can be seen (**Fig. 55**). Abductor tendon injuries of the hip most commonly occur in elderly women more than 65 years of age and are also sometimes found in high-level athletes. The exact cause of gluteus medius tendinopathy or tendon degeneration is uncertain. The gluteus medius and gluteus minimus tendon are consider as rotator cuff of hip. Gluteus minimus and medius lesions can be classified as tendinosis, partial tears, or full-thickness tears (**Fig. 56**) with or without tendon

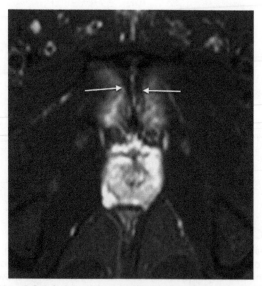

Fig. 53. Axial T2 FS-weighted image shows advanced osteitis pubis with articular surface irregularities and edema that involves both pubic bodies (*arrows*).

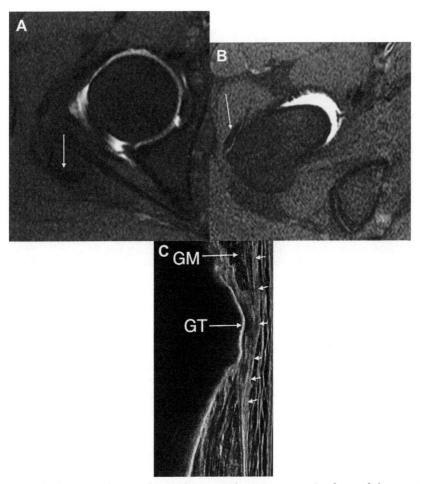

Fig. 54. (A) Gluteus medius tendon insertion on the superoposterior facet of the greater trochanter (*arrow*). (B) Gluteus minimus tendon insertion on the anterior facet (*arrow*). (C) Coronal ultrasound image shows greater trochanter (GT), gluteus medius (GM), and iliotibial band (*multiple small arrows*).

retraction. Bursitis is found in 40% or more of patients with abductor tendon conditions (**Fig. 57**). Some abductor avulsions have occurred as complications of total hip arthroplasty. Ultrasound can be performed as an office-based procedure with precise steroid or local anesthesia injection under ultrasound guidance.

ILIOPSOAS BURSITIS

The iliopsoas bursa is the largest bursa of the hip. In 15% of individuals with hip pathology, there is patent iliopsoas bursa communication with the hip. The hallmark of iliopsoas bursitis is enlargement of the iliopsoas bursa caused by either synovial

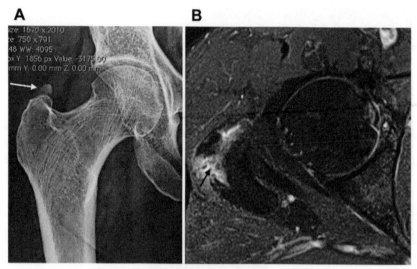

Fig. 55. (*A*) AP radiograph of the right hip shows calcification (*arrow*) adjacent to the greater trochanter. (*B*) Axial PD FS-weighted image shows greater trochanteric bursitis (*arrow*) and gluteus minimus tendonitis.

fluid or hypertrophic synovium. The 3 major causes of iliopsoas bursitis are rheumatoid arthritis, acute trauma, and overuse injury.[42] Overuse is a common cause of iliopsoas bursitis in the athletic population. Bursitis is the result of constant friction from the overlying iliopsoas tendon in overuse. Bursitis occurs commonly in individuals

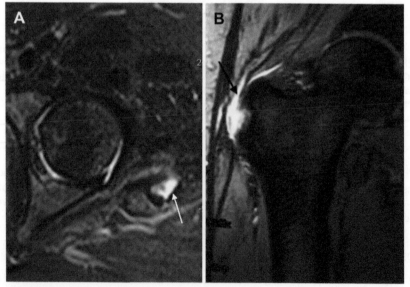

Fig. 56. (*A*) Axial PD FS-weighted image shows a gluteus medius tendon tear (*arrow*). (*B*) Greater trochanteric bursitis and gluteus medius tendon tear (*arrow*).

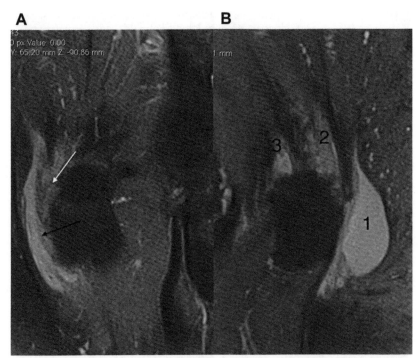

Fig. 57. (*A*) Coronal PD FS-weighted image shows greater trochanteric bursitis (*black arrow*) and gluteus medius tendon tear (*white arrow*). (*B*) Bursitis and gluteus tendinitis: (1) greater trochanteric bursitis, (2) subgluteus medius bursa, (3) subgluteus minimus bursa.

involved in strength training, rowing, uphill running, ballet, jumping, and competitive track and field.[42]

Diagnosing iliopsoas bursitis can be difficult clinically. Imaging is often required to differentiate bursitis from other causes of groin pain. MRI findings of iliopsoas bursitis (**Fig. 58**) are a focal or elongated fluid collection located anterior to the hip joint, posterior or posteromedial to the iliopsoas tendon, and lateral to the femoral vessels. The size and communication are best appreciated on MR. Iliopsoas bursitis is shown on ultrasound as elongated or focal anechoic or hypoechoic bursa when compared with the contralateral asymptomatic hip. Doppler analysis is useful in differentiating iliopsoas bursitis from a pseudoaneurysm of the femoral vessels.

SNAPPING HIP SYNDROME

The snapping hip syndrome or coxa saltans is characterized by a snapping or clicking sensation that occurs with movement of the hip. Three types have been identified[43]: external, internal, and intraarticular.

The most common type is external, related to friction from the posterior aspect of the iliotibial band as it slides over the greater trochanter as the hip extends from a flexed position. Friction from the anterior edge of the gluteus maximus may also contribute. MR images may show focal thickening of the iliotibial band, greater trochanteric bursitis, and soft tissue inflammation (**Fig. 59**). The internal snapping is related to snapping of the iliopsoas tendon over the iliopectineal eminence, femoral

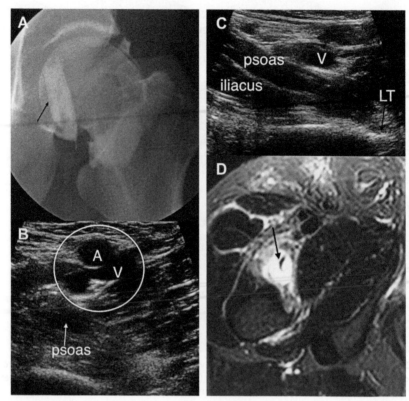

Fig. 58. (*A*) Left iliopsoas bursa (*arrow*) distension after hip arthrogram. (*B*) Transverse ultrasound image of distal iliopsoas tendon (*arrow*) and neurovascular structure (*circle*). (*C*) Oblique sagittal ultrasound image of distal iliopsoas tendon insertion on the lesser trochanter (LT) and relation to vein (V). (*D*) Axial T2 FS-weighted image of a patient with rheumatoid arthritis shows iliopsoas bursitis and a tendon tear (*arrow*).

head, or anterior capsule (**Fig. 60**). The intraarticular snapping can be caused by an abnormality in the joint itself, such as a labral tear or loose bodies (**Fig. 61**).

SACROILIAC JOINT DYSFUNCTION

Sacroiliac (SI) joint dysfunction is a poorly understood condition without imaging abnormality. The classic location for pain emanating from the SI joint is the sacral sulcus, the region medial to the posterior superior iliac spine. The pain from a symptomatic SI joint can also radiate to the groin, abdomen, thigh, and calf, making it difficult to distinguish from other conditions such as disc disease. The SI joint can be involved in a wide range of disorders such as traumatic sprain, osteoarthritis, ankylosing spondylitis, and sacroiliitis from other inflammatory arthritis or infection. Sacroiliitis-like changes can be seen in athletes.[44,45] Erosions and sclerosis involving the SI joint can be seen in athletes, particularly long-distance runners and soccer players (**Fig. 62**). The SI joint is similar to the pubic symphysis and the acromioclavicular joint; repetitive shear stress at these joints can lead to bone resorption. The mechanism for developing the erosions and sclerosis is unknown.

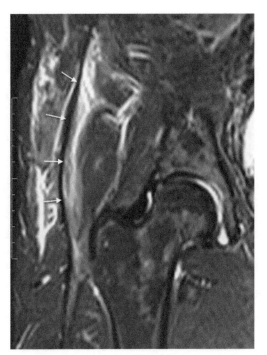

Fig. 59. Coronal T2 FS-weighted image shows iliotibial band strain (*arrows*) and surrounding soft-tissue edema.

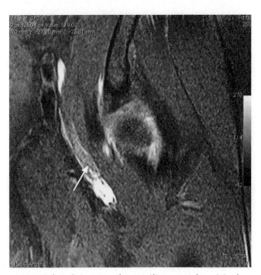

Fig. 60. Coronal T1 FS-weighted image shows iliopsoas bursitis (*arrow*) with snapping tendon.

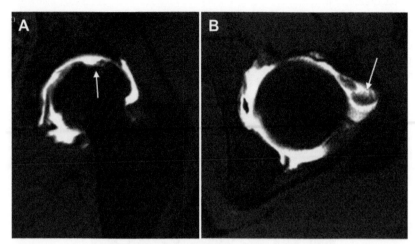

Fig. 61. (*A*) Coronal T1 FS-weighted image shows an osteochondral crater (*arrow*). (*B*) Axial T1 FS-weighted image shows loose bodies (*arrow*) along the anterior joint capsule.

PIRIFORMIS SYNDROME AND MUSCLE DENERVATION PATTERN

The piriformis syndrome, also known as pseudosciatica, wallet sciatica, hip socket neuropathy, deep gluteal syndrome, or neuritis of the proximal sciatic nerve, is secondary to nerve irritation or compression by the piriformis muscle. There are several developmental variations in the anatomic relationship between the sciatic nerve and piriformis. Trauma to the gluteal region and overuse in high-performance athletes are the most common cause of the piriformis syndrome. MRI may show piriformis hypertrophy and effacement of the fat in the greater sciatic foramen, tumor, abscess, or hematoma (**Fig. 63**).

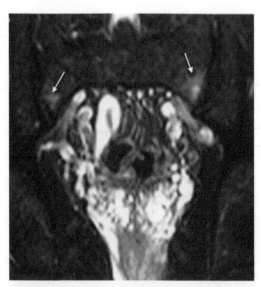

Fig. 62. Coronal STIR-weighted image of a 32-year-old female marathon runner shows sacroiliitis-like changes (*arrow*). Her arthritis workup was normal, and pubic symphysis showed similar changes.

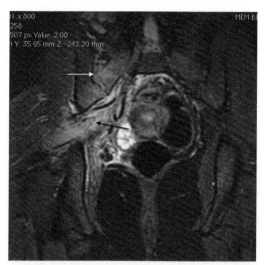

Fig. 63. Coronal STIR-weighted image in a young female after a snowboarding injury shows a right SI joint sprain (*white arrow*) and soft-tissue injury to piriformis muscle (*black arrow*) and sciatic nerve.

The sciatic, femoral, and obturator nerve around the pelvis may be injured. Knowledge of the relevant distribution of the nerve is helpful in understanding muscle denervation pattern. In the acute phase, muscles may show mild enlargement and diffuse edema, whereas in the chronic phase, muscle groups may show volume loss and fatty infiltration.

SUMMARY

The precise diagnosis of sports-related hip and groin injuries could be challenging given the complex anatomy and broad number of possible pain generators. This article reviews the spectrum of imaging appearance and techniques available to enable accurate diagnosis. Although radiographs of patients with FAI may initially appear normal, closer scrutiny reveals anatomic abnormalities that predispose to abnormal contact between the femur and the acetabulum. MRI protocols are modified according to clinical indication with small field-of-view high-resolution imaging of the symptomatic hip, pubic symphysis, or SI joint. Because of lack of ionizing radiation and low cost, ultrasound is an attractive first choice for imaging of superficial tendons and soft tissue but is operator dependent.

REFERENCES

1. Anderson K, Strickland SM, Warren R. Hip and groin injuries in athletes. Am J Sports Med 2001;29(4):521–33.
2. Lecouvet FE, Vande Ber BC, Malghem J, et al. MR imaging of the acetabular labrum: variation in 200 asymptomatic hips. AJR Am J Roentgenol 1996;167: 1025–8.
3. Bharam S. Labral tears, extra-articular injuries, and hip arthroscopy in the athlete. Clin Sports Med 2006;25:279–92.
4. Kavanagh EC, Koulouris G, Ford S, et al. MR imaging of groin pain in the athlete. Semin Musculoskelet Radiol 2006;10(3):197–207.

5. Konrath GA, Hamel AJ, Olson SA, et al. The role of the acetabular labrum and the transverse acetabular ligament in load transmission in the hip. J Bone Joint Surg Am 1998;80:1781–8.
6. Petersilge CA. MR arthrography for evaluation of the acetabular labrum. Skeletal Radiol 2001;30:423.
7. Abe I, Harada Y, Oinuma K, et al. Acetabular labrum: abnormal findings at MR imaging in asymptomatic hips. Radiology 2000;216:576.
8. Aydingoz U, Ozturk MH. MR imaging of the acetabular labrum: a comparative study of both hips in 180 asymptomatic volunteers. Eur Radiol 2001;11:567.
9. Dinauer PA, Murphy KP, Carroll JF. Sublabral sulcus at the posteroinferior acetabulum: a potential pitfall in MR arthrography diagnosis of acetabular labral tears. AJR Am J Roentgenol 2004;183(6):1745–53.
10. Lien LC, Hunter JC, Chan YS. Tubular acetabular intraosseous contrast tracking in MR arthrography of the hip: prevalence, clinical significance, and mechanism of development. AJR Am J Roentgenol 2006;187:807–10.
11. Blankenbaker DG, Davis KW, De Smet AA, et al. MRI appearance of the pectinofoveal fold. AJR Am J Roentgenol 2009;192:93–5.
12. Czerny C, Hoffman S, Neuhold A, et al. Lesions of the acetabular labrum: accuracy of MR imaging and MR arthrography in detection and staging. Radiology 1996;200(1):225–30.
13. Knuesel PR, Pfirrmannn CW, Noetzli HP, et al. MR arthrography of the hip: diagnostic performance of a dedicated water-excitation 3D double-echo steady-state sequence to detect cartilage lesions. AJR Am J Roentgenol 2004;183:1729–35.
14. Philippon MJ, Martin RR, Kelly BT. A classification system for labral tears of the hip. Arthroscopy 2005;21(Suppl):e36.
15. Czerny C, Hofmann S, Urban M, et al. MR arthrography of the adult acetabular capsular-labral complex: correlation with surgery and anatomy. AJR Am J Roentgenol 1999;173:345.
16. Anderson LA, Peters CL, Park BB, et al. Acetabular cartilage delamination in femoroacetabular impingement. Risk factors and magnetic resonance imaging diagnosis. J Bone Joint Surg Am 2009;91:305–13.
17. Ganz R, Parvizi J, Beck M, et al. Femoroacetabular impingement: a cause for osteoarthritis of the hip. Clin Orthop Relat Res 2003;417:112–20.
18. Tanzer M, Noiseux N. Osseous abnormalities and early osteoarthritis. Clin Orthop Relat Res 2004;429:170–7.
19. Kassarjian A, Yoon LS, Belzile E, et al. Triad of MR arthrographic findings in patients with cam-type femoroacetabular impingement. Radiology 2005;236(2):588–92.
20. Beck M, Kalhor M, Leunig M, et al. Hip morphology influences the pattern of damage to the acetabular cartilage: femoroacetabular impingement as a cause of early osteoarthritis of the hip. J Bone Joint Surg Br 2005;87:1012–8.
21. Notzli HP, Wyss TF, Stoecklin CH, et al. The contour of the femoral head-neck junction as a predictor for the risk of anterior impingement. J Bone Joint Surg Br 2002;84(4):556–60.
22. Tannast M, Siebenrock KA, Anderson SE. Femoroacetabular impingement: radiographic diagnosis–what the radiologist should know. AJR Am J Roentgenol 2007; 188:1540–52.
23. Anda S, Terjesen T, Kvistad KA, et al. Acetabular angles and femoral anteversion in dysplastic hips in adults: CT investigation. J Comput Assist Tomogr 1991;15:115–20.
24. Leunig M, Beck M, Kalhor M, et al. Fibrocystic changes at anterosuperior femoral neck: prevalence in hips with femoroacetabular impingement. Radiology 2005; 236:237–46.

25. Epstein HC. Traumatic dislocations of the hip. Clin Orthop 1973;92:116.
26. Larson CB. Fracture dislocations of the hip. Clin Orthop 1973;92:147.
27. Matheson GO, Clement DB, McKenzie DC, et al. Stress fractures in athletes: a study of 320 cases. Am J Sports Med 1987;15:46–58.
28. Wolff J. Das Gesetz der Transformation der Knochen. Berlin: Hirschwald; 1982.
29. Frostt HM. Wolff's law and bone's structural adaptations to mechanical usage: an overview for clinicians. Angle Orthod 1994;64:175–8.
30. Pentecost RL, Murray RA, Brindley HH. Fatigue, insufficiency, and pathologic fractures. JAMA 1964;187:1001–4.
31. Milgrom C, Giladi M, Stein M, et al. Stress fractures in military recruits: a prospective study showing an unusually high incidence. J Bone Joint Surg Br 1985;67:732–5.
32. Kiuru MJ, Pihlajamaki HK, Ahovuo JA. Fatigue stress injuries of the pelvic bones and proximal femur: evaluation with MR imaging. Eur Radiol 2003;13:605–11.
33. Soubrier M, Dubost JJ, Boisgard S, et al. Insufficiency fracture. A survey of 60 cases and review of the literature. Joint Bone Spine 2003;70:209–18.
34. Grangier C, Garcia J, Howarth NR, et al. Role of MRI in the diagnosis of insufficiency fractures of the sacrum and acetabular roof. Skeletal Radiol 1997;26:517–24.
35. Kiuru MJ, Pihlajamaki HK, Hietanen HJ, et al. MR imaging, bone scintigraphy, and radiography in bone stress injuries of the pelvis and the lower extremity. Acta Radiol 2002;43:207–12.
36. Robinson P, Salehi F, Grainger A, et al. Cadaveric and MRI study of the musculotendinous contributions to the capsule of the symphysis pubis. AJR Am J Roentgenol 2007;188:W440–5.
37. Gilmore J. Groin pain in the soccer athlete: fact, fiction, and treatment. Clin Sports Med 1998;17:787–93.
38. Irshad K, Feldman LS, Lavoie C, et al. Operative management of "hockey groin syndrome": 12 years of experience in National Hockey League players. Surgery 2001;130:759–64.
39. Joesting DR. Diagnosis and treatment of sportsman's hernia. Curr Sports Med Rep 2002;1:121–4.
40. Meyers WC, Lanfranco A, Castellanos A. Surgical management of chronic lower abdominal and groin pain in high-performance athletes. Curr Sports Med Rep 2002;1:301–5.
41. Cvitanic O, Henzie G, Skezas N, et al. MRI diagnosis of tears of the hip abductor tendon (gluteus medius and gluteus minimus). AJR Am J Roentgenol 2004;182(1):137–43.
42. Johnston CA, Wiley JP, Lindsay DM, et al. Iliopsoas bursitis and tendinitis. A review. Sports Med 1998;25(4):271–83.
43. Miller MD, Howard RF, Plancher KD. Treatment of snapping hip. Surgical atlas of sports medicine. Philadelphia: Saunders; 2003.
44. Brolinson PG, Kozar AJ, Cibor G. Sacroiliac joint dysfunction in athletes. Curr Sports Med Rep 2003;2(1):47–56.
45. Major NM, Helms CA. Pelvic stress injuries: the relationship between osteitis pubis (symphysis pubis stress injury) and sacroiliac abnormalities in athletes. Skeletal Radiol 1997;26:711–7.

Mechanics of Hip Arthroscopy

James R. Boyle, MD[a], Jason A. Silva, MD[b], Sean Mc Millan, DO[a],
Brian D. Busconi, MD[c],*

KEYWORDS
- Hip arthroscopy • Setup • Positioning

HISTORY

Burman[1] first discussed hip arthroscopy in the literature in 1931 when he said "it is manifestly impossible to insert a needle between the head of the femur and the acetabulum." Since that time, it has been proved that hip arthroscopy is, in fact, possible, and over the last 20 to 30 years, the indications and success of hip arthroscopy have grown significantly. Early hip arthroscopies involved only the central or intra-articular compartment. However, the introduction of the concept of femoroacetabular impingement by Dr Thomas Sampson,[2] along with the development of techniques to access the peripheral compartment (intracapsular/extra-articular) by Dienst and colleagues[3] from Germany, provided for the development of routine arthroscopy of the peripheral compartment of the hip.

ROOM SETUP AND EQUIPMENT

Safe and reliable arthroscopic access to the hip joint depends on several factors beyond surgical technique. Specially designed instruments, adequate fluoroscopic visualization, and an effective traction device are all necessary to work within the hip, specifically in the central intra-articular compartment.

When the patient is in the supine position (**Fig. 1**), the surgeon stands at the level of the operative hip, with the assistant and scrub technician on the same side. When the patient is in the lateral position (**Fig. 2**), the surgeon may stand in front or behind the patient, based on his or her preference. The scrub technician should be on the same side as the surgeon, and the position of the assistant is most often opposite

The authors have nothing to disclose.
[a] Division of Sports Medicine, Department of Orthopedics, University of Massachusetts Memorial Medical Center, 281 Lincoln Street, Worcester, MA 01605, USA
[b] Department of Orthopedics, University of Massachusetts Memorial Medical Center, 55 Lake Avenue North, Worcester, MA 01655, USA
[c] Department of Orthopedics and Physical Rehabilitation, University of Massachusetts Medical School, 281 Lincoln Street, Worcester, MA 01605-2192, USA
* Corresponding author.
E-mail address: brian.busconi@umassmemorial.org

Clin Sports Med 30 (2011) 285–292
doi:10.1016/j.csm.2010.12.005
0278-5919/11/$ – see front matter © 2011 Elsevier Inc. All rights reserved.

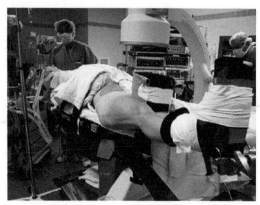

Fig. 1. The patient is positioned in the supine position. Note the perineal post is well padded with the leg abducted and slightly internally rotated.

the surgeon. The arthroscopic tower and pump are placed at the level of the head opposite the surgeon for an unobstructed view. The fluoroscope monitor is positioned at the patient's feet, where it can be seen by all members of the surgical team. The C-arm is positioned to provide an anteroposterior (AP) and a lateral view of the hip throughout the procedure to facilitate cannula placement, instrument use, and establishment of bony landmarks. When the patient is in the supine position, the fluoroscope can be positioned either between the patient's legs or entering from the nonoperative side. A free Mayo stand may be placed either over the patient at the shoulder level or behind the scrub nurse at the patient's feet for instrument passing. The back table is placed behind the surgeon and scrub nurse for convenient access throughout the procedure. The anesthesiologist is in the standard position at the patient's head.

ANESTHESIA

Hip arthroscopy is generally performed under general anesthesia because it is thought to provide the best environment available for muscle relaxation, which is critical for

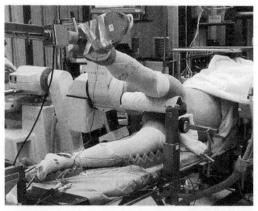

Fig. 2. The patient is positioned in the lateral decubitus position. Again note the perineal post is well padded with the leg abducted and slightly internally rotated.

distraction of the hip joint and access to the central compartment. Alternatively, spinal and/or epidural anesthesia with motor blockade may also provide adequate muscle relaxation for hip distraction. Every effort should be made to maintain the patient's systolic blood pressure below 100 mmHg in order to optimize visualization.

PATIENT POSITIONING

The 2 positions commonly used to access the hip joint arthroscopically with the assistance of distraction are the lateral decubitus and supine positions. Both approaches are technically feasible and provide access to all structures necessary in the course of arthroscopic hip surgery, and the choice is primarily the surgeon's preference. The supine approach to the hip was introduced first because it incorporated existing fracture tables, which were readily available to surgeons in most operating rooms.[4] The lateral position for hip arthroscopy was developed, in part, for the treatment of obese patients and was first reported by Glick and colleagues[5] from San Francisco and later adopted and developed further by McCarthy and colleagues[6] from Boston.

A routine fracture table or a specialized traction table may be used when the patient is placed in the supine position. Care must be taken to have a well-padded perineal post to limit the risk of pudendal nerve neuropraxia associated with traction. Most surgeons are familiar with the supine access to the hip area because of the treatment of hip fractures in this position. Other advantages of the supine position include the ease and reproducibility of positioning, accessibility of standard equipment, and the minimal amount of patient manipulation necessary. Some disadvantages of the supine position reported are limitations with obese patients and more difficult mobilization of the operative leg to reach the peripheral compartment.

A regular fracture table with attachments or a specialized traction table is used for the lateral position. The patient must be stabilized in the decubitus position, usually with a beanbag, posts, or a pegboard. Attention must be paid to padding downsided bony prominences and placing an axillary roll to support the down arm. A perineal post is placed between the legs to allow for distraction and a lateral vector to the operative leg. Advantages of the lateral position quoted are familiarity with the position because of hip arthroplasty, improved access for portal placement in obese patients, and easier access to the peripheral compartment because of better mobilization of the operative leg. Disadvantages discussed include potential extravasation of fluid into the abdomen and anesthesia concerns with the lateral decubitus position.[7,8]

ARTHROSCOPIC PORTALS

The 3 arthroscopic portals most commonly described for access of the central compartment of the hip are the anterolateral, anterior, and posterolateral portals.[9] Before creating the portals, the outline of the greater trochanter and the anterior superior iliac spine (ASIS) should be marked on the skin surface. A line is drawn distally along the thigh beginning at the ASIS. The safe zone for hip arthroscopy is the area between the posterior aspect of the greater trochanter and this vertical line extending from the ASIS. The sciatic nerve lies approximately 1.5 cm posterior to the posterior edge of the greater trochanter, whereas the femoral neurovascular structures lie medial to the ASIS. As the anterolateral portal lies in the middle of the safe zone, most hip arthroscopists choose it for the area of initial penetration into the joint.

The anterolateral portal (**Fig. 3**) is created just anterior and superior to the proximal tip of the greater trochanter. This pathway pierces the gluteus medius and enters the hip capsule at the lateral edge of the anterior margin. The superior gluteal nerve is the structure most at risk with the anterolateral portal. This nerve that supplies the gluteus

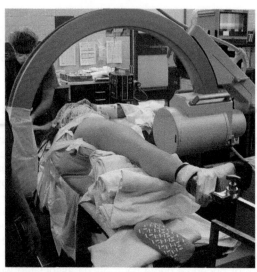

Fig. 3. Lateral decubitus patient positioning with the C-arm in the "over the top" position for intra-operative imaging.

medius, gluteus minimus, and tensor fascia lata exits the pelvis and travels posterior to anterior along the undersurface of the gluteus medius. The nerve is found an average of 4.4 cm above the level of the anterolateral arthroscopic portal.

The standard anterior portal is placed in line with the anterolateral portal at its intersection with the line drawn distal from the ASIS. This portal is often made slightly lateral to this intersection to avoid the branches of the lateral femoral cutaneous nerve (LFCN). The portal pathway is through the muscle belly of the sartorius and rectus femoris before entering the anterior hip capsule. Structures at risk when placing this portal include the LFCN, femoral nerve, and the lateral circumflex femoral artery. The LFCN usually branches proximal to the level of the anterior portal, but small lateral branches may be injured during portal placement. The femoral nerve is found an average of 3.2 cm medial to the location of the anterior portal. The ascending branch of the lateral circumflex artery is usually found approximately 3.6 cm distal to the anterior portal, but some terminal branches may lie in the area of the anterior portal.

The posterolateral portal is located 1 cm superior and posterior to the tip of the greater trochanter. This portal passes through both the gluteus medius and the gluteus minimus before entering the posterior edge of the lateral hip joint capsule superior and anterior to the piriformis tendon. The sciatic nerve is most at risk with this portal, as it lies approximately 2 to 3 cm posterior to the portal.[10–12]

There are many other described accessory portals used for access to the peripheral or lateral compartments. These portals should be placed under direct visualization on an as-needed basis.[10]

AUTHORS' EXPERIENCE

The authors' preferred technique uses the lateral position (**Fig. 4**) and general anesthesia. The patient is placed on a fracture table with a standard ski boot–type foot attachment positioned parallel to the floor. The patient's body is secured using a beanbag to maintain the lateral position. Special attention is paid to padding the

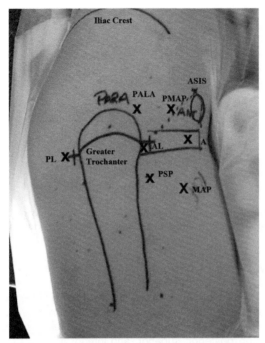

Fig. 4. A patient's right hip with commonly utilized portals denoted. From the posterior to anterior: A, anterior portal; AL, antero-lateral portal; MAP, mid-anterior portal; PL, postero-lateral portal; PSP, peritrochanteric space portal; PALA, proximal antero-lateral accessory portal; PMAP, proximal mid-anterior portal.

nonoperative leg, which rests free on the operating table and helps to stabilize the pelvis along with the patient's body weight. The use of an axillary roll under the patient and an arm holder for the arm on the operative side is also imperative. The foot of the operative leg is secured to the traction apparatus through the boot attachment.

The hip is positioned in neutral flexion to facilitate access into the hip joint at the beginning of the procedure. A series of rolled towels, secured with tape, is placed in the perineal area to serve as the post, which also protects the area and obtains 15° to 20° of abduction to facilitate access to the peripheral compartment of the hip without compromising the ability to access the central compartment of the joint. Neutral rotation of the leg is maintained to help protect the sciatic nerve and posterior structures by increasing the distance between these structures and the operative field. Traction is then applied to the operative leg through the boot attachment.

The C-arm is used to confirm acceptable distraction of the femoral head from the acetabulum with an AP view of the operative hip (**Fig. 5**). At least 8 mm of separation is needed for safe access to the central compartment of the joint without injuring the articular cartilage. If 8 mm of distraction is not achievable, the author inserts a spinal needle into the capsule to break the suction seal of the hip joint.

If the AP radiograph does not show adequate distraction, it has been the authors' experience that the attachment of the foot to the boot apparatus is most commonly the issue. The foot must be firmly secured to the boot to effectively distract the operative hip. A combination of Velcro straps associated with the boot and an overwrap of Coban (3M, St Paul, MN, USA) self-adherent elastic wrap are used to provide

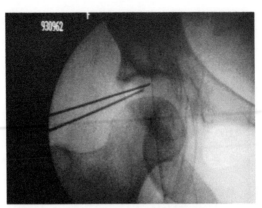

Fig. 5. An AP C-arm image demonstrating appropriate hip joint distraction, as well as fluoroscopic evidence of appropriate needle placement and air arthrogram.

additional security. Before tightening the straps, it is necessary to ensure that the dorsal surface of the foot is padded adequately.

The surgical site is prepared with Chloraprep (2% chlorhexidine gluconate/70% isopropyl alcohol). An area from the lower border of the ribs to the midthigh of the operative leg, from spine to umbilicus, is prepared. Four sterile towels are folded and placed at the anterior, posterior, superior, and inferior edges of the field to provide a first layer of drapes. A large drape with a central access hole is placed over the towels so as to cover the entire patient and table, including the traction boot. The center of the hole is placed on the greater trochanter of the operative leg and secured into place with an Ioban dressing (3M).

This drape has attached sterile plastic bags on the anterior and posterior surfaces, which help to control fluid overflow from the arthroscopic apparatus. The cables and tubes of the arthroscope and associated tools are connected, and the procedure is begun.

ARTHROSCOPIC TECHNIQUE

The authors establish the anterolateral portal, located at the anterior edge of the greater trochanter, initially. The first step in establishing the anterolateral portal is the introduction of a spinal needle at the anterior edge of the greater trochanter. The needle is guided into the hip joint using fluoroscopy. The proper path of the approach is parallel to the femoral neck, as close as possible to the femoral head, to avoid injuring the labrum. The tip of the needle should be rotated away from the femoral head to avoid scuffing the cartilage of the head with the tip of the needle. The tip of the needle should be used to penetrate the hip capsule without contacting the acetabular cartilage. Once the intra-articular location of the needle is established, the inner stylus is removed and a nitinol (flexible metal) guidewire is introduced through the needle. A cannulated switching stick is passed over the guidewire, and after the intra-articular position of the switching stick is confirmed, the guidewire is removed. A standard arthroscopic cannula is passed over the switching stick, and the switching stick is subsequently removed. A standard 4-mm 70° arthroscope is introduced into the cannula for visualization.

The anterior portal is established next. A 17-gauge spinal needle is passed through the skin at a point corresponding to the intersection of a vertical line extended from the

ASIS and a horizontal line extending from the anterolateral portal. The needle is visualized arthroscopically to ensure that the path taken does not injure the anterior labrum or articular cartilage. A nitinol wire is passed through the spinal needle in a fashion similar to the establishment of the anterolateral portal, and the needle is removed. A sharp-tipped dilator is then passed over the guidewire and used to create a capsulotomy. Care must be taken to direct the dilator away from the articular surface of the femoral head to prevent damage as it pierces through the anterior capsule. The dilator is removed, and a switching stick is placed over the guidewire, if needed, to switch to a more anterior viewing portal; otherwise, the anterior portal is used as a working portal for most of the procedure. The arthroscopic examination of the central compartment can now begin, including any indicated procedures. It has been the authors' experience that judiciously increasing the size of the anterior capsulotomy with either a small scalpel or a shaver may be of benefit and allow for more maneuverability within the joint. This process is most often done by removing tissue from the lateral edge of the capsulotomy, working back toward the anterolateral viewing portal.

Once the central compartment arthroscopy is finished, the traction is released and the leg is flexed to 50° to 80° to facilitate access to the peripheral compartment. Manual dynamic flexion and internal rotation are needed to identify the impingement and perform the decompression. Further debridement of the anterior capsule and synovium is often necessary for visualization of the anterior and lateral portions of the femoral head and femoral neck. Once the debridement is accomplished, fluoroscopy is used to confirm the position of the medial and lateral edges of the femoral neck to ensure full and accurate removal of any osteophytes or impinging tissues. For complex labral repairs or acetabuloplasty, a third posterolateral working portal is used. This posterolateral portal is craeted in an outside in fashion with spinal needle assistance while viewing from anterior to posterior. The use of an inferior accessory portal to assist with peripheral compartment work has also been described, but in most cases, it is possible to access the femoral neck using leg flexion and, if needed, a small degree of internal rotation, to find the area of impingement. Other accessory portals that have been described include the following: proximal anterolateral accessory portal (PALA), proximal mid-anterior portal (PMAP) and a peritrochanteic space portal (PSP).

After completion of all the necessary work, it is important to assess the need for capsular closure, which depends on the size of the capsulotomy performed. This procedure should be routinely done in individuals with lax ligaments.

Local anesthetics are used to assist with postoperative pain control. Before incision, the surgical site is anesthetized with a local anesthetic, through the skin and into the subcutaneous tissue. Once the procedure is completed, the hip joint proper is further anesthetized with a combination of long-acting local anesthetic and morphine. Hip arthroscopy is routinely performed as a day surgery procedure, and patients are discharged after a short stay in the recovery area once they obtain clearance from the anesthesia and nursing staff. Upon discharge, the patients are given a narcotic prescription for pain control, as well as a 14 day course of indomethacin for heterotrophic bone formation prevention.

COMPLICATIONS

The reported complication rate for hip arthroscopy is low, with 1 large series reporting 1.4%.[13] Some common complications encountered are neuropraxias of the LFCN secondary to anterior portal placement, pudendal nerve issues because of the perineal post, or iatrogenic damage to the articular cartilage during arthroscopy. With careful technique and accurate portal placement, many of these complications can be limited. Another known complication associated with hip arthroscopy is heterotrophic bone formation. In an effort to minimize this risk, the author recommends a 14 day post-operative course of indomethacin.

SUMMARY

In this article, the concepts important for hip arthroscopy are reviewed. Room setup, necessary equipment, and the basics of patient positioning are detailed, and the benefits of lateral versus supine positions are evaluated. The placement of common arthroscopic portals and the authors' preferred position and technique for hip arthroscopy are discussed. Also, the potential complications encountered are discussed.

REFERENCES

1. Burman MS. Arthroscopy or the direct visualization of joints: an experimental cadaver study. J Bone Joint Surg 1931;29:669–95.
2. Sampson TG. Arthroscopic treatment of femoroacetabular impingement. Tech Orthop 2005;20:56–62.
3. Dienst M, Godde S, Sell R, et al. Hip arthroscopy without traction: in vivo anatomy of the peripheral joint compartment. Arthroscopy 2001;17:924–31.
4. Eriksson E, Arvidsson L, Arvidsson H. Diagnostic and operative arthroscopy of the hip. Orthopedics 1986;9:169–76.
5. Glick JM, Sampson TG, Gordon RB, et al. Hip arthroscopy by the lateral approach. Arthroscopy 1987;3:4–12.
6. McCarthy JC, Day B, Busconi B. Hip arthroscopy: applications and techniques. J Am Acad Orthop Surg 1995;3:115–22.
7. Bartlett CS, DiFelice GS, Buly RL, et al. Cardiac arrest as a result of intraabdominal extravasation of fluid during arthroscopic removal of loose body from the hip joint of a patient with an acetabular fracture. J Orthop Trauma 1998;12:294–9.
8. Sampson TG. Complications of hip arthroscopy. Clin Sports Med 2001;20:831–6.
9. Byrd JWT, Pappas JN, Pedley MJ. Hip arthroscopy: an anatomic study of portal placement and relationship to extraarticular structures. Arthroscopy 1995;11:418–23.
10. Kelly BT, Philippon MJ, editors. Arthroscopic techniques of the hip: a visual guide. Thorofare (NJ): SLACK; 2010. p. 1–26.
11. Miller MD, Cole BJ, editors. Textbook of arthroscopy. Philadelphia: Elsevier; 2004. p. 429–42.
12. Andrews JR, Timmerman LA, editors. Diagnostic and operative arthroscopy. Philadelphia: WB Saunders Company; 1997. p. 209–24.
13. Clarke MT, Arora A, Villar RN. Hip arthroscopy: complications in 1054 cases. Clin Orthop 2003;406:84–8.

The Labrum of the Hip: Diagnosis and Rationale for Surgical Correction

Michael T. Freehill, MD, Marc R. Safran, MD*

KEYWORDS

• Labrum • Acetabulum • Impingement • Femoroacetabular

The treatment of labral pathologic condition of the hip has become a topic of increasing interest. In patients undergoing hip arthroscopy, tears of the acetabular labrum are the most commonly found pathologic condition and the most common cause of mechanical symptoms. Although a labral tear may occur with a single traumatic event, often another underlying cause may be already present, predisposing the individual to injury. In one study of patients undergoing hip arthroscopy for an atraumatic labral tear, 87% demonstrated radiographic evidence of an osseous abnormality, including femoroacetabular impingement (FAI), arthritis, or hip dysplasia.[1]

Although the number of diagnoses of labral tears of the acetabulum seems to be on the increase, there still remains debate on the function and importance of this structure. There have been 2 important points that have emerged regarding the repair of the labrum and the greatest chance of a successful outcome. First, labral repair is performed not only to relieve pain and mechanical symptoms but also to attempt the avoidance or delay of an accelerated rate of degeneration of the hip. Second, it is important to address the underlying cause of the labral tear and any other cause of dysfunction of the hip at the same time because it increases the chances for improved outcome (resolution of symptoms) and reduces the likelihood of recurrence. Most commonly, these problems include FAI, hip dysplasia, and hip instability. This article discusses the structure and function of the acetabular labrum, the diagnosis of labral injury through physical examination and imaging modalities, and the current treatment options, including labrectomy, labral repair, and reconstruction.

ACETABULAR LABRUM ANATOMY

The acetabular labrum is a fibrocartilaginous structure at the free margin of the bony acetabulum of the pelvis. The labrum is divided into capsular and articular sides. The

Department of Orthopaedic Surgery, Stanford University, 450 Broadway Street, Redwood City, CA 94063, USA
* Corresponding author.
E-mail address: msafran@stanford.edu

Clin Sports Med 30 (2011) 293–315
doi:10.1016/j.csm.2010.12.002
0278-5919/11/$ – see front matter © 2011 Elsevier Inc. All rights reserved.

capsular side of the labrum is thicker and composed of dense connective tissue, whereas the articular side of the labrum is composed of type II collagen fibrocartilage.[2] Although the labrum is attached to the articular rim similar to the glenoid of the shoulder, the structure is more of a horseshoe shape. This shape is due to the inferior portion of the acetabulum being composed of the transverse acetabular ligament. The labrum does run in continuity with the transverse acetabular ligament because it is a fibrous band connecting the anterior and posterior portions of the labrum. The cross section of the acetabular labrum is triangular, similar to a meniscus. The osseous rim of the acetabulum penetrates into this triangle for attachment to the labrum (**Fig. 1**). A type of pincer FAI lesion could be present when this bony protrusion into the labrum is too prominent or steep.

The hip capsule with its inherent ligaments does not insert directly into the labrum as it does in the shoulder. The physician must remain aware of this physiologic structural difference, because a cleft between the capsule and labrum may be apparent on advanced imaging modalities and could be confused with a labral tear.

There is no intrinsic blood supply present in the acetabular labrum.[3] An anastomotic ring surrounding the capsular attachment of the labrum provides the blood supply to the labrum. Because the capsule attaches directly to the supraacetabular bony area and is higher on the capsular side of the labrum, it makes sense that there is a significant diminution of vascular density moving toward the articular surface and the free edge of the labrum.[2] This vascular pattern was confirmed by Kelly and colleagues,[4] who reported that the overall mean vascularity of the labrum was greater at the capsular portion attached to the osseous acetabulum. The healing potential is greatest at the peripheral capsulolabral junction, where the blood supply is greatest, an important factor when considering whether a labral tear is repairable. The anastomotic ring

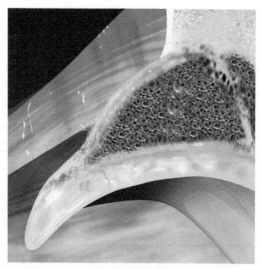

Fig. 1. Acetabular labrum and relationship of the capsule. The labrum is a triangular fibrocartilage with bony protrusion of the acetabulum within its substance. The capsule attaches proximal to the labrum, leaving a cleft between the 2 structures. Blood supply to the labrum comes mostly from the capsule, with some penetration into the capsular side of the labrum, mostly near the acetabular attachment. Also note that the labrum usually is in continuity with the articular cartilage of the acetabulum. (*Courtesy of* Marc R. Safran, MD.)

is composed of contributories from the superior and inferior gluteal arteries, the obturator artery, and an ascending branch of the medial femoral circumflex artery.[5]

Recent studies have confirmed that the radial branches of a periacetabular periosteal vascular ring supply the labrum. These branches travel on the periosteal surface and penetrate the joint capsule near its insertion and continue within a loose connective tissue layer on the capsular surface of the labrum. No contribution from the hip capsule, synovial lining, or osseous acetabular rim could be demonstrated.[6]

There are a multitude of nerve endings present in the acetabular labrum. Kim and Azuma[7] identified both corpuscular receptors responsible for pressure, deep sensation, and temperature in the labrum, as well as free nerve endings. The free nerve endings of the labrum originate from the obturator nerve and a branch of the nerve to the quadratis femoris.[5] The presence of these free nerve endings is responsible for the pain in case of a torn labrum. The proprioceptive function of the labrum is an area devoid of current research. More unmyelinated nerve endings are found in the anterior and superior portions of the labrum and, coincidentally, these are the labral locations most commonly torn.

ACETABULAR LABRUM FUNCTION

Similar to the labrum of the glenoid, the acetabular labrum increases articular surface area and socket depth. Konrath and colleagues[8] performed a biomechanical study to assess the role of the acetabular labrum in load transmission. After complete removal of the labrum in 9 hips, no significant changes were detected with regard to contact area, load, and mean or maximum pressure in the anterior or superior aspects of the acetabulum in a single leg stance phase. Since then, new studies have proven the importance of an intact and functioning labrum.

The acetabular labrum has been shown to possess important biomechanical properties. First, the intact labrum creates a seal between the central and peripheral compartments, opposing the flow of synovial fluid from the central compartment. The central compartment contains the intra-articular portion of the labrum, the articular surfaces of the acetabulum, and most of the femoral head. An intact labrum allows the maintenance of the synovial fluid flow within the central compartment, achieving a negative pressure within the joint with increased stability and resistance of distraction of the femoral head.[9,10]

Safran and colleagues[11] have shown that in a cadaveric model with passive ranges of motion, the femoral head moves relative to the acetabulum when all the soft tissues are intact. This translation of the head relative to the acetabulum is greater when the muscle and skin are removed, even more so when the capsule is partially resected. Loss of the labrum, or at least its function, may also result in increased translation of the femoral head, which may result in instability and/or accelerated degeneration of the hip. Other investigators have shown the stabilizing effect of the labrum as well. Crawford and colleagues[12] have shown that less force is required to distract the femur by 3 mm after creating tears in the labrum when compared with the intact state. Dy and colleagues[13] demonstrated that abduction with external rotation (ER) produces anterior translation of the femoral head, resulting in additional forces to the anterior capsule and labrum.

The second function of the labrum, also achieved by creating a central compartment seal, is the uniform distribution of synovial fluid, providing nutrition to the articular cartilage and a smooth gliding surface between the femoral head and the acetabulum.[14] Loss of this seal secondary to a disrupted labrum could result in higher forces experienced by the cartilage and subsequent chondral injury. Song and colleagues[14] demonstrated that resistance to rotation, when the hip loaded progressively, increased after partial resection of the labrum. Therefore, the intact labrum maintains a low-friction environment, which may slow chondral wear. In addition, Ferguson and colleagues[15–17] have shown that cartilage consolidation and deformation is greater when there is a labral tear. It may be that the labrum slows exudation of the synovial fluid from within the articular cartilage with joint loads. The labrum can function as a barrier to the fluid from being compressed out of the articular cartilage as determined by the reduced cartilage compressibility with joint loads when the labrum is intact.

Furthermore, the proprioceptive mechanoreceptors in the labrum may be important in hip function and possibly stability. Thus, the labrum has several important properties that are key to appropriate hip function and, possibly, the prevention of degenerative changes of the hip.[18]

DIAGNOSIS
History

The diagnosis of acetabular labral tears may be difficult for the physician. A thorough background, including a history of hip dysplasia, slipped capital femoral epiphysis, Legg-Calvé-Perthes, or previous trauma, can be associated with labral tears. FAI is likewise common with labral pathologic condition and is potentially responsible for the injury; however, many patients may not know they possess these osseous abnormalities at baseline. The mechanism of injury is commonly reported as a sudden twisting or pivoting motion, with a "pop," "click," "catching," or "locking" possibly occurring. Pain is most often described as insidious in onset, followed by a low-energy acute injury. In a study by Burnett and colleagues,[19] in a cohort of patients with a labral tear documented at arthroscopy, pain was usually located in the groin (92%) and exacerbated by activity (92%), as well as sitting, arising from the seated position, or descending stairs. Less commonly, pain may be located at the lateral hip or posteriorly. Not uncommonly, patients present with fairly long-standing groin pain that also develop into lateral hip pain secondary to hip abductor weakness, resulting in trochanteric bursitis and posterior hip pain caused by piriformis weakness. These developments seem to be secondary to the altered mechanics associated with the long-standing groin pain. Discomfort is exacerbated with motion into a flexed or internally rotated position or extension from a flexed position (hip extension test).[20]

When FAI co-exists, most patients describe an insidious onset of hip pain in the groin, with some remembering the general time frame of the beginning of the discomfort. Patients often state that they do not have trouble with activities of daily living except in sitting positions or when donning their socks and/or shoes; however, they do usually experience an exacerbation of their symptoms with sporting activities or an inability to perform these sports secondary to pain. FAI with a labral tear is more likely in young active adults who describe intermittent pain and exacerbation of symptoms with prolonged walking or sitting. Hip arthritis is frequently associated with labral tears as part of the pathologic condition. The physician must remain conscientious of other potential diagnoses that may mimic hip labral pathologic condition. These musculoskeletal causes include lower back disk pathologic condition or sacroiliitis, proximal femoral stress fractures, pubic rami fractures, psoas or rectus femoris tendinitis, or abductor muscle pathologic condition. Furthermore, genitourinary and gastrointestinal problems, including inguinal and sports hernias, may result in groin pain and should be kept in mind when evaluating a patient with hip or groin pain. However, physicians must also be aware that any of these causes could co-exist with a labral tear or may be the primary diagnosis.

Physical Examination

The physical examination should allow the physician to observe bilateral lower extremities. The presence of pelvic obliquity can be determined by placing the index fingers on the iliac crests and both thumbs on the posterior superior iliac spines (PSISs) (**Fig. 2**). The height of the index fingers should be symmetric for equal leg lengths. Hip abductor weakness is assessed with the Trendelenburg sign, in which the examiner's thumbs are level on the PSISs and move up when the patient stands on the contralateral leg. Gait should be observed, and an antalgic gait should be differentiated from a Trendelenburg gait observed with abductor muscle weakness or hip dysplasia. Leg lengths can be measured from the anterior superior iliac spines to the medial malleolus (or more accurately using a scanogram, if necessary).

In the supine position, the hip is taken through a range of motions. Flexion is measured, and although often not appreciably decreased, a torn labrum elicits pain at the extremes of flexion. The Thomas test is used to assess for a flexion contracture. At 90° flexion, ER and internal rotation (IR) are measured. IR in a patient with a torn labrum is often decreased and creates discomfort when in position. IR is also reduced in FAI or osteoarthritis (OA), whereas ER may be reduced in OA or adhesive capsulitis

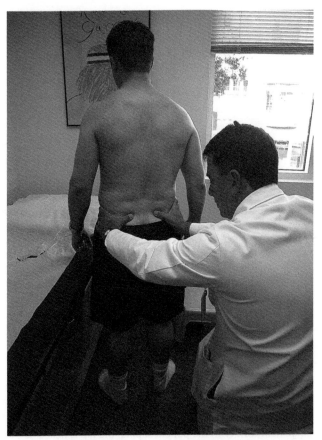

Fig. 2. Examination of the patient for leg length discrepancy and hip abductor weakness using the Trendelenburg test. (*Courtesy of* Marc R. Safran, MD.)

of the hip. The impingement test is performed with the hip flexed to 90°, maximum IR, and moving the hip into adduction (flexed-adducted-internally rotated [FADIR]) (**Fig. 3**). Although this test was originally described for dysplasia of the hip,[21] it is also affective for diagnosis of FAI with potentially associated labral pathologic condition and other sources of intra-articular pain. The labrum can be evaluated for catching the labral tear in a manner similar to the McMurray maneuver for the knee. The hip is started in a position of flexion, abduction, and ER and then brought in adduction and (IR), while extending the hip (**Fig. 4**). This maneuver is then repeated by starting in the FADIR position and moving into ER, abduction, and extension. This maneuver may reproduce the pain associated with a labral tear and/or a catch or clunk of the labrum. Labral tears may also be associated with iliopsoas pathologic condition, and thus, assessing for iliopsoas weakness by resisting hip flexion while seated can be useful. Internal snapping hip caused by iliopsoas tightness or weakness is often associated with intra-articular pathologic condition, including labral tears. Internal snapping hip may also be elicited by having the patient actively move their hip from a position of flexion, abduction, and ER to adduction and IR, while extending the hip. Alternatively,

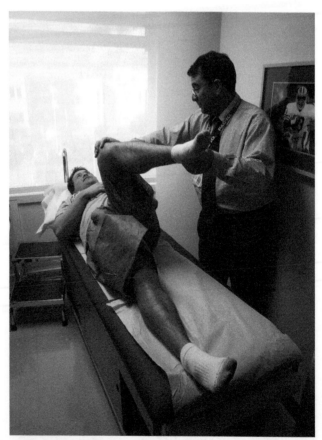

Fig. 3. Hip impingement test. With the patient supine, the hip is flexed 90°, adducted, and internally rotated. This maneuver may produce pain and is associated with intra-articular hip pain, although not specifically FAI. (*Courtesy of* Marc R. Safran, MD.)

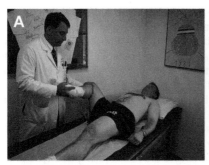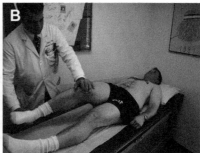

Fig. 4. (*A, B*) Labral stress test. The patient is placed supine, and the hip brought into flexion, abduction, and ER. Then the extremity is extended as it is adducted and internally rotated. This maneuver may reproduce pain and/or cause a clunk of a labral tear. (*Courtesy of* Marc R. Safran, MD.)

having the patient lift their leg 12 in from the examination table and moving from abduction-ER to adduction-IR may also elicit deep hip snapping.

Because hip instability may also be a cause of labral tears, evaluation for this problem should also be studied. This study includes an assessment of generalized ligamentous laxity as well as evaluation of hip rotation in flexion and in extension. While the patient lays supine, passive ER position of the feet should be evaluated for excessive ER, which may be a clue to iliofemoral ligament insufficiency. Furthermore, with the patient supine and the leg placed in a figure-of-4 position, the distance of the lateral knee to the examination table should be compared side to side and it may be an indicator of excessive hip ligamentous laxity.

Instability and labral pathologic condition may also be tested with the hyperextension ER test. Having the patient lay at the end of the examination table holding on to 1 knee (with hip and knee flexed) while the other extremity is hanging over the end of the table in hyperextension, the examiner externally rotates the leg in neutral abduction-adduction and in adduction. Posterior pain should alter the examiner to consider the possibility of posterior hip impingement, while anterior or groin pain may be elicited in the case of hip instability and/or labral tear.

Resisted straight leg testing can also provide a clue of hip pain by loading the joint. Abductor strength is tested by abduction resistance against the examiner's hand with the patient testing in the side-lying position. With the patient lying lateral, the Ober test is performed, and the inability to lower the leg below neutral (extension, adduction, inferiorly) position demonstrates the presence of a tight iliotibial (IT) band. A standard neurovascular examination of baseline strength, including bilateral iliopsoas, quadriceps, hamstrings, tibialis anterior, extensor hallucis longus, and gastrocnemius-soleus, as well as symmetry of dorsalis pedis and posterior tibial arterial pulses, evaluation of back range of motion and tenderness, and Lasègue' sign should be performed.

Imaging

Although the acetabular labrum cannot be visualized on roentgenograms, findings of FAI, OA, dysplasia, or other associated pathologic conditions of the hip could provide a clue to the potential of labral pathologic condition. Furthermore, calcification of the labrum, either partial or complete, may be visualized. The standard plain radiographic set includes an anteroposterior (AP) pelvis with cross-table lateral radiographs. A well-centered AP pelvis can be obtained by ensuring that the coccyx is midline and

1 to 3 cm superior to the symphysis pubis. A true AP is essential because rotation or tilting of the pelvis could alter the angles and version being radiographically determined. Hip structures that must be visualized include the femoral head shape and contour, acetabulum (particularly both the anterior and posterior walls as well as the cotyloid fossa and floor), the lateral edge of the acetabulum, the ilioischial line, the joint space, the sourcil, femoral neck-shaft, and the ischial spine.

Degenerative OA of the hip is most commonly graded using the Tonnis classification.[22] The Tonnis classification has been most commonly used and is specific for the hip; however, its utility has recently come into question because of its insensitivity to lesser degrees of degeneration and lack of relationship to prognosis or guiding treatment. In grade 0, no arthritic changes are present; in grade 1, sclerosis, minimal joint space narrowing, and minimal osteophytes are present; in grade 2, a moderate amount of joint space narrowing and small cystic changes are present; and in grade 3, moderate to complete joint space narrowing and large cysts are present. The femoral head should be evaluated for sphericity. Lack of sphericity or chronic changes present laterally could represent a history of Legg-Calvé-Perthes disease, slipped capital femoral epiphysis, or FAI.

Abnormal version of the acetabulum is determined by the presence of the crossover sign (for relative cranial acetabular retroversion), the posterior wall sign (for posterior wall insufficiency), and the ischial spine signs. Originally described by Reynolds and colleagues,[23] a crossover sign is when the anterior and posterior proximal acetabular edges cross before meeting together superiorly and laterally without crossing over. This sign represents retroversion of the superior acetabulum such that the anterior superior acetabulum is more lateral than the posterior superior acetabulum and is associated with FAI pincer anatomy. It has also been suggested that the projection of the ischial spines into the pelvis on the AP indicates retroversion.[24] A posterior wall sign is present when the rim of the posterior wall is medial to the center of the femoral head. This wall sign is important for surgical planning because there may be a need to address a deficiency of acetabulum posteriorly. Excessive posterior acetabular wall (significantly lateral to the center of the femoral head) may be due to excessive anteversion or osteophytic change that may result in posterior hip impingement.

FAI can be thought of as a morphologic condition that predisposes to intra-articular damage, which later becomes painful. There are 2 main categories of bony abnormalities based on location of impingement that are present in FAI: a femoral-sided cam lesion and an acetabular-sided pincer lesion. The cam lesion is commonly a bump on the anterior, lateral, or anterolateral femoral head-neck junction, with loss of femoral head-neck offset creating what is often referred to as a pistol grip deformity. The lateral contour takes on a flat or convex extension at the neck junction. This type of bony abnormality results in decreased range of motion before abutment occurs with the acetabular rim and can create the symptoms of FAI by initially separating the labrum from the acetabular rim/chondral junction, damaging the articular cartilage or causing synovial irritation. This impingement is because the femoral head possesses an increased radius of curvature, which distorts the articulation with the acetabulum. A short or thick femoral neck, residuals of slipped capital femoral epiphysis, deformity from Legg-Calvé-Perthes, or fracture malunion may also result in cam-type FAI. Thus, the unique pattern of labral pathologic condition associated with cam-type FAI is a labral-chondral separation.

The pincer type of FAI is present with overcoverage of the acetabulum relative to the femoral head. This presence of pincer type of FAI may be the result of relative retroversion, true retroversion, cranial retroversion, or a deep socket, as seen with coxa profunda, coxa protrusio, and/or a center-edge angle of more than 40°. Radiographically, coxa profunda is when the floor of the acetabulum reaches the ilioischial line, whereas protrusio occurs when the femoral head reaches the ilioischial line.[25] There is overcoverage and abutment occurring with the femoral head-neck junction early, causing impingement-type symptoms. This type of impingement results in a crushing of the labrum, resulting in intrasubstance degeneration. Most patients have components of both types of impingement.

In both types of FAI, the labrum becomes impinged and can subsequently degenerate or tear. Generally, the pincer type causes labral failure earlier through the direct crushing mechanism, whereas in the cam type, it occurs later, as a labral-chondral separation occurs early, sparing the labral substance initially. Patients with FAI present 86% of the time with a mixed type of impingement assessed on radiographs.[26]

The cross-table lateral view allows for assessment of the proximal femur, including the head-neck junction, as well as lateral view of the acetabulum, allowing for assessment of anterior coverage. Thus cam lesions, both anterior and lateral, can be assessed on the AP pelvis and lateral films; however, true anterolateral prominences may be underappreciated.

Fibrocystic changes causing herniation pits can often be seen in the region of a cam lesion and are thought to be secondary to the chronic abutment with the superior rim. These changes have been reported in 33% of hips with FAI.[27] The center-edge angle is determined by a longitudinal line through the center of the femoral head perpendicular to the teardrop or ischial tuberosities and a line from the center of the femoral head to the lateral edge of the acetabulum. A normal angle is greater than 20° to 25°. An angle less than this value represents undercoverage of the acetabulum, and an angle more than 35° to 40° could represent overcoverage and possible presence of a pincer lesion.

Advanced Imaging

It has been shown that a large field-of-view (FOV) magnetic resonance imaging (MRI), that is, an MRI of the pelvis, has the ability to detect a labral tear less than 10% of the time.[28] A small FOV MRI of the hip can detect a labral tear 25% of the time. However, a small FOV MRI arthrogram of the hip can detect a labral tear greater than 90% of the time. As such, an MRI arthrogram is the authors' imaging modality of choice. More recently, it has been found that 3T MRI without contrast may be as good as arthrography.[29] A long-acting anesthetic is added with the contrast agent when performing hip MR arthrography. This addition of the anesthetic allows assessment to determine if the pain is intra-articular or not. This technique is elucidated further later.

The coronal and axial sequences are excellent for visualization of the acetabular labrum. On MRI, the normal acetabular labrum appears as a triangular structure with low signal intensity and sharp margins. There is often a recess between the outer margin of the labrum and the joint capsule, the cleft as described earlier, which should not be confused with a labral tear. With degeneration of the labrum, there is increased signal on T2 fat suppression (FS) images (**Fig. 5**A). Labral-chondral separation can be identified as a fluid-filled cleft at the base of the labrum adjacent to the acetabular cartilage (see **Fig. 5**B). Because chronic labral tears may produce paralabral cysts, T2-weighted sequences that demonstrate extra-articular fluid collections, such as paralabral cysts, may provide a clue of a labral tear.

Thus, the advanced imaging modality of choice to detect a symptomatic labral tear is MR arthrography. This technique is effective in the evaluation of labral pathologic condition and femoral head-neck abnormalities. MRI is still not optimized to evaluate for articular cartilage damage in the hip, and arthrography does not improve the ability

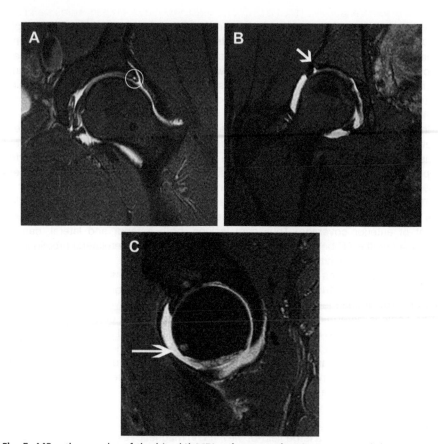

Fig. 5. MR arthrography of the hip. (*A*) MRI arthrogram showing a torn and degenerative labrum with contrast within the substance of the labrum. The area of interest is encircled. (*B*) Coronal MRI arthrogram showing fluid between the labrum and acetabular rim (*arrow*), consistent with a labral-chondral separation. Also note in (*B*) that the labrum is rounded and not a sharp triangle, also consistent with labral damage. (*C*) An inclusion cyst (*arrow*) at the femoral head-neck junction, consistent with FAI. (*Courtesy of* Marc R. Safran, MD.)

much. MRI is also advantageous because it can not only detect labral and sometimes cartilage damage but also assess the extent and severity of the abnormality. Furthermore, MRI is beneficial in ruling out other uncommon causes of hip pain, including stress fractures, musculotendinous injuries, avascular necrosis, hernias, and tumors. The sensitivity and accuracy of MR arthrography for the diagnosis of acetabular labral tears has been reported as 100% and 94%, respectively.[30]

Leunig and colleagues[31] reported that the type of pathologic condition observed on MR arthrography can aid in determining the cause responsible for the abnormal acetabular labrum. In both developmental dysplasia of the hip and FAI, disorders of the labrum were most common in the anterosuperior quadrant; however, the labrum was enlarged in the dysplastic hips and not the FAI hips. In cam-type FAI, repetitive shear forces to the anterosuperior acetabulum produce an outside-in abrasion of the acetabular cartilage or avulsion of the labrum from the acetabular rim. In pincer impingement, there is intrasubstance damage to the labrum. In both types of FAI, inclusion cysts of the femoral head-neck region can be found as a result of the abutment (see **Fig. 5C**).

Although the assessment of the articular surface is improved with this imaging modality, intraoperative evaluation arthroscopically is still the gold standard. Nonetheless, information regarding the articular surface is essential in operative planning when a bony remodeling procedure is expected.

The alpha angle described by Notzli and colleagues,[32] is an adjuvant measurement for diagnosis of FAI on MRI. On the axial views, the angle is determined by the intersection of lines from the center of the femoral head to the center of the femoral neck and a line from the center of the femoral head to the point on the neck where the contour changes from a predrawn circle around the femoral head. Notzli and colleagues[32] reported a mean alpha angle of 74° in patients with symptoms of FAI, as opposed to a mean of 42° in controls. Most clinicians use an alpha angle of greater than 55° as being consistent with FAI. However, there are many problems with the alpha angle. First, the loss of offset may not be anteriorly located, because different patients have different areas in which cam lesions are present. Second, it has been shown there is an unacceptably high interobserver variability in this measurement.[33] Also, the outcome of FAI surgery does not correlate with the restoration of the alpha angle to normal values.[34]

The authors have found the use of computed tomography (CT) scans, particularly 3-dimensional CT scan reconstructions, useful for enhanced evaluation of concomitant bony anatomy. This modality is found particularly in preoperative surgical planning, when concomitant bony surgery is planned with the labral surgery.

Fluoroscopic Injections

Injection into the hip joint under fluoroscopy is a proven way to distinguish intra-articular and extra-articular conditions because not all labral tears (or other imaging identified pathologic condition) are symptomatic or the source of the patient's pain. Patients are instructed to move their hips into the positions that hurt before the injection, and then again after the injection, assessing the degree of pain relief. The reasons that patients with intra-articular pathologic condition do not get pain relief include (1) the pain is not coming from inside the joint; (2) the injection was not into the joint; and (3) there was a traumatic injection (multiple or prolonged attempts to get the injection in the joint), and in some situations, there is no relief when associated with gadolinium, although the reasoning is not clear.

Anesthetic medications are injected and relief of symptoms subjectively reported by the patient is 90% reliable as an indication the abnormality is intra-articular.[35] Corticosteroids can also be added to help with discomfort from a co-existing degenerative process and could be a therapeutic treatment.

Classification of Labral Tears

There are different classification systems for acetabular labral tears based on anatomic location, cause, histology, magnetic resonance arthrography (MRA), arthroscopy, and those correlating with chondral damage. However, classification systems are only useful if they help provide prognosis or guide treatment, which few do. Tears of the labrum have been classified by location, dividing the acetabulum in 3 quadrants or defining the acetabulum as a clock face. Labral damage based on cause has been classified as traumatic, degenerative, FAI, capsular/laxity and hip hypermobility, dysplasia, and idiopathic. Seldes and colleagues[36] described 2 types of tears according to a histologic evaluation: the first type is a detachment of the labrum from the articular surface (labral-chondral separation), the second type is intrasubstance injury, composed of one or more cleavage planes within its substance. However, when evaluating this classification in the face of knowledge about FAI, a type-1 tear is a labral-chondral separation in which the labrum is spared and is more typical with cam-type impingement. Type 2 tears are intrasubstance cleavage tears of variable depths and are more typical of pincer-type impingement.

Lage and colleagues[37] devised an arthroscopic classification system for the description of labral tears and identified 4 types of tears: radial flap, radial fibrillated, longitudinal peripheral, and abnormally mobile. The first type (radial flap) was the most common (56.8%), involving a disruption of the free margin of the labrum. The radial fibrillated tears (21.6%) were associated with degenerative articular cartilage. Longitudinal peripheral tears (16.2%) were present at the junction of the acetabular rim. The fourth type, the abnormally mobile tear, was found in 5.4% of patients.

McCarthy and colleagues[38] underscored the correlation between articular cartilage damage and labral tears in different stages. In stage 0, there is a contusion of the labrum with adjacent synovitis. In stage 1, there is a small free margin tear of the labrum with intact articular cartilage surfaces of the acetabulum and femoral head. Stage 2 is defined by a visible labral tear with focal articular damage of the adjacent femoral head but with normal acetabular cartilage. In stage 3, there is also a labral tear but with adjacent focal acetabular articular cartilage damage with or without femoral head articular cartilage chondromalacia. Stage 3 is subdivided according to the involvement of the acetabular articular cartilage: 3A, when the lesion is less than 1 cm; 3B, when it is greater than 1 cm. Stage 4 is identified by extensive acetabular labral tearing with associated diffuse arthritic articular cartilage alterations in the joint.

Czerny and colleagues[39] described a classification according to MRA findings in labral pathologic condition. Stage 0 is the normal labrum. Stage IA is defined as the labrum showing increased signal that does not extend to the margin, whereas stage IB demonstrates a thicker labrum, and the labral recess is not visible because this space is filled by the enlarged labrum. In stage IIA, contrast material extends into the substance of the labrum, while the labral attachment and recess are still preserved. Stage IIB (as compared with stage IIA) is defined by a thicker labrum with no labral-chondral recess visible. In stage IIIA, the labrum is detached from the acetabulum, maintaining its triangularity. Stage IIIB is identified by a labral detachment with a thickened and rounded labrum.

The Multicenter Arthroscopic Hip Outcomes Research Network (MAHORN) group has proposed a classification system to study labral tears to determine if there is a prognostic difference of different types of tears with regard to outcomes (**Box 1**).

Thus, several classification systems exist that are descriptive in nature. However, as noted earlier, the importance of a classification system should be for prognostic purpose or to guide treatment. Although helpful in descriptive terms, none of the classification systems described earlier fulfills the key criteria for a useful classification system. It remains to be seen, but the Seldes classification, although simple, may hold promise regarding differentiating reparable from nonreparable labral tears, because vascularity from the acetabulum may allow the repair of labral-chondral separations, whereas intrasubstance tears, without inherent blood supply within the substance of the labrum, may not necessarily be reparable with current technology. Thus, this classification may be useful in that it may guide treatment.

Treatment

The treatment of labral tears and their associated disorders is important to relieve pain and may help in the preservation of the hip of young and active adults. Labral tears can be caused by several factors, including trauma, FAI, hip dysplasia, instability, psoas impingement, and degenerative arthritis. Nonoperative management is the initial treatment of all conditions of the hip. These efforts include physical therapy,

---

Box 1
Proposed MAHORN classification of labral tears

I Normal

II Hypoplastic/Hyperplastic

III Tear

    IIIA Complex/Degenerative

    IIIB Labral-chondral separation

    IIIC Partial

    IIID Complete

    IIIE Flap

IV Intrasubstance changes

    IVA Mucinoid/Yellow

    IVB Floppy

    IVC Bruising

    IVD Ossified

    IVE Calcific

---

antiinflammatory medications, rest, and activity modification. Physical therapy in the face of FAI, unless the impingement is caused by an anteverted pelvis, is usually unsuccessful.[40] An experimental study has shown that the labrum can partially heal and regenerate and thus is worthy of an attempt of conservative management.[41] However, labral pathologic condition with associated osseous abnormalities, particularly FAI or dysplasia, may continue to produce symptoms because the underlying cause of the labral tear has not been addressed, either inhibiting healing or causing a healed tear to retear. In addition, symptomatic improvement, although likely for only a short time, may be achieved with an intra-articular injection of corticosteroids.

Candidates for arthroscopic intervention are those who have exhausted nonoperative means, with persistent hip pain for more than 1 month, positive reproducible examination findings, pain relief with intra-articular anesthetic injection, and MRI results consistent with labral pathologic condition. Surgical intervention is aimed at addressing the labral pathologic condition and its underlying cause.

The natural history or consequence of an acetabular labral tear is still debated. Labral tears have been identified to occur in locations of localized hip arthritis. As a result, it has been theorized that labral tearing occurs early in the osteoarthritic hip. However, no definitive study has demonstrated whether labral tears ultimately result in arthritis or the arthritis causes the tears.

The femoral head does not have a constant center of rotation with motion, thus, it moves relative to the acetabulum during the range of motion.[11] Although small amounts of motion are expected and the articular cartilage can handle these forces, increased translations of the femoral head within the acetabulum could result in greater shear forces. Articular cartilage is optimally configured to resist compressive forces and, to a lesser degree, shear forces. Thus, increased translation of the femoral head with resultant shearing may result in accelerated wear of the cartilage. Alterations of the soft tissue could potentially produce or accentuate this environment. Crawford and colleagues[12] created labral tears in cadaveric specimens and determined that it increased femoral head motion within the acetabulum. After venting of the capsule, forces to distract the femur 3 mm decreased 43% and then further to 60% after creation of a labral tear. Furthermore, the greater friction associated with labral tearing, as well as cartilage consolidation, may also result in accelerated breakdown of articular cartilage, resulting in degenerative arthritis.

Secondary to its tenuous blood supply and pattern of vascularity, the acetabular labrum possesses a limited capacity to heal. Thus, the traditional procedure of debridement of the torn labrum and partial labrectomy, in an effort to remove unstable portions, potentially alleviates the risk of propagation and relieves associated pain. Labral tears were initially treated with open techniques; however, significant morbidity was associated with these procedures. Advances in hip arthroscopy have both decreased the morbidity associated with these procedures and increased the ability to visualize and adequately address labral pathologic condition.

Current techniques to treat unreparable labral tears include removal of the loose torn tissue (**Fig. 6**A). This procedure may be performed using a mechanical suction-shaver, meniscus-like biters (see **Fig. 6**B), or radio frequency ablation. There have been no studies comparing the efficacy or safety of these devices for labral surgery, and each have their advantages and disadvantages. For instance, a radio frequency device is often smaller and longer, and some devices have bendable ends, making their use easier due to enhanced maneuverability, but the risk of these thermal devices to the articular cartilage (directly or through increased joint temperature) and the remaining/nonablated tissue must be taken into account. The key to performing partial labrectomy is to leave as much normal tissue as possible while removing the damaged torn ends. The goal is to have stable edges to reduce the risk of retearing or propagation of the labral tear, while attempting to leave as much labrum intact as possible. Although the labrum has circumferential fibers, and thus partial labrectomy may affect some of this function, that the labrum has bony attachment along the majority of the labrum would suggest that the remaining labrum may still provide function, as suggested by Safran and Giordano.[42] Furthermore, it is important to treat the associated pathologic condition, as is discussed later.

The earliest literature on hip arthroscopy with labral debridement alone demonstrated widely varying results at short-term follow-up. The overall range of good to excellent results was 67% to 93%.[43–48] The largest study of 58 hips by Santori and Villar[43] reported 67% good to excellent results at mean 42 months. Byrd and Jones[44] reported the highest good to excellent results of 93% at 26 months mean follow-up. Shindle and colleagues[49] performed a meta-analysis evaluating outcomes of studies

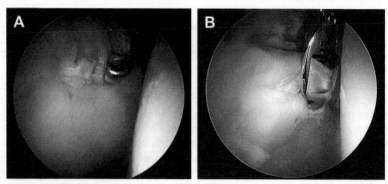

Fig. 6. (A) Arthroscopic view of a 43-year-old male patient with a degenerative labral tear treated with arthroscopic partial labrectomy. (B) Another patient undergoing partial labrectomy with a meniscal-like biter. (*Courtesy of* Marc R. Safran, MD.)

of partial labrectomies. They noted a resolution of mechanical symptoms and reduction of hip pain in 91% of cases at a mean follow-up of 2.5 years. They also noted in the studies using modified Harris Hip Scores,[44] an improvement of 31% to 40% at follow-up of 2 to 3.5 years.[49]

The early literature, however, is limited by several confounding problems. First, most studies reporting the treatment of labral tears were likely not truly treating isolated labral pathologic condition. Many associated pathologic conditions, including arthritis, were either treated or existed in the patients studied for the outcome of labral debridement. Labral tears are often associated with chondral lesions, and the most recent literature has shown that chondral damage is a negative prognostic finding in hip arthroscopy for many pathologic conditions, including labral tears and FAI. In addition, most of the studies were performed before FAI was described, and thus the co-existence of untreated FAI must be taken into account (as discussed later). In the subgroup of patients with moderate chondral damage with labral pathologic condition, Farjo and colleagues[47] reported 32% of these patients having a bad result. In fact, Farjo and colleagues[47] reported that their good to excellent results with labral debridement alone dropped from 71% in patients with no preoperative arthritis to 21% in those who possessed degenerative changes. Another confounding problem is the lack of a validated outcome score for active patient with nonarthritic hip problems. The Harris Hip Score was developed for the evaluation of individuals undergoing arthroplasty for hip arthritis, and suffers from a ceiling effect for the younger active patient. As such, the Harris Hip Score is suboptimal and may not be sensitive enough to have value to study the effects of labral surgery.

The confounding effect of FAI in labral pathologic condition cannot be understated and has been evaluated in several ways, confirming the need to address concomitant pathologic condition with the labral tear. Tanzer and Noiseaux[50] concluded that FAI is a common cause responsible for anterior groin pain, labral tearing, chondral damage, and eventual arthritis of the hip. In a group of patients with labral tears, a cam FAI deformity was present 97% of the time. These 38 patients were treated arthroscopically for the labral tears alone with partial labrectomy and not addressing the co-existing FAI. Mechanical symptoms completely resolved in all the patients; however, only 25% reported relief from their pain. Thus, the investigators concluded that the continued presence of FAI despite resection of the torn labrum resulted in residual symptoms and suggest that the FAI must also be addressed. In another study, a comparison was made of patients who were treated with arthroscopic partial labrectomy and excision of the FAI lesion (study group) versus those with hip arthroscopic partial labrectomy only (control group). Bardakos and colleagues[51] demonstrated that the pain in patients can be improved in the short term without removing the impingement lesion; however, those patients who had the impingement removed did better. Modified Harris Hip Scores were higher in those in those in whom the cam-type lesion was removed compared with those who only had arthroscopic labral surgery, although not significant. The trend was supported by the significant percentage of excellent/good postoperative scores in the study group (83%) versus the control group (60%).

Kim and colleagues[52] retrospectively evaluated 43 patients with early OA and acetabular labral tears treated arthroscopically. The labral tears were addressed with debridement (labrectomy) and not repair. At mean follow-up of 50 months, they reported satisfactory results in patients with early OA; however, clinical improvement when additional FAI was present was insufficient. No patient with FAI improved, and the investigators concluded that the arthroscopic debridement of the hip (labrectomy) with early OA fails if detectable FAI is present.

Thus, it can be reasoned that labrectomy alone produces suboptimal results in the face of co-existing FAI. The poor outcomes from these early studies of partial labrectomy may have been the result of unrecognized and untreated FAI. Surgically addressing the osseous abnormality restores more normal hip mechanics and potentially prevents or delays the progression of degenerative arthritis.

However, debridement of the labrum alone, even when a cheilectomy of the cam deformity is performed, still may result in increased femoral head motion within the acetabulum and the potential loss of the central compartment seal, which could result in a focal area of cartilage consolidation and increased chondral strain. Greaves and colleagues[53] showed that cartilage consolidation in the femoral head is increased with labral tear and restored with labral repair. Therefore, it seems appropriate to attempt labral repair whenever possible, along with correction of the FAI for maximum benefit and results.

On the other hand, labral tears in the face of hip dysplasia often signify decompensation of the hip. The distribution of weight-bearing forces is shared more significantly by the labrum because of the deficient acetabulum in hip dysplasia. As a result, when the labrum becomes torn, it cannot share the loads as effectively, if at all, and the shallow acetabulum must bear the brunt of the load. This scenario leads to accelerated wear of the articular cartilage at the acetabular rim. Removal of the torn labrum results in further decompensation and may result in an accelerated deterioration of the joint. The underlying problem is the deficiency of bony support. Not addressing the bony issue, such as with a periacetabular osteotomy, may result in rapid deterioration of the patient's symptoms. The same can be said for labral repair in the face of hip dysplasia. If a surgeon attempts to repair the labrum, if the bony deficiency is not corrected, the repair will not be successful as a result of the excessive forces that caused the labrum to fail in the first place.

Restoration and maintenance of the labrum seems appropriate with the knowledge that it possesses important mechanical properties at the hip. Chondrolabral tears (Type I) would be most likely to heal because of the increased vascularity on the capsular side. Studies have demonstrated that healing does take place in this setting. Philippon and colleagues[54] reported on labral repairs in an ovine model. A 1.5-cm labral-chondral separation was created in 10 mature female sheep and was arthroscopically repaired with 1 suture anchor and simple loop stitch. Histology demonstrated that the labrum was stable and grossly healed in all models 12 weeks after repair. However, the labral healing was found to be incomplete in all specimens, and it was concluded that although these lesions are capable of healing, the process of healing is via fibrovascular tissue or reattachment with new bone formation.

Conceptually, repair should be undertaken to restore the suction seal and the biomechanical environment of negative intra-articular pressure, seal to exudation of joint fluid for a reduced friction-bearing surface as well as limit cartilage consolidation, maintain stability and provide proprioceptive input.[18] However, there are no clinical studies in the literature that studied the isolated repair of labrum of the hip, and therefore, debate still remains.

Scientific evidence supporting any particular technique of labral repair is lacking. Most surgeons use suture anchors to perform labral repair, similar to shoulder surgery; however, there are several important differences. When performing a labral repair, the acetabular rim needs to be cleared of soft tissue and the bone abraded for soft tissue healing to the acetabular rim. The anchor needs to be placed on the acetabular rim. Because of the greater curvature of the acetabulum as compared with the glenoid, the drill guide must come from a portal more distal than the usual central compartment arthroscopic portals, which helps avoid penetration of the joint by the drill or anchor

(**Fig. 7**). The anchor should be placed as close to the acetabular rim as possible without penetrating the joint to attempt to restore the labral function/labral seal on the femoral head. The sutures have generally been passed around the labrum as a simple repair. However, the authors have found that this pattern does not restore the normal labral function and think this may be because of the eversion of the edge of the labrum by the suture (**Fig. 8**A). As a result, the authors have used a vertical mattress suture, passing one limb of the suture behind the femoral head and one limb through the substance of the labrum, from anterior to posterior, approximately middle distance between the labral free edge and acetabular edge (see **Fig. 8**B). This construct pushes the labrum toward the femoral head, restoring the seal. The knot is tied on the capsular side of the labrum to avoid abrasion against the femoral head (**Fig. 9**). Because the labrum is subject to strain of varying degrees dependent on the range of motion, the patients are placed in a hip brace postoperatively, limiting particular motions based on the location of the tear/repair using the data from the authors' cadaveric study of hip labral strain.[55]

Espinosa and colleagues[56] retrospectively reviewed 60 hips in patients who underwent arthrotomy and surgical dislocation for acetabuloplasty and chielectomy associated with FAI. In the first 25 hips, the labrum was resected and in the next 35, the remaining labrum was reattached to the acetabular rim. At 2-year follow-up, the resection group had 28% excellent results and the labral reattachment group 80% excellent results. Radiographic signs of OA were significantly more prevalent in the labral resection group. However, this was a consecutive series, which suffered methodologically from other factors, such as improved surgical technique, rehabilitation, potentially earlier diagnosis (with earlier recognition of this diagnosis), and/or less damage to the labrum.

Philippon and colleagues[57] reported on the outcomes of hip arthroscopy for FAI with associated chondrolabral dysfunction. They studied 58 patients who underwent labral repair versus 54 with debridement alone. The multivariate analysis predictors of

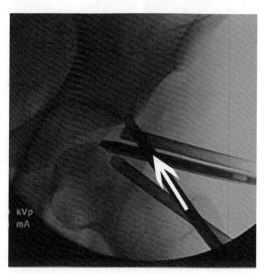

Fig. 7. Fluoroscopic image during a labral repair. The 3 standard hip arthroscopy portals with cannulas are in place, along with a more distal portal for the drilling and introduction of an acetabular labral repair anchor (*arrow*), demonstrating the path that diverges from the joint surface. (*Courtesy of* Marc R. Safran, MD.)

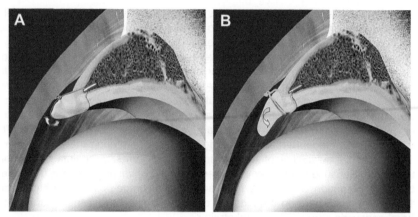

Fig. 8. Labral repair. (*A*) Effect of a simple suture around the labrum. The suture pulls the labral edge away from the femoral head, everting it (*arrow*). This suture may result in a reduced suction seal. (*B*) Effect of a vertical mattress suture, allowing the free edge of the acetabular labrum to fall normally toward the femoral head (*arrow*), allowing restoration of the seal. (*Courtesy of* Marc R. Safran, MD.)

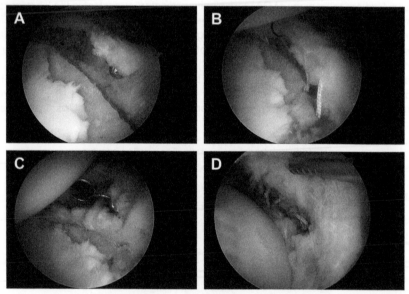

Fig. 9. Labral repair in 23-year-old professional basketball player with combined-type FAI. (*A*) Labrum elevated/retracted after acetabuloplasty and chondroplasty. (*B*) Acetabular rim after the placement of 4 suture anchors. The sutures have already been passed in a vertical mattress manner. One limb of the suture comes from the anchor behind the labrum, while the other comes in front of the labrum (articular side) then through the substance of the labrum toward the capsular side to produce a vertical mattress pattern. (*C*) Central compartment view after the sutures have been tied. Notice the free edge of the labrum is leaning toward the joint, while the acetabular edge is tightly adhered to the acetabular rim. (*D*) View from the peripheral compartment; the shaver is pulling the capsule (*upper right*) up to demonstrate the sutures (*blue and white*) on the capsular side of the labrum, away from the femoral head. The labrum is lying on the femoral head (to the left) restoring the seal. (*Courtesy of* Marc R. Safran, MD.)

better outcome were higher preoperative Harris Hip Scores, 2 mm or more of joint space narrowing, and repair of the labrum versus resection. However, because this was nonrandomized retrospective study, the individuals who had labral repair may have possessed less pathologic condition or damage to the joint, making the labrum more amenable to repair, whereas those with partial labrectomy may have had more damage to the labrum and the rest of the joint and this could influence the results.

Larson and Giveans[58] reported on 36 consecutive hips in which the acetabular labrum was debrided and 39 in which refixation was performed in patients with FAI. Mean follow-up of 21.4 and 16.5 months, respectively, demonstrated Harris Hip Scores significantly better in the refixation group. Good to excellent results were 67% in the debridement group versus 90% in the refixation group. Again, being a retrospective consecutive series study, there are methodological challenges that prevent an absolute conclusion that labral repair is better than partial labrectomy.

Thus, the 3 studies that currently exist comparing partial labrectomy with labral repair all suggest the repair is better than debridement. However, all 3 studies have methodological problems limiting the power of their conclusion, and each was studied in patients with FAI and were not patients with isolated labral repairs. As such, although it seems that labral repairs may be better, and conceptually, it makes sense to repair the labrum to maintain its function (which has yet to be shown), randomized controlled studies are lacking for the optimal treatment of labral tears, in the face of FAI, dysplasia, or in an isolated situation.

A comprehensive review of the treatment of labral pathologic condition would not be complete without a discussion of labral reconstruction. Philippon and colleagues[59,60] described a reconstruction procedure using IT band autograft in which the labrum cannot be repaired secondary to lack of adequate or quality tissue. A piece of fascia lata is rolled up and inserted into the joint and attached to the acetabular rim with labral repair techniques. Early outcomes for regaining function and satisfaction from their series are satisfactory. Because of no comparison group and the short-term follow-up, it remains to be seen if these results hold up or restore long-term function. However other investigators have started to report early results using other graft sources, such as semitendinosus (Dean Matsuda, MD, personal communication, 2010) or rectus femoris (Thomas Sampson, MD, personal communication, 2010).

SUMMARY

The importance of the labrum and its function continue to be reported in the literature. Diagnosing labral tears of the hip remains challenging in the face of many other potential or co-existing diagnoses. When conservative management fails, arthroscopic intervention can be performed. Labral repair is conceptually superior to debridement alone. There is limited scientific evidence suggesting that labral repairs can heal and result in improved clinical outcomes. Thus, labral repair should be considered when possible, particularly for labral injuries at the labral-chondral junction with good labral substance. In addition, the importance of addressing associated bony pathologic condition, particularly FAI when present, is paramount in a successful outcome. Adhering to these treatment principles allows the young and active adults the best chance at recovery and delay in a degenerative process. At present, labral reconstruction is being studied and may be a viable option when labral repair is not possible.

REFERENCES

1. Wenger DE, Kendall KR, Miner MR, et al. Acetabular labral tears rarely occur in the absence of bony abnormalities. Clin Orthop Relat Res 2004;426:145–50.

2. Petersen W, Petersen F, Tillmann B. Structure and vascularization of the acetabular labrum with regard to the pathogenesis and healing of labral lesions. Arch Orthop Trauma Surg 2003;123(6):283–8.

3. McCarthy J, Noble P, Aluisio FV, et al. Anatomy, pathologic features, and treatment of acetabular labral tears. Clin Orthop Relat Res 2003;406:38–47.

4. Kelly BT, Shapiro GS, Digiovanni CW, et al. Vascularity of the hip labrum: a cadaveric investigation. Arthroscopy 2005;21(1):3–11.

5. Putz R, Schrank C. Anatomy of the labor-capsular complex. Orthopade 1998; 27(10):675–80 [in German].

6. Kalhor M, Horowitz K, Beck M, et al. Vascular supply to the acetabular labrum. J Bone Joint Surg Am 2010;92(15):2570–5.

7. Kim YT, Azuma H. The nerve endings of the acetabular labrum. Clin Orthop Relat Res 1995;320:176–81.

8. Konrath GA, Hamel AJ, Olson SA, et al. The role of the acetabular labrum and the transverse acetabular ligament in load transmission in the hip. J Bone Joint Surg Am 1998;80(12):1781–8.

9. Takechi H, Nagashima H, Ito S. Intra-articular pressure of the hip joint outside and inside the limbus. Nippon Seikeigeka Gakkai Zasshi 1982; 56(6):529–36.

10. Terayama K, Takei T, Nakada K. Joint space of the human knee and hip joint under a static load. Eng Med 1980;9:66–74.

11. Safran MR, Zaffagnini S, Lopomo N, et al. The influence of soft tissues on hip joint kinematics: an in vitro computer assisted analysis. Poster Presentation at the 55th Annual Meeting of the Orthopaedic Research Society. Las Vegas (NV), February 22–25, 2009.

12. Crawford MJ, Dy CJ, Alexander JW, et al. The 2007 Frank Stinchfield Award: the biomechanics of the hip labrum and the stability of the hip. Clin Orthop Relat Res 2007;465:16–22.

13. Dy CJ, Thompson MT, Crawford MJ, et al. Tensile strain in the anterior part of the acetabular labrum during provocative maneuvering of the normal hip. J Bone Joint Surg Am 2008;90(A):1464–72.

14. Song Y, Safran MR, Ito H, et al. Poster 1153: articular cartilage friction increases in hip joints after partial and total removal of the acetabular labrum. Presented at the 55th Annual Meeting of the Orthopaedic Research Society. Las Vegas (NV), February 22–25, 2009.

15. Ferguson SJ, Bryant JT, Ganz R, et al. The influence of the acetabular labrum on hip joint cartilage consolidation: a poroelastic finite element model. J Biomech 2000;33:953–60.

16. Ferguson SJ, Bryant JT, Ganz R, et al. The acetabular labrum seal: a poroelastic finite element model. Clin Biomech (Bristol, Avon) 2000;15:463–8.

17. Ferguson SJ, Bryant JT, Ganz R, et al. An in vitro investigation of the acetabular labral seal in hip joint mechanics. J Biomech 2003;36:171–8.

18. Safran MR. The acetabular labrum: anatomic and functional characteristics and rationale for surgical intervention. J Am Acad Orthop Surg 2010;18: 338–45.

19. Burnett RS, Della Rocca GJ, Prather H, et al. Clinical presentation of patients with tears of the acetabular labrum. J Bone Joint Surg Am 2006;88(7): 1448–57.

20. McCarthy JC, Noble PC, Schuck MR, et al. The Otto E. Aufranc award: the role of labral lesions to development of early degenerative hip disease. Clin Orthop Relat Res 2001;393:25–37.

21. MacDonald SJ, Garbuz D, Ganz R. Clinical evaluation of the symptomatic young adult hip. Semin Arthroplasty 1997;8:3–9.
22. Tönnis D. [Eine neue form der huftfan- nenschwenkkung durch dreifachos- teostomiezur ermoglichung spoterer hufprothesenversorgung]. Orthop Praxis 1979; 15:1003–5 [in German].
23. Reynolds D, Lucas J, Klaue K. Retroversion of the acetabulum: a cause of hip pain. J Bone Joint Surg Br 1999;81:281–8.
24. Kalberer F, Sierra RJ, Madan SS, et al. Ischial spine projection into the pelvis: a new sign for acetabular retroversion. Clin Orthop Relat Res 2008;466: 677–83.
25. Beck M, Leunig M, Parvizi J, et al. Anterior femoroacetabular impingement: part II. Mid-term results of surgical treatment. Clin Orthop Relat Res 2004; 418:67.
26. Beck M, Kalhor M, Leunig M, et al. Hip morphology influences the pattern of damage to the acetabular cartilage: femoroacetabular impingement as a cause of early osteoarthritis of the hip. J Bone Joint Surg Br 2005;87:1012–8.
27. Leunig M, Beck M, Kalhor M, et al. Fibrocystic changes at anterosuperior femoral neck: prevalence in hips with femoroacetabular impingement. Radiology 2005; 236:237–46.
28. Toomayan GA, Holman WR, Major NM, et al. Sensitivity of MR arthrography in the evaluation of acetabular labral tears. AJR Am J Roentgenol 2006;186(2): 449–53.
29. Sundberg TP, Toomayan GA, Major NM. Evaluation of the acetabular labrum at 3.0-T MR imaging compared with 1.5-T MR arthrography: preliminary experience. Radiology 2006;238(2):706–11.
30. Chan YS, Lien LC, Hsu HL, et al. Evaluating hip labral tears using magnetic resonance arthrography: a prospective study comparing hip arthroscopy and magnetic resonance arthrography diagnosis. Arthroscopy 2005;21:1250.
31. Leunig M, Podesywa D, Beck M, et al. Magnetic resonance arthrography of labral disorders in hips with dysplasia and impingement. Clin Orthop Relat Res 2004; 418:74–80.
32. Nötzli HP, Wyss TF, Stoecklin CH, et al. The contour of the femoral head-neck junction as a predictor for the risk of anterior impingement. J Bone Joint Surg Br 2002;84:556–60.
33. Lohan DG, Seeger LL, Motamedi K, et al. Cam-type femoral-acetabular impingement: is the alpha angle the best MR arthrography has to offer? Skeletal Radiol 2009;38(9):855–62.
34. Brunner A, Horisberger M, Herzog RF. Evaluation of a computed tomography–based navigation system prototype for hip arthroscopy in the treatment of femoroacetabular cam impingement. Arthroscopy 2009;25(4):382–91.
35. Byrd JW, Jones KS. Diagnostic accuracy of clinical assessment, magnetic resonance imaging, magnetic resonance arthrography, and intra-articular injection in hip arthroscopy patients. Am J Sports Med 2004;32:1668–74.
36. Seldes RM, Tan V, Hunt J, et al. Anatomy, histologic features and vascularity of the adult acetabular labrum. Clin Orthop Relat Res 2001;382:232–40.
37. Lage LA, Patel JV, Villar RN. The acetabular labral tear: an arthroscopic classification. Arthroscopy 1996;12:269–72.
38. McCarthy J, Wardell S, Mason S, et al. Injuries to the acetabular labrum: classification, outcome, and relationship to degenerative arthritis. Presented at the Annual Meeting of the American Academy of Orthopaedic Surgeons. San Francisco (CA), February 13–17, 1997.

39. Czerny C, Hofmann S, Neuhold A, et al. Lesions of the acetabular labrum: accuracy of MR imaging and MR arthrography in detection and staging. Radiology 1996;200:225–30.
40. Jager M, Wild A, Westhoff B, et al. Femoroacetabular impingement caused by a femoral osseous head-neck bump deformity: clinical, radiological, and experimental results. J Orthop Sci 2004;9:256–63.
41. Miozzari HH, Clark JM, Jacob HA, et al. Effects of removal of the acetabular labrum in a sheep model. Osteoarthritis Cartilage 2004;12:419 30.
42. Safran MR, Giordano G, Lindsey DP, et al. Effect of acetabular labrum tears and resection on labral strain. Transactions of the 55th Annual Meeting of the Orthopaedic Research Society. Las Vegas (NV), February 22–25, 2009.
43. Santori N, Villar RN. Acetabular labral tears: result of arthroscopic partial limbectomy. Arthroscopy 2000;16(1):11–5.
44. Byrd JW, Jones KS. Prospective analysis of hip arthroscopy with 2-year follow-up. Arthroscopy 2000;16(6):578–87.
45. McCarthy J, Barsoum W, Puri L, et al. The role of hip arthroscopy in the elite athlete. Clin Orthop Relat Res 2003;406:71–4.
46. Potter BK, Freedman BA, Andersen RC, et al. Correlation of short form-36 and disability status with outcomes of arthroscopic acetabular labral debridement. Am J Sports Med 2005;33:864–70.
47. Farjo LA, Glick JM, Sampson TG. Hip arthroscopy for acetabular labral tears. Arthroscopy 1999;15(2):132–7.
48. O'Leary JA, Berend K, Vail TP. The relationship between diagnosis and outcome in arthroscopy of the hip. Arthroscopy 2001;17(2):181–8.
49. Shindle MK, Voos JE, Nho SJ, et al. Arthroscopic management of labral tears in the hip. J Bone Joint Surg Am 2008;90(Suppl 4):2–19.
50. Tanzer M, Noiseaux N. Osseous abnormalities and early osteoarthritis: the role of hip impingement. Clin Orthop Relat Res 2004;429:170–7.
51. Bardakos NV, Vasconcelos JC, Villar RN. Early outcome of hip arthroscopy for femoroacetabular impingement. The role of femoral osteoplasty in symptomatic improvement. J Bone Joint Surg Br 2008;90(12):1570–5.
52. Kim KC, Hwang DS, Lee CH, et al. Influence of femoroacetabular impingement on results of hip arthroscopy in patients with early osteoarthritis. Clin Orthop Relat Res 2007;456:128–32.
53. Greaves LL, Gilbart MK, Yung AC, et al. Effect of acetabular labral tears, repair and resection on hip cartilage strain: a 7 T MR study. J Biomech 2010;43:858–63.
54. Philippon MJ, Arnoczky SP, Torrie A. Arthroscopic repair of the acetabular labrum: a histologic assessment of healing in an ovine model. Arthroscopy 2007;23(4):376–80.
55. Giordano G, Lindsey DP, Gold G, et al. Strains within the intact acetabular labrum during passive range of motion. Transactions of the 55th Annual Meeting of the Orthopaedic Research Society. Las Vegas (NV), February 22–25, 2009.
56. Espinosa N, Rothenfluh DA, Beck M, et al. Treatment of femoro-acetabular impingement: preliminary results of labral refixation. J Bone Joint Surg Am 2006;88(5):925–35.
57. Philippon MJ, Briggs KK, Yen YM, et al. Outcomes following hip arthroscopy for femoroacetabular impingement with associated chondrolabral dysfunction: minimum two-year follow-up. J Bone Joint Surg Br 2009;91(1):16–23.
58. Larsen CM, Giveans MR. Arthroscopic debridement versus refixation of the acetabular labrum associated with femoroacetabular impingement. Arthroscopy 2009;25:369–76.

59. Philippon MJ, Briggs KK, Hay CJ, et al. Arthroscopic labral reconstruction in the hip using iliotibial band autograft: technique and early outcomes. Arthroscopy 2010;26(6):750–6.
60. Philippon MJ, Schroder e Souza BG, Briggs KK. Labrum: resection, repair, and reconstruction sports medicine and arthroscopy review. Sports Med Arthrosc 2010;18(2):76–82.

Acetabular Labral Tears: Diagnosis, Repair, and a Method for Labral Reconstruction

Leandro Ejnisman, MD[a], Marc J. Philippon, MD[a,b,c],*,
Pisit Lertwanich, MD[a]

KEYWORDS

- Labral tears • Labral reconstruction • Hip pain

Acetabular labral tears are a common cause of hip pain.[1–3] In athletes, hip injuries represent 3.1% to 8.4% of sports injuries in recent reports.[4,5] The prevalence of labral tears in patients with hip complaints has been reported from 22% to 55%.[6,7] The understanding of labral tears has greatly evolved in the past few years, and there now is better understanding of labral anatomy, function, disease and treatment. Hip arthroscopy has played an important role in the development of this knowledge, and has been established as a treatment option for the treatment of labral pathology. The goals of this article are to describe labral anatomy, to explain clinical presentation of labral pathology, and to provide guidelines in arthroscopic treatment.

ANATOMY

The acetabular labrum is a triangular fibrocartilaginous structure located circumferentially around the bony acetabulum, which becomes attached to the transverse

In 2010/2011 Leandro Ejnisman was a Visiting Scholar in Hip Arthroscopy and Biomechanics. Scholarship provided with grants from the Instituto Brasil de Tecnologias da Saúde.
Financial Disclosures: Board member/owner/officer/committee appointments: Arthrocare (MJP). Royalties: Smith & Nephew, Arthrocare, DonJoy, Bledsoe (MJP). Paid consultant or employee: Smith & Nephew (MJP). Research or institutional support from companies or suppliers: Smith & Nephew, Ossur, Arthrex, Siemens (MJP, LE).
[a] Steadman Philippon Research Institute, 181 West Meadow Drive, Suite 1000, Vail, CO 81657, USA
[b] The Steadman Clinic, Vail, CO, USA
[c] Department of Surgery, McMaster University, Hamilton, Ontario, Canada
* Corresponding author. Steadman Philippon Research Institute, 181 West Meadow Drive, Suite 1000, Vail, CO 81657.
E-mail address: karen.briggs@sprivail.org

Clin Sports Med 30 (2011) 317–329
doi:10.1016/j.csm.2010.12.006
0278-5919/11/$ – see front matter © 2011 Elsevier Inc. All rights reserved.

acetabular ligament posteriorly and anteriorly.[8] There is no distinction between the labrum and the transverse acetabular ligament, and they appear to be a continuous structure.[9] Histologically, the labrum merges with the acetabular cartilage through a transition zone of 1 mm to 2 mm.[9] A recent study in human embryos showed that the chondrolabral junction is not uniform throughout the acetabulum and may have an anterior zone with weaker attachment to the bony acetabulum.[10] This zone was also described by McCarthy and colleagues[6] as the most frequent location of labral tears. Lower biomechanical properties in the anterosuperior region of the labrum compared with other regions may be a contributing factor of higher prevalence of labral tears at this area.[11]

The labrum plays a crucial role in normal hip mechanics. Crawford and colleagues,[12] using a three-dimensional motion analysis system, demonstrated labral tears lead to increased femoral head displacement in cadaveric hips. Fergunson and colleagues[13,14] demonstrated that the labrum provides a suction seal, keeping the synovial fluid inside the hip joint, which would help in pressure distribution and joint lubrication (**Fig. 1**).

Free nerve endings can be found in the acetabular labrum, and they may be involved in pain and proprioceptive sensation of the hip joint.[4] The labrum receives blood supply from branches of the obturator artery, superior gluteal artery and inferior gluteal artery. The articular side of the labrum is relatively avascular, compared with the capsular side, which is surrounded by highly vascularized synovium.[15] There are no specific areas of relative hypovascularity in the labrum. Labral tears seems to have a healing potential, as neovascularization occurs in labral tears studied histologically.[9] It also has been shown in an ovine model that labral repairs are capable of healing via fibrovascular repair tissue and/or direct reattachment via new bone formation.[16]

CLASSIFICATION OF LABRAL TEARS

Acetabular labral tears have been known for decades. Labral pathology has been described in trauma,[17] Perthes disease,[18] and acetabular dysplasia.[19] Labral tears also have been recognized as an early event in the development of hip osteoarthritis.[20]

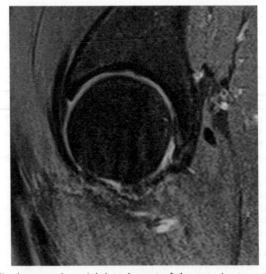

Fig. 1. A longitudinal tear and partial detachment of the anterior to anterolateral labrum.

Seldes and colleagues[9] described two different histologic types of labral tears. Type 1 is a detachment of the labrum from the articular surface at the transition zone between the fibrocartilaginous labrum and the articular hyaline cartilage. Type 2 consists of one or more cleavage planes of variable depth within the substance of the labrum. Lage and colleagues[21] developed a classification based on the etiology of the labral tear and divided the tears into 4 categories: traumatic, degenerative, idiopathic, and congenital. Recently, femoroacetabular impingement (FAI) has been described as another cause of labral damage. This condition is an abnormal contact between the femoral head–neck junction and the acetabular rim caused by abnormal bony morphology.[22] In addition, capsular laxity and psoas impingement can result in labral tears. Therefore, the authors have included all of these conditions in a classification of labral tears summarized in **Table 1**.

The bony abnormalities in Cam and Pincer FAI, cause different patterns of labral tears.[20] Most commonly they are combined; if not combined, cam is more common. Cam impingement is characterized by abnormal femoral head–neck offset. This produces shear forces that create a primary lesion at the chondrolabral junction separating the labrum from the articular cartilage. Pincer impingement results from overcoverage of the acetabulum. In this type of impingement, the labrum is crushed between the acetabular rim and the femoral neck, causing degeneration of the labrum with intrasubstance ganglion formation.

Capsular laxity can be caused by congenital disorders and acquired conditions. Elher-Danlos syndrome, Marfan syndrome, and Down syndrome are common congenital causes of capsular laxity. Repetitive rotational sporting activities stress the capsule, resulting in attenuation of the iliofemoral ligament.[2] This capsular laxity leads to rotational instability, which results in increased pressure on the anterior superior labrum as the head rides anterior in the joint.[23]

A tight psoas tendon can compress the anterior capsulolabral complex and cause atypical anterior labral tears. Patients with labral tears require thorough evaluation for all possible causes that must be treated concurrently with arthroscopic labral treatment. This is crucial for good clinical outcomes, protection of labral healing, and prevention of labral reinjuries.

CLINICAL PRESENTATION

A detailed history and physical examination are essential to correctly diagnose labral tears, its causes, and concomitant disorders. Many remote conditions can present with referred pain to hip and groin areas,[8] such as the lumbar spine, sacroiliac joint,

Table 1	
Labral tear classification	
Type	**Base Condition**
1. Morphologic alterations	A) Femoroacetabular impingement Cam Pincer Mixed-type B) Dysplasia
2. Functional alterations	A) Instability B) Iliopsoas impingement
3. Trauma	Traumatic
4. Degeneration	Hip degenerative disease

or intrapelvic structures. Examination of the pubic region is important especially in athletes, since athletic pubalgia is an important differential diagnosis that can exist alone or in conjunction with labral tears. The term sports hip triad has been coined by Feeley and colleagues[4] to describe athletes presenting with a labral tear, adductor strain, and a rectus strain.

Patients with labral tears typically complain of anterior groin pain, but pain also can be referred to the buttock, greater trochanter, thigh, and medial knee. Other symptoms include clicking, locking, catching, instability, giving way, and stiffness.[24] The duration of symptoms must be evaluated and are extremely variable. A recent publication has shown as many as 45% of patients presenting with a sudden onset of symptoms.[25] Sports practiced by the patients and specific positions must be interrogated, as some types of sports are more prone to labral injuries, such as golf and ice hockey.[26]

Physical examination must be thorough; attention must be given to the patient gait, lower abdomen, lumbar spine, sacroiliac joints, and knees. Martin and colleagues[27] analyzed physical examinations of the hip performed by 6 hip specialists and found enough commonality to form the basis of recommended examination maneuvers in the evaluation of hip pain. Physical examination for labral tears superimposes with FAI examination, as these pathologies have a strong association. Hip examination must address motor strength, range of motion, points of tenderness, presence of limping, and Trendelenburg test. Hip motion is decreased in FAI, especially in cam impingement.[24,28,29] The most reliable specific test is the impingement test, which is done by flexion-adduction-internal rotation of the hip. This test is positive when it elicits anterior hip pain.[24] Forced external rotation with extension also can trigger hip pain related to acetabular labral tears.[9] The flexion-abduction-external rotation (FABER) test is a useful provocative maneuver. The affected leg is placed in a figure of four position so that the ipsilateral ankle is positioned proximal to the contralateral knee. The clinician should evaluate the presence of anterior hip pain, as well as the vertical distance between the lateral genicular line and the examination table, which is typically increased compared with the contralateral side in FAI patients.[24] A resisted leg raise in the supine position is another test used to elicit mechanical symptoms attributable to intra-articular abnormalities,[11] as well as an assessment of hip flexor strength.[27]

IMAGING

Plain radiographs remain the mainstay in evaluating hip pain. Many radiographic views can be used in the hip pain workup including an anteroposterior (AP) view of the pelvis, a cross-table lateral view, 45° and 90° Dunn view, a frog leg lateral view, and a false profile view.[30] The senior author (MJP) routinely uses an AP view of the pelvis, a cross-table lateral view, and a false profile view. It is crucial to assess proper patient positioning during radiographs to correctly determine osseous anatomy, especially acetabular rim morphology. Wenger and colleagues[31] reviewed hip radiographs of patients with labral tears and found that 87% of these patients had at least one bony abnormality.

Pincer impingement is characterized by acetabular overcoverage that can be either global or focal. Acetabular global overcoverage can happen in cases of coxa profunda or protusio acetabuli.[22] Focal overcoverage happens in a retroverted acetabulum, represented by the crossover sign,[24] the posterior wall sign, and a prominent ischial spine.[32] The amount of acetabular coverage of the femoral head can be measured by the center edge (CE) angle of Wiberg.[33] Increased angles are related to pincer impingement, while decreased angles are related to acetabular dysplasia. In some patients, paralabral cysts can be observed associated with labral tears. The femoral head–neck offset can be evaluated by measuring the alpha angle in the cross-table lateral view.

Other radiographic modalities are usually required to further delineate intra-articular hip pathology. Three-dimensional computed tomography can be employed to assess the extent of osseous resection that should be done during a hip arthroscopy. Magnetic resonance imaging (MRI) provides the most detailed images of intra-articular hip pathology, showing with great details labral anatomy and femoral and acetabular cartilage. The alpha angle is measured in the axial oblique sequences to evaluate the femoral head–neck junction.[24]

TREATMENT OF LABRAL TEARS

The initial treatment for labral tears should be conservative, consisting of physical therapy, anti-inflammatory medication, and activity modification. If patients have persistent pain after 4 weeks of treatment, they are candidates for hip arthroscopy.[2] Recent data suggest that early intervention in labral pathology leads to better results. Philippon and colleagues[26] showed that hockey players with labral tears who underwent arthroscopic treatment within 1 year from the time of injury returned to sports earlier than patients who had surgery more than 1 year after injury.

SURGICAL TECHNIQUE: LABRAL REPAIR

Hip arthroscopy may be performed in either the supine or lateral position depending on surgeon preference. The senior author (MJP) performs hip arthroscopy with patients in the modified supine position.[2] After placement of an extra wide post to protect the perineum, the hip is placed in a position of 10° flexion, 15° internal rotation, 10° lateral tilt, and neutral abduction. Traction is applied in the operative limb between 10 to 25 kg of force, with gentle countertraction applied to the contralateral limb. After traction, the leg is placed in slight adduction over the post, which forces the femoral head laterally. The leg is internally rotated to bring the femoral neck parallel to the floor. Traction is controlled with fluoroscopy, with the goal of a minimum of 8 mm to 10 mm of distraction.

Adequate portal placement is of paramount importance to hip arthroscopy, as a wrong portal placement can lead to neurovascular injury and inadequate joint visibility. The anterolateral portal is established 1 cm proximal and 1 cm anterior to the tip of the greater trochanter. The midanterior portal is made 6 cm to 7 cm from the anterolateral portal, at a 45° to 60° angle with respect to the longitudinal line passing through the anterolateral portal. This location should be half way between the longitudinal lines passing through the anterior superior iliac spine and the anterolateral portal. The latter portal is established with direct visualization from the anterolateral portal, with the 70° arthroscope.

After portal placements, a small capsulotomy is performed to facilitate mobility of the arthroscopic instruments and visualization of the joint. The labral tear is then assessed by location and size (**Fig. 2**). The labral tissue quality is evaluated, as well as the labral size. Labral tear treatment can be done either by débridement or repair. In the light of current understanding of the labral function and importance, it is important to make an effort to preserve as much labral tissue as possible. Clinical outcomes comparing débridement versus refixation have shown better results with labral repair.[25,34,35] Moreover, an experiment using ovine model showed the capacity of labral tears to heal after arthroscopic repair.[16] Therefore, the authors' approach is to preserve the labrum whenever possible. Labral débridement is limited to patients with a small peripheral tear that after resection retains enough tissue to maintain normal labral function.

To perform labral repair, the labral tear is first débrided of fraying and unhealthy tissue, with the goal of leaving only viable tissue with good healing capacity. Then, the acetabular rim is trimmed to a bleeding bed with a motorized burr. The labrum

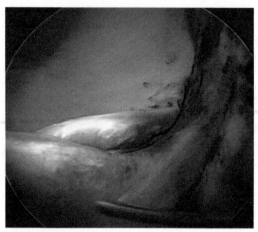

Fig. 2. Arthroscopic view of labral tear.

is repaired to the acetabular bone with the use of suture anchors (**Fig. 3**). They are drilled approximately 2 mm to 3 mm below the cartilage surface. Special care is taken not to penetrate the articular surface with the anchor. Typically, the most anterior part of the labral tear will be addressed first, with the anchors being delivered through the midanterior portal. Then, sequential anchors are placed along the labral tear to achieve adequate stability. More posterior anchors are placed through the anterolateral portal. The knots must be placed at the capsular side of the labrum, as failure to do so may cause an iatrogenic injury to the adjacent cartilage by the knot (**Fig. 4**).

The anchor suture can be looped around the labrum or passed through it. This decision is based on tissue quality and the position desired for the labrum. A hypotrophic labrum is not a good candidate for sutures to be passed through, as the tissue may be ripped as an arthroscopic penetrator is used to pass the suture through the labrum. Sutures looped around the labrum usually tend to evert it, while sutures passed through the labrum tend to invert it. This characteristic can be used to better restore the labral suction seal, as the labrum needs to sit correctly on the femoral head to act as a gasket for the joint. To make sure the suction seal has been restored, traction is released after anchor placement, and a dynamic examination is then performed

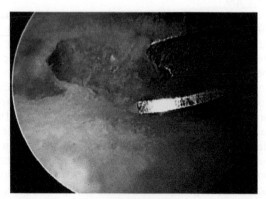

Fig. 3. Suture anchor placement in the acetabular rim close to the surface.

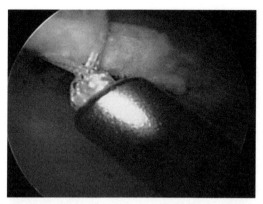

Fig. 4. The suture knots are on the capsular side of the labrum to avoid the knots rubbing on the cartilage surface.

(**Fig. 5**). The hip is brought through a complete range of motion to ensure adequate sealing by the labrum. If any labral area seems unstable, additional anchors can be placed. It is very important to make sure the labrum is stable at the time zero, so that there is no risk of labral retear during early postoperative rehabilitation.

Addressing associated conditions is essential for good surgical outcomes. Bony abnormality such as femoroacetabular impingement must be corrected to protect the labrum from new injuries. One study of revision hip arthroscopy showed that the most common reason patients returned for revision hip arthroscopy was persistent impingement.[36] To correctly address the pincer impingement, sometimes it is necessary to detach the labrum from the acetabular rim using an arthroscopic knife (**Fig. 6**). Then, the detached labrum is treated as a regular labral tear and is repaired to the trimmed rim as the technique described using suture anchors.

The pincer lesion also can be evaluated without labral detachment. In this situation, the bony overhang is trimmed over the labrum until the chondro–labral junction is reached. This method can create zones of labral instability, and these unstable areas

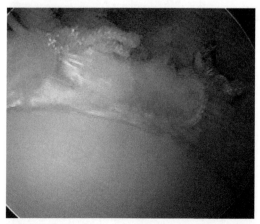

Fig. 5. The labrum is tightly sealed to the femoral head when the hip is moved through normal range of motion.

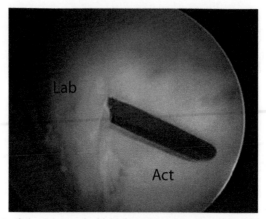

Fig. 6. Detachment of the labrum (Lab) before rim trimming. This allows for refixation of the labrum (Lab) on the new acetabular (Act) rim following trimming.

should be treated with anchor placement. It is important to evaluate the CE angle before performing the acetabular trimming to avoid situations of hip dysplasia and instability. It is estimated that 1 mm of bony resection at the acetabular rim decreases 2.4° of the CE angle, while 5 mm of rim resection cause a 5° change of the CE angle.[37] Cam impingement can be evaluated and treated in the peripheral compartment.

Tight psoas tendon that causes psoas impingement of the labrum can be released using a transcapsular approach. A small capsulotomy is made at the anterior part of the capsule, corresponding to the psoas valley of the acetabular rim (**Fig. 7**). The tendinous part of the iliopsoas muscle can be identified and then released using an arthroscopic knife. Psoas tendon release should be performed as the last step of the surgery, so that the risk of intra-abdominal fluid extravasation is diminished. In the end of the procedure, the capsule is closed with a number 2 Vicryl suture, (Ethicon,

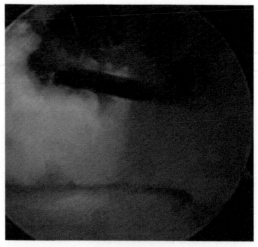

Fig. 7. A small capuslotomy showing the psoas tendon release.

Somerville, NJ, USA) and platelet-rich plasma is injected into the joint. For patients with capsular laxity, the capsule should be plicated to restrain the capsule and restore stability.

LABRAL RECONSTRUCTION

When treating labral tears, the authors' main objective is to preserve the labrum. This is not always possible, however. For cases that the labrum is deemed not amenable to repair, the senior author (MJP) has developed a method for labral reconstruction with the iliotibial band autograft.[38] Indications for labral reconstruction are hypotrophic labrum and complex tears. The authors define hypotrophic labrum by a width of 5 mm, and opt to reconstruct when it is less than 3 mm. Hypotrophic labrum can be caused by an anatomic variation or by previous labral débridment. Complex tears are defined as tears that completely disrupt the longitudinal fibers of the labrum. In these situations, there is not enough healthy tissue for a labral repair, and a labral reconstruction is the authors' method of choice for treatment.

Patient positioning and portal placement are similar to the aforementioned. When a labral tear is considered unrepairable, it is débrided until only healthy tissue is left. At this time, the acetabular rim is trimmed for an acetabular overhang if existent or just as a bleeding bed for the graft. Then the labral deficiency is measured using the tip of a motorized burr as a reference.

The iliotibial band is used as the graft donor site. The operative leg is taken out of traction, and it is straightened and internally rotated. An incision is done just distal to the anterolateral portal over the greater trochanter. The iliotibial band is exposed, and the graft is harvested at the junction between the anterior two-thirds and posterior one-third. The graft is retrieved as a rectangle with 15 mm to 20 mm in width, and it should be 30% to 40% longer than the actual defect to guarantee adequate length to restore the labrum.

The graft is taken to the back table and prepared while the defect in the iliotibial band and the incision are closed after a trochanteric bursectomy is performed if indicated. The graft is kept moist and cleared of all soft tissue attached to it. Number 2 Vicryl sutures (Ethicon, Somerville, NJ, USA) are used to capture both extremities of the graft. The graft is placed in a Graftmaster (Smith & Nephew, Andover, MA, USA) using the sutures in its extremities and is now tubularized using 2–0 Vicryl stitches. A suture loop of number 2 Vicryl is made at the thickest lateral end of the graft to facilitate later maneuverability. Platelet-rich plasma is injected in the graft to enhance cellular healing potential.

Traction is now reestablished. An anchor is placed at the most anterior part of the defect through the midanterior portal. One of the limb sutures is passed through the graft outside the joint with a free needle. A knot then is made and pushed with a knot pusher at the same time when the graft is introduced into the joint through a plastic canula (**Fig. 8**). The other suture limb of the suture anchor can be passed through the native labrum to create a side-to-side anastomosis between the graft and native labrum. Then, a second suture anchor is placed at the most posterior part of the defect, and the graft is fixed using the suture loop to aid in control and anchoring the graft. After the knot placement, the graft is addressed as a regular bucket–handle labral tear. Additional suture anchors are placed approximately 1 cm apart along the midportion of the graft until stable fixation is achieved (**Fig. 9**).

Traction is released, and the hip is evaluated with dynamic examination in all planes of motion to assess the fixation and position of the graft. The graft should resemble the native labrum and should recreate the suction seal of the hip joint. A flexible

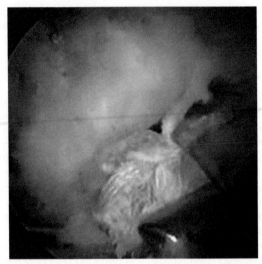

Fig. 8. Iliotibial band graft entering the joint through the midanterior portal.

radiofrequency device can now be used to make the graft and the native labrum smooth, by removing fraying edges to ensure good visualization of the reconstruction.

Clinical Outcomes of Labral Reconstruction

The authors' clinical experience with labral reconstruction has now reached over 150 procedures, and results are promising.[38] Second-look arthroscopies have been done in several patients to treat adhesions and residual chondral lesions, and in all cases the graft was incorporated and the suction seal well maintained. Modified Harris Hip Score raised from 62 to 85, and the median patient satisfaction was 8 out of 10 after an average follow-up time of 18 months. Hip replacement was performed in 9% of cases. Joint narrowing was a predictor of lower satisfaction, and age below 30 years old was a predictor of better patient satisfaction after labral reconstruction.

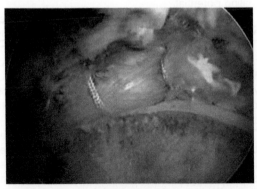

Fig. 9. The labral reconstruction is complete with the graft secured and with a tight seal to the femoral head during dynamic examination.

POSTOPERATIVE PROTOCOL

Protocols are the same for labral repair and labral reconstruction. The authors like patients to get on a stationary bike with no resistance within 4 hours after surgery, and to use a continuous passive motion (CPM) machine until 2 to 3 weeks after surgery. Patients are kept at 10 kg of flat-foot weight for 2 to 3 weeks also. This time is increased to 8 weeks if a microfracture procedure was performed. Patients are advised to wear an antirotational bolster and a hip brace to prevent stress in the repaired capsule. In order to prevent flexor contracture, patients should lay prone for 2 hours per day. All these measures are done with the objective of preventing capsular adhesions, which is one of common reasons for revision arthroscopy.[36]

SUMMARY

Labral tears are the most common finding in hip arthroscopies. The acetabular labrum is essential for adequate joint mechanics, so preserving the labrum and its function as a suction seal is mandatory to keep the hip stable and delay the development of joint degeneration. Labral repair is the preferred method to treat labral tears, and when this is not possible to do, labral reconstruction with the iliotibial band graft is an alternative treatment with promising early outcomes.

REFERENCES

1. Fitzgerald RH. Acetabular labrum tears. Diagnosis and treatment. Clin Orthop Relat Res 1995;311:60–8.
2. Kelly BT, Weiland DE, Schenker ML, et al. Arthroscopic labral repair in the hip: surgical technique and review of the literature. Arthroscopy 2005;12:1496–504.
3. Kim YT, Azuma H. The nerve endings of the acetabular labrum. Clin Orthop Relat Res 1995;320:176–81.
4. Feeley B, Powell J, Muller M, et al. Hip injuries and labral tears in the national football league. Am J Sports Med 2008;36:2187–95.
5. Borowski L, Yard E, Fields S, et al. The epidemiology of US high school basketball injuries, 2005–2007. Am J Sports Med 2008;36:2328–35.
6. McCarthy JC, Noble PC, Schuck MR, et al. The Otto E. Aufranc award: the role of labral lesions to development of early degenerative hip disease. Clin Orthop Relat Res 2001;393:25–37.
7. Narvani AA, Tsiridis E, Kendall S, et al. A preliminary report on prevalence of acetabular labrum tears in sports patients with groin pain. Knee Surg Sports Traumatol Arthrosc 2003;11:403–8.
8. Shindle MK, Voos JE, Nho SJ, et al. Arthroscopic management of labral tears in the hip. J Bone Joint Surg Am 2008;90(Suppl 4):2–19.
9. Seldes RM, Tan V, Hunt J, et al. Anatomy, histologic features, and vascularity of the adult acetabular labrum. Clin Orthop Relat Res 2001;382:232–40.
10. Cashin M, Uhthoff H, O'Neill M, et al. Embryology of the acetabular labral–chondral complex. J Bone Joint Surg Br 2008;90:1019–24.
11. Smith CD, Masouros S, Hill AM, et al. A biomechanical basis for tears of the human acetabular labrum. Br J Sports Med 2009;43:574–8.
12. Crawford MJ, Dy CJ, Alexander JW, et al. The 2007 Frank Stinchfield award. The biomechanics of the hip labrum and the stability of the hip. Clin Orthop Relat Res 2007;465:16–22.

13. Ferguson SJ, Bryant JT, Ganz R, et al. The acetabular labrum seal: a poroelastic finite element model. Clin Biomech 2000;15:463–8.
14. Ferguson SJ, Bryant JT, Ganz R, et al. An in vitro investigation of the acetabular labral seal in hip joint mechanics. J Biomech 2003;36:171–8.
15. Kelly BT, Shapiro GS, Digiovanni CW, et al. Vascularity of the hip labrum: a cadaveric investigation. Arthroscopy 2005;21:3–11.
16. Philippon MJ, Arnoczky SP, Torrie A. Arthroscopic repair of the acetabular labrum: a histologic assessment of healing in an ovine model. Arthroscopy 2007;23:376–80.
17. Hall RL, Scott A, Oakes JE, et al. Posterior labral tear as a block to reduction in an anterior hip dislocation. J Orthop Trauma 1990;4:204–8.
18. Grossbard GD. Hip pain during adolescence after Perthes' disease. J Bone Joint Surg Br 1981;63:572–4.
19. McCarthy JC, Lee J-A. Acetabular dysplasia: a paradigm of arthroscopic examination of chondral injuries. Clin Orthop Relat Res 2002;405:122–8.
20. Ganz R, Parvizi J, Beck M, et al. Femoroacetabular impingement: a cause for osteoarthritis of the hip. Clin Orthop Relat Res 2003;417:112–20.
21. Lage LA, Patel JV, Villar RN. The acetabular labral tear: an arthroscopic classification. Arthroscopy 1996;12:269–72.
22. Beck M, Kalhor M, Leunig M, et al. Hip morphology influences the pattern of damage to the acetabular cartilage: femoroacetabular impingement as a cause of early osteoarthritis of the hip. J Bone Joint Surg Br 2005;87:1012–8.
23. Philippon MJ. The role of arthroscopic thermal capsulorrhaphy in the hip. Clin Sports Med 2001;20:817–29.
24. Philippon MJ, Maxwell RB, Johnston TL, et al. Clinical presentation of femoroacetabular impingement. Knee Surg Sports Traumatol Arthrosc 2007;15:1041–7.
25. Philippon MJ, Briggs KK, Yen YM, et al. Outcomes following hip arthroscopy for femoroacetabular impingement with associated chondrolabral dysfunction: minimum two-year follow-up. J Bone Joint Surg Br 2009;91:16–23.
26. Philippon M, Weiss D, Kuppersmith D, et al. Arthroscopic labral repair and treatment of femoroacetabular impingement in professional hockey players. Am J Sports Med 2010;38:99–104.
27. Martin HD, Kelly BT, Leunig M, et al. The pattern and technique in the clinical evaluation of the adult hip: the common physical examination tests of hip specialists. Arthroscopy 2010;26:161–72.
28. Johnston TL, Schenker ML, Briggs KK, et al. Relationship between offset angle alpha and hip chondral injury in femoroacetabular impingement. Arthroscopy 2008;24:669–75.
29. Beaule PE, O'neill M, Rakhra K. Acetabular labral tears. J Bone Joint Surg Am 2009;91:701–10.
30. Clohisy J, Carlisle J, Beaule P, et al. A systematic approach to the plain radiographic evaluation of the young adult hip. J Bone Joint Surg Am 2008;90(Suppl 4):47–66.
31. Wenger DE, Kendell KR, Miner MR, et al. Acetabular labral tears rarely occur in the absence of bony abnormalities. Clin Orthop Relat Res 2004;426:145–50.
32. Kalberer F, Sierra RJ, Madan SS, et al. Ischial spine projection into the pelvis: a new sign for acetabular retroversion. Clin Orthop Relat Res 2008;466:677–83.
33. Wiberg G. Studies on dysplastic acetabula and congenital subluxation of the hip joint with special reference to the complication of osteoarthritis. Acta Chir Scand 1939;83(Suppl 58):4–196.

34. Espinosa N, Rothenfluh DA, Beck M, et al. Treatment of femoro–acetabular impingement: preliminary results of labral refixation. J Bone Joint Surg Am 2006;88:925–35.
35. Larson CM, Giveans MR. Arthroscopic debridement versus refixation of the acetabular labrum associated with femoroacetabular impingement. Arthroscopy 2009;25:369–76.
36. Philippon MJ, Schenker ML, Briggs KK, et al. Revision hip arthroscopy. Am J Sports Med 2007;35:1918–21.
37. Philippon MJ, Wolff AB, Briggs KK, et al. Acetabular rim reduction for the treatment of femoroacetabular impingement correlates with preoperative and postoperative center-edge angle. Arthroscopy 2010;26:757–61.
38. Philippon M, Briggs K, Dewing C, et al. Arthroscopic labral reconstruction in the hip using iliotibial band autgraft: technique and early outcomes. Arthroscopy 2010;26:750–6.

Arthroscopic Treatment for Chondral Lesions of the Hip

Thomas G. Sampson, MD

KEYWORDS

- Arthroscopic surgery • Chondral lesions of the hip
- Femoroacetabular impingement • Acetabular articular cartilage

Arthroscopic treatment of chondral lesions of the hip is very challenging. William Hunter FRS (23 May 1718–30 March 1783), a Scottish anatomist and physician, said "if we consult the standard chirurgical writers from Hippocrates down to the present age, we shall find, that an ulcerated cartilage is universally allowed to be a very troublesome disease; that it admits of a cure with more difficulty than carious bone; and that, when destroyed, it is not recovered."

Understanding the etiology is paramount not only in treating hip chondral damage but also in mitigating the cause, using arthroscopic means. For the purposes of this article, the authors address chondral lesions of the hip caused by either injury or morphologic conflicts such as seen in femoroacetabular impingement (FAI). Fractures, aseptic necrosis, and metabolic or immunologic damage are not addressed. Only those methods using arthroscopic surgery for the treatment of chondral lesions are presented here.

THE CHALLENGE OF HIP ARTHROSCOPY

The treatment of chondral lesions of the hip joint presents many difficulties, considering the hip joint is deep in the body and is a spherical joint. Although modern instruments can gain access to most of the hip joint, the treatment of chondral lesions is limited to excision, debridement, microfracture, and radiofrequency treatment. Because cartilage is friable, it does not lend itself to suturing techniques to repair it back to bone unless in the case of acetabular articular cartilage, when it is intact at the labrocartilage junction. In the latter, the cartilage may be repaired, demonstrated later in this article. Advanced methods of repair involve rim trimming and labral refixation to the rim, and relocation to cover articular defects.

Financial Disclosures: Consultant: Conmed. Former Consultant: Stryker Endoscopy. Smith & Nephew Endoscopy.

Department of Orthopaedics, University of California, 2299 Post Street, Suite 107, San Francisco, CA 94115, USA

E-mail address: tgsampsonmd@hotmail.com

Clin Sports Med 30 (2011) 331–348
doi:10.1016/j.csm.2010.12.012
0278-5919/11/$ – see front matter © 2011 Elsevier Inc. All rights reserved.

Access to the entire hip has not always been achieved even with high-angle scopes and steerable instruments, because of the variance in morphology and stiffness of the capsule and muscles. Therefore, this article discusses only the arthroscopic treatment of those areas that are accessible using current methods.

Joint Preservation

Hip preservation has become one of the hottest topics in orthopedics today as we have become aware of small changes in the normal anatomy of the hip that may lead to labral and chondral damage. Although joint preservation has been advocated in the young and active for many years, with the recognition of morphologic conflicts such as FAI, and the acknowledgment that FAI may cause early arthritis and lead to early total hip replacement, the role of both open and arthroscopic treatment of the hip have become a mainstay in attempting to correct either injurious or pathologic problems of the hip joint early in its disease. Of note, there are no publications available in the literature nor are there any presentations given at conferences to demonstrate any procedure that is able to mitigate or repair chondral damage and restore a "normal state of being."

Since the author's group developed the "lateral approach to hip arthroscopy" in 1984, it has used arthroscopic means to treat chondral damage to the hip joint.[1] The author has never been able to show with certainty that treatments reverse the affects of damage of the articular surface. Many cases, however, have shown improvement of pain and function and the lack of progression of the arthritis on radiographs. The arthroscopic results dramatically improved once the concept of changing the morphologic effects of impingement were initiated in 2002.[2,3]

This article should be considered as a guide to evaluating chondral defects of both the acetabulum and the femoral head, and give direction on various treatment methods for chondral damage of the hip.

Special Anatomy

When treating chondral lesions in the hip, there should be consideration of the influences of the nearby structures including the labrum, the notch with its transverse ligament, the ligamentum teres, and the fovea.

Ferguson and colleagues[4] have shown that the labrum acts as a fluid seal to enable nourishment to the articular cartilage. In a finite element analysis they found that the labrum seal maintains the pressure of the synovial fluid that prevents loss of boundary lubrication or solid-on-solid contact. The loss of that seal apparently leads to further damage of the articular surface.

A poster presentation at the 2010 International Society for Hip Arthroscopy by Field and colleagues showed with a flexed hip how the synovial fluid traveled from the low-pressure peripheral compartment to the high-pressure central compartment beneath the transverse ligament and notch, with the zona orbicularis acting as a bellow.

In a biomechanical study of the notch, it was found that the size of the acetabular notch with relationship to the femoral head allows for the head to consistently seat in the horseshoe-shaped acetabulum allowing for appropriate contact forces. Moreover, with concentric narrowing of the notch such as from osteophytes or excessive volume of the notch such as congenital anomalies, the femoral head cartilage might wear prematurely, due to the increased force contact on the articular surface.[5] There are entities in which absence of complete closure of the triradiate cartilage, leaving chondral defects and abnormalities such as a keyhole deformity or stellate lesions, may be associated with chondral injury and premature damage of the head (**Fig. 1**).

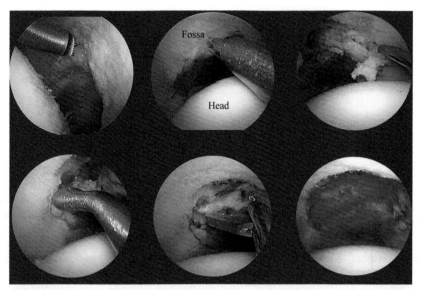

Fig. 1. Head damage and notch osteophyte excision. The head appears damaged by the fossa osteophyte. The radiofrequency (RF) probe is used to remove the soft tissue of the notch. A combination of arthroscopic burrs, curettes, and microfracture awls are used to remove the osteophyte and deepen the fossa.

The Anatomy of Cartilage of the Hip

The anatomy of the cartilage in the hip is not different from cartilage in any other joint with the exception of a variation of thickness of the acetabular and femoral sides. In addition, the thickness varies over the surface of the acetabulum and over the femoral head.[6] Hyaline cartilage is divided into 3 layers. The most superficial layer or tangential layer comprises 10% to 20% of the cartilage, with fibers arranged in arcuate layers. The next layer beneath is the middle zone that provides the bulk of the articular volume at 40% to 60%. The fibers are radially oriented. The deepest layer comprises 30% of the bulk of the cartilage and is just superficial to the tidemark of calcified cartilage, which is laminated to the subchondral bone. Many if not most of the lesions seen in the hip are at the level of the tidemark.

Types of Chondral Injury to the Hip Joint

The femoral head

In the absence of fractures of the hip joint, injuries may occur to the articular cartilage, with hip dislocation and impaction injuries sustained, for example, by an athlete when falling on his or her side, causing an osteochondral lesion of the femoral head, as shown by Byrd.[7] The lesion may be mistaken for aseptic necrosis.

Arthroscopic excision of the fragment may be all that is necessary; however, the long-term result of leaving the defect in the head is unknown. With large defects, some have considered filling with osteochondral plugs or partial head replacements (**Fig. 2**).

The acetabulum

From 1984 to 2002, most chondral lesions treated with hip arthroscopy by the author's group were debrided, excised, or abraded (**Fig. 3**). In the early years, many chondral lesions were mistaken for labral lesions. When looked at retrospectively there are

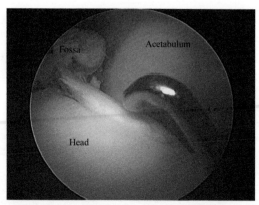

Fig. 2. Head osteochondrosis. An example of an osteocartilaginous defect of the femoral head.

reports on labral lesions and tears that are actually peripheral articular cartilage lesions or tears of the labrocartilage junction of the acetabulum.

Since 2002, with the advent of arthroscopic treatment for FAI, most chondral lesions are seen to be arise as a result of morphologic conflicts between an aspherical head and an overcovered rim. Prior to 2002 similar lesions were regarded as due to osteophytes and "rim syndrome."[8] The author has since more precisely recognized the fine details involved with damage at the labrocartilage junction of the acetabulum, discussed later in this article (**Fig. 4**).

History and physical examination

Cartilage lesions may be diagnosed prior to any diagnostic imaging by taking a proper history and doing a proper physical examination. There also needs to be an understanding of Hilton's law, which essentially states that the sensation of a joint is transmitted through the muscles that cross the affected joint. An understanding of Hilton's

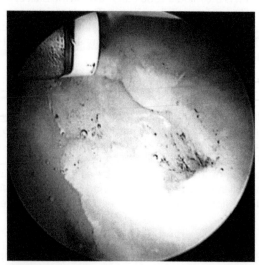

Fig. 3. Acetabular debridement with RF probe. The RF probe is used to stabilize full-thickness articular cartilage delamination as part of the abrasion chondroplasty.

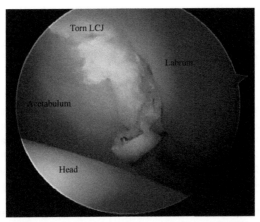

Fig. 4. Torn labrocartilage junction (LCJ). The RF probe is used to remove and stabilize the junctional tear.

law will explain why hip joint pain is referred to many areas about the hip. Most chondral and labral lesions may be felt as anterior groin pain; however, it also may be felt as pain referred to the trochanter and to the buttock area. On occasion it may be felt medially and along the adductor muscles and be mistaken for an inguinal hernia.

Chondral lesions may cause pain during certain activities or positions of the hip, similar to pain from labral lesions. Many patients complain of groin pain while sitting, felt anteriorly, and there may be some posterior lateral sensation of pain as well. With partial delamination or blistering of the articular cartilage of the acetabulum, the patient may feel a pinch anteriorly as seen with FAI or pain on rising from a seated position to a standing position. With blister-type delamination or full-thickness acetabular articular cartilage delamination defects, patients may complain of popping or clunking perceived anteriorly or anterior-laterally over the tensor fascia lata. The clunking or pop may be confused with a snapping iliopsoas. The difference between the two is that the iliopsoas will usually snap 100% of the time, whereas a cartilage defect will only intermittently snap or pop. The snapping iliopsoas will nearly always occur when bringing the flexed hip into extension, with hearing and feeling a pop or snap.

Patients with cartilage delamination or peel-off chondral lesions causing a large flap may occasionally feel a buckling or locking of the hip.

During the physical examination of the hip for chondral lesions, the workup may be confused by labral lesions. Conflicts between the femoral head and acetabulum may reveal a reduction in rotational movements, especially internal rotation. With partial-thickness cartilage lesions on the femoral head or acetabulum a "straight leg raising against resistance test" (which causes large compressive force across the articular surfaces) is usually negative, causing no groin pain. When there is a full-thickness articular cartilage defect down to subchondral bone, the same test may be quite painful in the groin. The patient feels the compressive forces that are not buffered by intact articular cartilage.

When performing the "impingement test," which consists of flexion of the hip to approximately 90° and rotating the hip from external to internal rotation and adduction, the lesion may be mapped out showing the extent of the acetabular articular cartilage defect. The patient is asked to complain at the onset of pain with flexion and internal rotation. In most cases on a right hip, the lesions occur from 1 to 4 o'clock or in zones 1 and 2. With intact blistered articular cartilage, the pain may be reproduced by bringing the hip down to more extension and internally rotating it at 6 o'clock, bringing it back up to 12 o'clock, and the patient will complain of pain at about 4 o'clock. When the articular cartilage is fragmented or there are flaps, often the pain is felt more clockwise than counterclockwise, or vice versa, depending on the flap orientation (**Fig. 5**).

Imaging

Radiographs are routinely obtained as the first study. The amount of acetabular coverage or dysplasia as well as conflicts with the head-neck junction may be evaluated with simple radiographs. These images include a low anteroposterior (AP) radiograph of the pelvis, with the coccyx seen to be less than 2 cm away from the pubic symphysis for proper pelvic orientation. A proper analysis of the joint spaces as well as the acetabular orientation and coverage may be determined. In addition, frog-leg and/or across-table laterals may show abnormalities of the head-neck junctional morphology.

Computed tomography (CT) is useful to map bony typographical anatomy, especially when treating FAI. The author cautions the use of CT because of the radiation exposure, though newer CT scanners lessen this concern. CT is beneficial, however, when looking for osteochondral lesions of the femoral head and loose bodies.

The author's group consistently uses magnetic resonance imaging (MRI) with and without arthrography for evaluating the articular cartilage as well as labral lesions. Subtle damage to the chondral surfaces may be seen with either test, depending on the conspicuity of the study. Use of at least a 1.5-T MRI scanner with the use of surface coils over the affected hip is advised so as to demonstrate all chondral lesions. The use of gadolinium may enhance visualization of cartilage lesions, and the use of intra-articular anesthetics may further delineate the hip joint as being the source of the hip pain if the symptoms are abated while anesthesia is present.

At present, new techniques in MRI such as the dGEMRIC (delayed gadolinium-enhanced MRI of cartilage) may emerge as a reliable method to better define cartilage defects.

Surgical mapping of chondral lesions

There are several methods with which to map chondral lesions in the hip. The author uses either a simple clock face or a zone method. The clock face anatomically has the 12 o'clock position directly lateral or at the apex position of the notch and the 6 o'clock

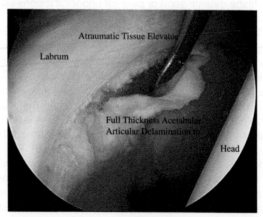

Fig. 5. Carpet delamination. The atraumatic tissue elevator is used to probe a full-thickness delamination defect that the labrocartilage junction.

position at the midpoint of the transverse ligament. The 3 o'clock position is medial on a right hip and lateral on a left hip, and 9 o'clock lateral on a right hip and medial on a left hip (**Fig. 6**).

The use of regional zones such as proposed by Ilizaliturri and colleagues[9] allows for precise description of a lesion's position. The author has found that most cartilage lesions from direct damage due to morphologic conflicts resulting from FAI are in zones 1, 2 and 3, whereas the indirect damage is in zones 4 and 5, such as a counter-coup lesions associated with Cam type FAI (**Fig. 7**).

Classification of femoral head lesions

In the author's opinion, there are no consistent practical classifications of femoral head lesions of the articular cartilage other than those used for avascular necrosis; however, most damage occurs in zones 2 and 3 near the fovea and superiorly. The damage may be caused from impaction of the head to the notch and/or damage seen from dislocation. Other lesions seen in the femoral head are consistent with damage caused by demarcation zones from FAI, damage from loose bodies, and damage from subchondral cysts secondary to FAI (**Fig. 8**A, B).

The author's group has proposed a new method of classifying femoral head cartilage lesions. Higher grades correlate with greater damage and a poorer prognosis. There are 2 special classifications, which include traumatic defects and demarcation zones, of damage from FAI (**Box 1**).

The prognosis for outcomes after repair is best at the lower grades. More aggressive treatment is necessary as the grade of damage increases. An example is an HC2 lesion, which may be treated with simple whisking of the fibrillated cartilage or thermal debridement, whereas an HC4 may require curettage and microfracture (**Fig. 9**).

Classification of acetabular chondral lesions

The Outerbridge classification[10] of chondral damage has often been used to describe chondromalacic defects in the hip. Beck and colleagues[11] have classified damage of the acetabular articular cartilage (**Box 2**); however, the author believes it does not guide treatment options.

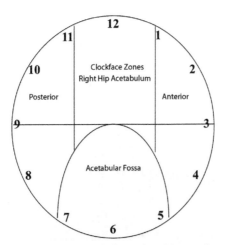

Fig. 6. Clock zones method of a right acetabulum. The oldest and most common method of describing locations on the acetabulum is the use of a clock face. The disadvantage of the system is that right and left hips will have different locations on the clock face with regard to the anterior and posterior positions of the defects.

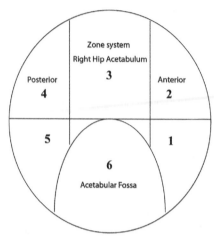

Fig. 7. Zones system of the acetabulum. The advantage is that description of a particular zone is identical for both right and left hips.

The author's group has proposed a classification for acetabular articular cartilage lesions in an effort to create an algorithm for treatment (**Box 3**).

Most lesions may be classified as either substance loss of the articular cartilage (partial or full thickness) or delamination. Both types are influenced as to whether there are labrocartilage junction defects or tears. With an intact labrocartilage junction, the cartilage may be repaired with the labrum back to bone as a flap. When the junction is torn the labrum may be repaired, although the cartilage may need excision.

As with the head classification, the higher is the grade of acetabular damage, the more aggressive the treatment. An example of a lower grade defect with an antici-pated good outcome is an AC1wD, which the author also calls a "full-thickness acetabular articular cartilage delamination defect" (FAACD). This defect may be treated by elevation of the cartilage defect with a flap of intact labrum, microfracture of the articular sided base bone to stimulate cartilage bonding along with labral refix-ation to the rim, and trimmed if needed to address a pincer lesion. Although this appears to be a lot of damage, its outcome is probably better than an AC4 where

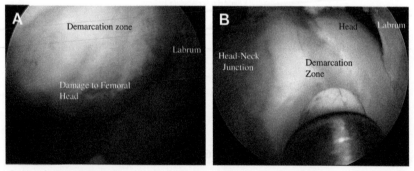

Fig. 8. Head demarcation zones. (*A*) The femoral head articular cartilage is damaged in the area of metaplastic bone overgrowth due to FAI. (*B*) Specific damage to the femoral head articular cartilage is caused by acetabular rim overgrowth impacting in the area of femoral head neck overgrowth, leaving a trough in the femoral head-neck junction.

Box 1
Proposed classification of femoral head cartilage lesions

Intact head substrate bone with chondral damage (no avascular necrosis)

    HC 0 = no damage

    HC 0T = uniform thinning (T)

    HC 1 = softening

    HC 2 = fibrillation

    HC 3 = exposed bone

    HC 4 = any delamination

Special class:

    HTD = traumatic defect (size in mm)

    HDZ = demarcation zone from FAI

Abbreviations: HC, femoral head cartilage; T, thinning; TD, traumatic defect; DZ, demarcation zone from FAI.

---

a large area of exposed bone may require rim trimming to reduce the size of the defect, and microfracture that typically produces fibrocartilage and labral relocation into the defect. The outcome of the latter is usually poorer and less predictable (**Fig. 10**).

With full-thickness articular cartilage loss that is less than 1 cm², microfracture alone may be of benefit. The author has found that if the cartilage loss is greater than 1 cm², then microfracture may be less effective and the hip will require rim trimming to reduce the size of exposed acetabular subchondral bone. The technique involves

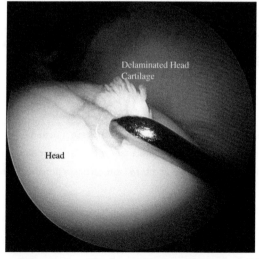

Fig. 9. Head cartilage delamination. The femoral head with nearly full-thickness delamination and fibrillation of the articular cartilage shows the full extent of the damage by probing.

> **Box 2**
> **Beck classification of damage to cartilage**
>
> Description criteria
>
> Normal: macroscopically sound cartilage
>
> Malacia: roughening of surface, fibrillation
>
> Debonding: loss of fixation to the subchondral bone, macroscopically sound cartilage; carpet phenomenon
>
> Cleavage: loss of fixation to the subchondral bone; frayed edges, thinning of the cartilage, flap
>
> Defect: full-thickness defect

translocation of the labrum into the defect to reduce the surface area required for filling of fibrocartilage.

Arthroscopic Management of Chondral Lesions

The usual arthroscopic setup and portals are the same for either supine or lateral approaches.[1,12] The author advocates the use of an extensive capsulotomy similar to open surgery extending from the base of the neck anterolateral, to proximally on the ileum adjacent to the labrum from the 12 o'clock to 4 o'clock positions. The capsular portion of the labrum is incised so as to leave a small cuff if reattachment becomes necessary (**Fig. 11**).

Distraction with a capsulotomy requires less force, and the scope may be driven into the central compartment under direct view, which minimizes risk of iatrogenic labral or chondral damage. The lesions are identified and may be palpated with a blunt probe or an atraumatic tissue elevator. Once the lesion is graded, appropriate treatment may be initiated.

The following are examples of methods used by the author's group to treat chondral lesions.

> **Box 3**
> **Classification for acetabular articular cartilage lesions**
>
> AC 0 = no damage
>
> AC 1 = softening no wave sign
>
> AC 1w = softening with wave sign intact labrocartilage junction
>
> AC 1wTj = softening with wave sign and torn labrocartilage junction
>
> AC 1wD = softening with wave sign and intact labrocartilage junction with delamination
>
> AC 1wTjD = softening with wave sign and torn labrocartilage junction with delamination
>
> AC 2 = fibrillation
>
> AC 2Tj = fibrillation with torn labrocartilage junction
>
> AC 3 = exposed bone small area <1 cm^2
>
> AC 4 = exposed bone large area >1 cm^2
>
> *Abbreviations:* A, acetabulum; C, cartilage defects; D, with delamination; Tj, Torn labrocartilage junction; w, with wave sign.

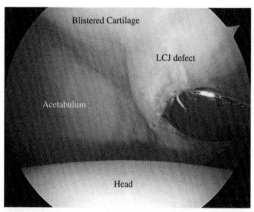

Fig. 10. Blistered articular cartilage with LCJ defect. The atraumatic tissue elevator is used to probe effect at the labrocartilage junction. While pushing on the defect, the blistered cartilage elevates off the substrate bone causing a "wave effect."

Head chondral lesions

HC0 to HC1 may require little to no treatment. HC2 (fibrillation) is treated with debridement. If there are notch osteophytes causing damage to the femoral head, they are removed with a combination of curettes, a long 4-mm hip burr, and microfracture awls (**Fig. 12A**).

HC4 delamination is treated with debridement and microfracture. Unfortunately, this lesion is difficult to treat because most awls cannot reach the entire lesion the prognosis is poor (see **Fig. 12B**).

HTD (traumatic defects) are usually the result of a fall on the side of the hip, and may be mistaken for aseptic necrosis. Simple excision of the loose fragment may be all that is necessary (**Fig. 13A–D**).

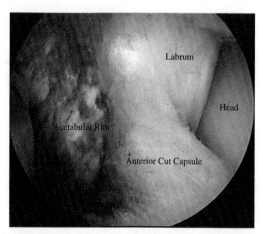

Fig. 11. Hip capsulotomy. A capsulotomy similar to an open procedure is done submuscularly using an RF probe; the capsule is incised from the base of the neck near the trochanteric line to proximal cephalad to the labrum on the acetabular rim. The capsulotomy is extended lateral and medial to give exposure to the anterior labroacetabular junction external to zones 1, 2, and 3.

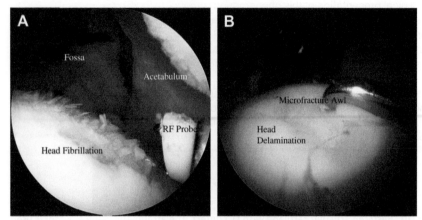

Fig. 12. Head fibrillation debridement and notch. (*A*) The fibrillated head is associated with mild to moderate arthritic changes of the hip. The RF probe is used to remove an abrasion by damaged cartilage. (*B*) The full-thickness articular cartilage delamination of the head is treated with abrasion chondroplasty and microfracture with a curved awl.

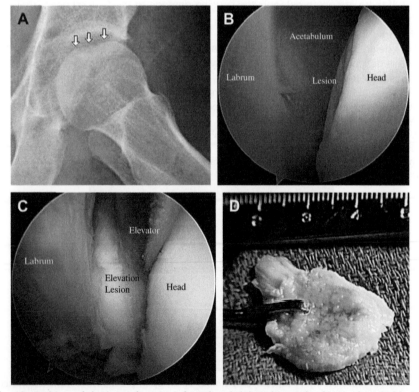

Fig. 13. Excision of the loose fragment from head. (*A*) Radiograph of osteochondral lesion femoral head from impaction injury of left hip (*arrows*). (*B*) Arthroscopic view of the femoral head and depression at the osteochondral defect. (*C*) The osteochondral patient has been elevated with an atraumatic tissue elevator. (*D*) The excised fragment.

The damage to the femoral head causing a demarcation zone is attributed to FAI. Treating the Cam bump may need to be extended to the lesion more medially in order to remove the defect (**Fig. 14**).

Acetabular chondral lesions

AC0 to AC1 essentially require no treatment. AC1w to AC1wTjD are repaired in an almost identical manner with minor variations. The concept is to identify the true lesion, which is a FAACD, first, and then create a milieu that allows for the substrate bone to heal and anneal to the separated cartilage. The same procedure may be done with or without tearing of the labrocartilage junction, except that with the latter, a stable flap of articular cartilage must be established to withstand compression and shearing of the head without being fully fixed (**Fig. 15A–J**).

AC2 lesions are debrided or excised to bone and may require microfracture. If it is associated with FAI, treatment of the Cam bump may prevent the recurrence and allow for healing.

If the labrocartilage junction is intact then there are several ways to treat this. Tzaveas and Villar[13] have shown that this may be treated by injecting fibrin glue beneath the defect, causing adherence. There have been some reports that the defect may benefit from microfracture through the articular cartilage to obtain a healing response. The author has found that by elevating the full-thickness defect, curetting and microfracturing the acetabular subchondral bone, one may stimulate a fracture healing response beneath the full-thickness cartilage. On a second look at approximately 1 year, improvement of the "wave affect" and the articular cartilage was seen. Symptomatically, patients generally improve with this technique (**Fig. 16A–C**).

With labrocartilage junction tear and AC2Tj (fibrillation), close attention is required to evaluate for the pincer effect, and excess rim requires rim trimming and labral refixation in addition to debridement.

In the event of the labrocartilage junction being torn, there is one report of sewing the articular cartilage back to the labrum. The author's group has treated this by excising the unstable portion of the articular cartilage flap and microfracturing behind the remaining flap, as well as performing rim trimming and refixation of the labrum.

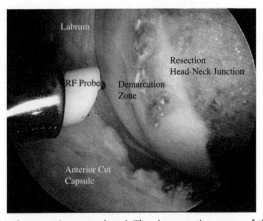

Fig. 14. Treating the demarcation zone head. The demarcation zone of the femoral head is caused by impaction of the acetabular rim on the head-neck junction. This zone is associated with FAI and is treated with resection osteoplasty. The RF probe is used to remove soft tissue before using the arthroscopic burr.

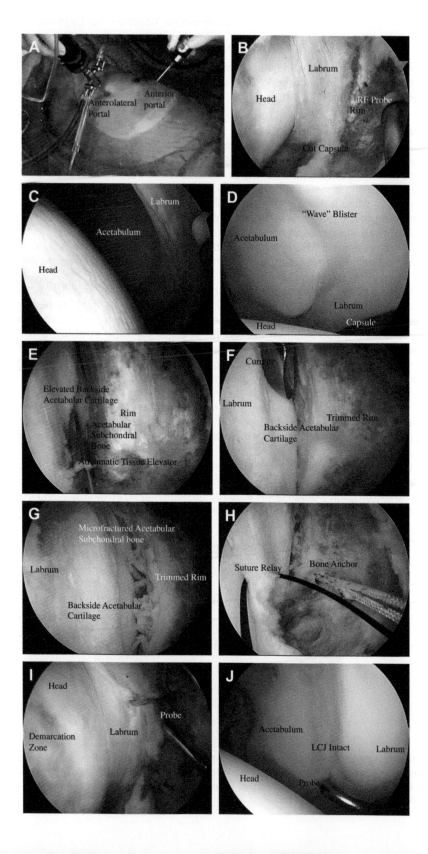

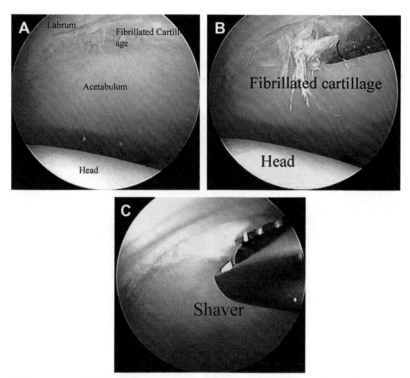

Fig. 16. Treatment of AC2 fibrillation defect. (*A*) Arthroscopic view of central compartment of right hip joint showing fibrillated cartilage at the periphery of the acetabulum at the labrocartilage junction. (*B*) Probing the fibrillated cartilage at the periphery. (*C*) Debridement of the fibrillated cartilage with the shaver.

Fig. 15. Treatment of FAACD with and without LCJ tear. (*A*) Outside view showing the arthroscope is in the anterolateral portal and the shaver is in an anterior portal. (*B*) Arthroscopic view showing the RF probe taking capsule off the anterior acetabular rim. (*C*) Arthroscopic view into the central compartment with a distraction. Note the darkened area of cartilage adjacent to the entry labrum, which is the area of full-thickness delamination of the cartilage. (*D*) Arthroscopic view of the blistered type wave effect. Note the change in color of the articular cartilage at the junction between the blister and the normal cartilage. (*E*) Arthroscopic view showing the atraumatic tissue elevator elevating the full-thickness acetabular articular cartilage delamination defect away from the subchondral bone. (*F*) Curettage is used to remove the calcific layer of the subchondral bone. (*G*) The area of subchondral bone is microfractured to promote healing, to be backside of the acetabular articular cartilage. (*H*) Using bone anchors and suture relay technique the intact labrocartilage junction is sutured to the acetabular rim at the labrocapsular junction. (*I*) View from the peripheral compartment after the labrocartilage junction has been refixed to the rim of the acetabulum. Note the demarcation zone of the femoral head that previously impacted the excess rim. (*J*) Second look in the central compartment. Note a slight bulge in the area of the blister that is now backed up by bone graft from microfracture. The labrocartilage junction remains intact after the procedure.

In most cases there is a mixture of a full-thickness cartilage loss and a full-thickness articular cartilage delamination, which can be repaired in similar fashion to the previous techniques (**Fig. 17**A–F).

AC3 and AC4, or less than 1 cm^2 of exposed bone may be treated with debridement, and more than 1 cm^2 may be treated with microfracture; in the latter it may

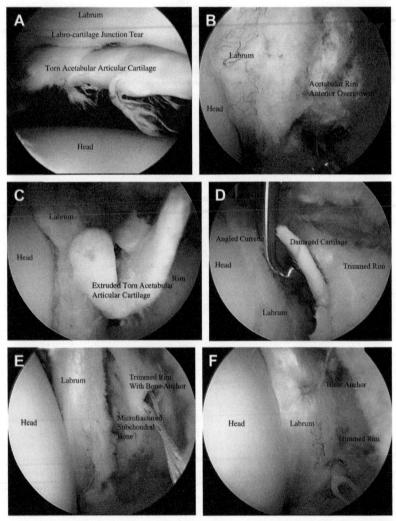

Fig. 17. Debridement of acetabular fibrillation, rim trimming, and labral refixation. (*A*) Arthroscopic view of right hip showing torn acetabular articular cartilage at the labrocartilage junction. (*B*) View from the peripheral compartment through a capsulotomy showing the excess bone of the anterior acetabulum before rim trimming. (*C*) Profile view after rim trimming of labral detachment showing extruded cartilage coming out of the central compartment. (*D*) Damaged articular cartilage being curetted away before microfracture and labral refixation. (*E*) View from the peripheral compartment before translocating the labrum into the acetabular chondral defect. (*F*) View from the peripheral compartment showing that the labrocartilage junction has been refixed back to the rim using bone anchors.

be necessary to relocate the labrum into the defect after rim trimming to reduce the overall size of the lesion (**Fig. 18**).

Postoperative protocol

Most specialists advocate a strict postoperative rehabilitation program with non–weight bearing for 6 to 8 weeks. The author has found no difference in mobilizing the patient immediately and progressing their weight bearing as tolerated, with many off crutches within 2 weeks. Only those physical therapists who have knowledge of conservative hip surgery should be involved. Range of motion, stretching, and core strengthening of the hip are essential; however, it takes weeks to months to reach a steady state. The bone needs a minimum of 6 weeks to primarily heal, and the articular cartilage may take 6 months to 2 years before either fibrocartilage or hyaline cartilage is present and durable enough for sports. Many patients return to some form of recreational activity within 6 months to 1 year; however, absolute pain relief may never be achieved in the majority of patients.

COMPLICATIONS

Although complications, such as infections, fractures, neuropraxias, and avascular necrosis (0.4%), are very low in hip arthroscopic surgery, many clinicians associate poor outcomes with complications. Because we are treating damaged cartilage, which in the purest sense may be considered varied degrees of arthritis of the hip, we must expect older age of an individual to be related to poorer outcome as well as shorter duration of symptom relief after arthroscopy. In fact, most failures that progressed to total hip replacements were anticipated, with the arthroscopic surgery acting as a bridge for those individuals who either did not have enough damage or had a high modified Harris Hip Score. The author's group treated 2 patients who developed acute chondrolysis, one probably from overload and one due to undiagnosed rheumatoid arthritis.

OUTCOMES

The author's group has attended to more than 1200 cases with some form of articular cartilage treatment over 26 years. The procedures done currently are vastly different to

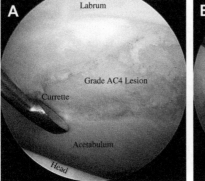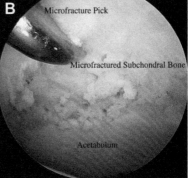

Fig. 18. Microfracture small and large defect with and without labral relocation. (*A*) Arthroscopic view of left hip central compartment showing a grade AC4 lesion before being curetted. (*B*) Microfracture of the articular cartilage defect.

those done initially. Because of the recognition of FAI and the ability to reshape abnormal morphology, this group is taking on more challenging cases with more damage to the hip joint. The results should be considered anecdotal, and at each period they are checked the average preoperative modified Harris Hip Score is 72 with a postoperative average score of 92. Less than 10% have gone on to total hips occurring 4 months to 7 years after the hip arthroscopy, the average being 53 months.

SUMMARY

The treatment of chondral lesions of the hip are difficult and may not ever reestablish normal chondral anatomy; however, the methods described will predictably improve pain and function of damaged hips. A new method of classifying and treating full-thickness acetabular articular cartilage defects is described, offering a good solution for cartilage repair while attempting to preserve most of the cartilage matrix in the process. It is the author's belief that the goal should be cartilage preservation, which in turn should lead to a healthier hip joint.

REFERENCES

1. Glick JM, Sampson TG, Gordon RB, et al. Hip arthroscopy by the lateral approach. Arthroscopy 1987;3(1):4–12.
2. Sampson T. Hip morphology and its relationship to pathology: dysplasia to impingement. Oper Tech Sports Med 2005;13(1):37–45.
3. Sampson T. Arthroscopic treatment of femoroacetabular impingement. Tech Orthop Hip Arthroscopy 2005;20(1):56–62.
4. Ferguson SJ, Bryant JT, Ganz R, et al. The influence of the acetabular labrum on hip joint cartilage consolidation: a poroelastic finite element model. J Biomech 2000;33(8):953–60.
5. Daniel M, Iglic A, Kralj-Iglic V. The shape of acetabular cartilage optimizes hip contact stress distribution. J Anat 2005;207(1):85–91.
6. Kurrat HJ, Oberlander W. The thickness of the cartilage in the hip joint. J Anat 1978;126(Pt 1):145–55.
7. Byrd JW. Hip arthroscopy for posttraumatic loose fragments in the young active adult: three case reports. Clin J Sport Med 1996;6(2):129–33 [discussion: 133–4].
8. Klaue K, Durnin CW, Ganz R. The acetabular rim syndrome. A clinical presentation of dysplasia of the hip. J Bone Joint Surg Br 1991;73(3):423–9.
9. Ilizaliturri VM Jr, Byrd JW, Sampson TG, et al. A geographic zone method to describe intra-articular pathology in hip arthroscopy: cadaveric study and preliminary report. Arthroscopy 2008;24(5):534–9.
10. Outerbridge RE. The etiology of chondromalacia patellae. J Bone Joint Surg Br 1961;43-B:752–7.
11. Beck M, Kalhor M, Leunig M, et al. Hip morphology influences the pattern of damage to the acetabular cartilage: femoroacetabular impingement as a cause of early osteoarthritis of the hip. J Bone Joint Surg Br 2005;87(7):1012–8.
12. Byrd JW. Hip arthroscopy utilizing the supine position. Arthroscopy 1994;10(3):275–80.
13. Tzaveas AP, Villar RN. Arthroscopic repair of acetabular chondral delamination with fibrin adhesive. Hip Int 2010;20(1):115–9.

Hip Instability: Anatomic and Clinical Considerations of Traumatic and Atraumatic Instability

Beatrice Shu, MD[a], Marc R. Safran, MD[b],*

KEYWORDS

- Hip instability • Iliofemoral ligament • Hip anatomy
- Hip arthroscopy • Hip capsulorrhaphy

Hip instability is uncommon because of the substantial conformity of the osseous femoral head and acetabulum. It can be defined as extraphysiologic hip motion that causes pain with or without the symptom of hip joint unsteadiness. The cause can be traumatic or atraumatic, and is related to both bony and soft tissue abnormality. Gross instability caused by trauma or iatrogenic injury has been shown to improve with surgical correction of the underlying deficiency. Subtle microinstability, particularly from microtraumatic or atraumatic causes, is an evolving concept with early surgical treatment results that are promising.

ANATOMY

The hip joint has traditionally been modeled as a highly restrained and concentric ball and socket joint that is inherently stable because of the osseous anatomy.[1] However, anatomic and finite element analysis studies have suggested that the relationship may not be perfectly congruent or spherical, may be incongruous because of size and/or shape, and, under physiologic load, may flatten the weight-bearing surface and widen the circumference at the level of the labrum enhancing a friction fit.[2,3] Gliding and rolling would then occur, and translation of the hip joint center may be as much as 2 to 5 mm in flexible hips.[2,4–6]

The authors have nothing to disclose.

[a] Department of Orthopaedic Surgery, Stanford Hospital and Clinics, Edwards Building, R144, M/C 5343, 300 Pasteur Drive, Stanford, CA 94302, USA

[b] Department of Orthopaedic Surgery, Stanford University, 450 Broadway Street, Redwood City, CA 94063, USA

* Corresponding author.

E-mail address: msafran@stanford.edu

Clin Sports Med 30 (2011) 349–367

doi:10.1016/j.csm.2010.12.008

0278-5919/11/$ – see front matter © 2011 Elsevier Inc. All rights reserved.

Osseous acetabular coverage over the femoral head is estimated at nearly half or almost 40% of a complete sphere,[7,8] providing 170 degrees of hemispherical coverage.[9] This coverage is increased by the labrum, which in one cadaveric study can vary in width from approximately 3 to 8 mm, increasing the surface area of the acetabulum on average by more than 25% and the volume by almost 20%.[10] Inferiorly, the labrum merges with the transverse acetabular ligament to provide a complete and full seal.

The intact labrum is in continuity with the bony acetabulum and creates a suction cup effect by resisting fluid flow from between the femoral head and acetabulum, thereby increasing intra-articular hydrostatic fluid pressure. The labrum may also aid in distributing stresses to the joint during loading, and both laboratory and clinical reports suggest that labral damage adversely affects stability.[11–13] The labrum may also function as a seal, separating the central compartment (the area within the confines of the labrum/acetabulum) from the peripheral compartment (the intracapsular area outside the acetabulum/along the femoral neck). The labrum may help maintain the negative intra-articular pressure that exists within the hip, as in other joints. Despite the prevalence of labral tears in asymptomatic adult patients, a correlation does exist between labral disorders and instability.[14]

In a biomechanical study of cadaveric hips, femoral subluxation with venting of the labral seal with a 20-gauge needle averaged 1 mm with internal rotation and 0.5 mm with abduction. There was no change when repeated with a 15-mm labral tear cut and repaired with a single suture and cyanoacrylate glue. However, maximal range of motion at a set torque did change with external rotation at 30 degrees flexion and abduction between intact, vented, and labral incised specimens in a significant fashion.[11] However, perhaps more importantly, these investigators showed that, after venting of the capsule, forces to distract the femur 3 mm decreased 43% and the force to distract the same amount decreased to 60% after creation of a labral tear.[11]

The capsuloligamentous complex is composed of circular and longitudinal fibers. The circular fibers, or zona orbicularis, are more substantive posterior and inferior and then blend into the deep iliofemoral ligament (ILFL). The longitudinal fibers are ample anteriorly and reinforced by distinct bands, which are the named ligaments and include the iliofemoral, pubofemoral, and ischiofemoral ligaments (ISFLs). The capsule inserts proximal to the labrum by a few millimeters, creating a recess.[7] In contrast, the capsule attaches proximal to the intertrochanteric line posteriorly, but at the more distal intertrochanteric line anteriorly. The anterosuperior capsule is thick and taut; inferoposteriorly it is thinner and more capacious.[7,9]

Our group has quantitatively studied the gross anatomy of the hip capsular ligaments, including the insertions (Telleria JJM, Lindsey DP, Giori NJ, et al. A quantitative assessment of the insertional footprints of the hip capsular ligaments and their spanning fibers. Submitted for publication).[15] The strongest ligament of the body is the ILFL or Y ligament of Bigelow, so named because of its shape and fiber orientation. The ILFL is shaped like an inverted Y and distally split into 2 distinct arms; the mean area is 34.6 cm[2] (Fig. 1). The single proximal attachment abuts the base of the anterior inferior iliac spine (AIIS) like a crescent, and extends to within a few millimeters of the acetabular rim (mean distance from rim = 2.9 mm) and has a mean footprint area of 4.2 cm[2]. The most superomedial aspect of the proximal ILFL footprint was, on average, 12.7 mm inferoposterior to the AIIS. The lateral arm crosses the joint obliquely and inserts on the anterior prominence of the greater trochanteric crest, just superior to the origin of the intertrochanteric line; the footprint is shaped like an elongated oval with a mean area of 3.1 cm[2]. The medial arm of the ILFL travels almost vertically inferior and inserts on a subtle angulated prominence of the anterior femur at

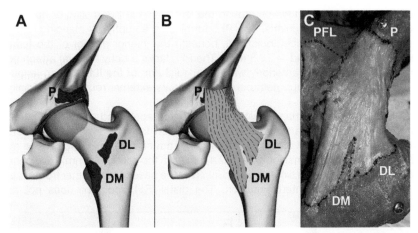

Fig. 1. The ILFL. Computer model of the 3 ILFL attachment footprints (*A*) and whole ILFL (*B*) showing the ligamentous anatomy of the anterior hip. (*C*) The ILFL in situ from a cadaveric specimen. Proximally the ILFL can be seen blending with the PFL. P, proximal; DL, distal lateral; DM, distal medial; PFL, pubofemoral ligament. (*Courtesy of* Marc R. Safran, MD.)

the level of the lesser trochanter; the footprint is circular and has a mean area of 4.8 cm^2. The medial and lateral arms are 2.3 mm apart on intertrochanteric line and diverge 56.8 mm distal to the most superior aspect of the proximal attachment, approximately 71% of the way down the ligament. The widths of the medial and lateral ILFL arms at the divergence point are 22.2 mm and 25.1 mm, respectively. Its role in preventing anterior translation with the hip in extension is important; it also primarily limits external rotation. Flexion with adduction tensions the iliofemoral lateral band, whereas abduction also tightens the medial band of the pubofemoral ligament. Thus the ILFL controls external rotation in flexion and both internal and external rotation in extension.

The pubofemoral ligament (PFL) has a mean total area of 13.0 cm^2 and originates on the iliopectineal eminence of the superior pubic ramus (**Fig. 2**). The proximal footprint of the PFL is triangular and has an average mean area of 1.4 cm^2, the most distal inferomedial aspect of the footprint is 2.1 mm from the acetabular rim and the most superolateral aspect is 37.9 mm from the AIIS. The PFL courses inferoposteriorly

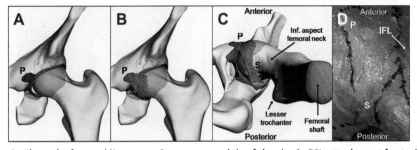

Fig. 2. The pubofemoral ligament. Computer models of the single PFL attachment footprint (*A*) and whole PFL (*B*) viewed anteriorly. Model of PFL sling (*C*) wrapping around the femoral head, viewed from an inferior position looking upwards at the inferior aspect of the femoral head. P, proximal. (*D*) The PFL in situ from a cadaveric specimen viewed from an inferior position looking upwards at the inferior aspect of the femoral head, similar to the computerized demonstration in (*C*). (*Courtesy of* Marc R. Safran, MD.)

under the medial ILFL and wraps around the femoral head like a sling or hammock, proximal to the zona orbicularis. The PFL terminates abruptly by blending with the proximal ISFL, near the acetabular rim, beneath the inferior aspect of the femoral neck (mean length of blend = 16.8 mm). The PFL lacks a bony femoral attachment. Fibers of the PFL blends anteriorly with the medial arm of the ILFL (mean length of blend = 26.8 mm). The pubofemoral ligament limits external rotation, especially in extension.[16]

The ISFL resembles a triangle with a long tapered apex, and has a mean area of 18.4 cm^2. The ISFL has a broad triangular origin on the ischial acetabular margin, beginning near the root of the ischial ramus, with a mean area of 6.4 cm^2. The most lateral aspect of the proximal footprint is 2.4 mm from the acetabular rim. The ligament spirals superolaterally as a single band to insert at the base of the greater trochanter at the femoral neck-trochanteric junction. The distal ISFL footprint does not have

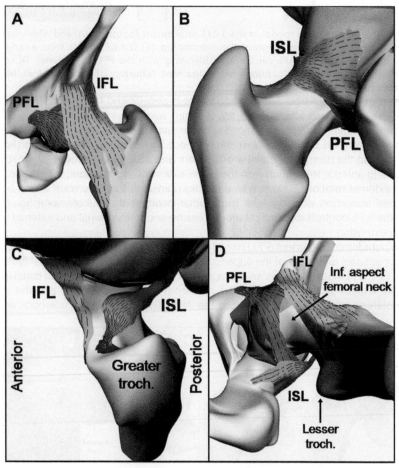

Fig. 3. Ligamentous relationships of the hip capsule. Computer model showing the anterior blend of the PFL and IFL (*A*) and the posterior blend of the PFL and ISL (*B*). (*C*) Shows a superior view looking down on the hip demonstrating the ISL inserting medial to the greater trochanter on the superior/lateral femoral neck, while (*D*) is an inferior position looking upwards at the inferior aspect of the femoral head. PFL, pubofemoral ligament; IFL, iliofemoral ligament; ISL, ischiofemoral ligament. (*Courtesy of* Marc R. Safran, MD.)

a consistent shape, but has a mean area of 1.2 cm^2. The distal ISFL and distal lateral ILFL footprints are separated by 6.5 mm of capsular tissue and do not blend into each other. The distal PFL blends with the proximal ISFL (**Fig. 3**). Internal rotation (in flexion and extension) and posterior translation are restricted by the ISFL, a fan-shaped band of fibers that spirals laterally and blends with the zona orbicularis.[7,16]

The zona orbicularis exists inside of the capsule and has been widely used as a landmark in hip arthroscopic surgery. Although most capsular fibers run longitudinally parallel to the femoral neck, fibers of the zona orbicularis encircle the femoral neck (**Fig. 4**).[17,18] This condensed group of circular fibers has been reported to wrap around the femoral neck and constitute the narrowest area within the capsule, which reinforces its stabilizing function.[17] We have shown that the zona orbicularis is important in resisting axial distraction of the hip.[19] The helical orientation of the capsuloligamentous fibers creates a screw-home effect as the hip moves into extension. In this position, the ILFL is on tension and offers the maximum stability by close packing the joint. It follows that the hip is loose packed as the capsuloligamentous fibers untwist and slacken in flexion external rotation, and the inherent osseous stability of this position predominates. According to Philippon,[9] the hip is at greatest risk for traumatic dislocation in flexion and adduction because of the absence of both osseous congruity and close-pack positioning.

The ligamentum teres is intra-articular, but extracapsular, and varies greatly in size as well as presence. The ligamentum teres is pyramidal and somewhat flattened, and gradually becomes round or oval in cross section and has a mean length between 30 mm and 35 mm. It has a broad origin, blending with the entire transverse ligament of the acetabulum, is attached to the ischial and pubic sides of the acetabular notch by 2 bands, and its insertion is into the fovea capitis femoris. The fovea capitis is an area of the femoral head devoid of cartilage, lying slightly posterior and inferior to its center. The ligamentum teres is tightest in adduction, flexion, and external rotation of the hip. Because this is the position in which the joint is least stable, a mechanical role for the ligamentum teres has been proposed in contributing to the stability of the hip, but science confirming this is limited.[20] The ligamentum teres does limit axial distraction,

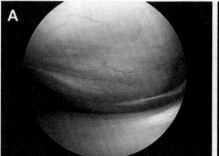 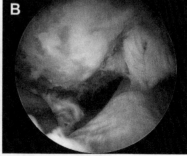

Fig. 4. The zona orbicularis is a condensed group of circular fibers within the capsule that wraps around the femoral neck and constitutes the narrowest area within the capsule. (*A*) Arthroscopic view of the peripheral compartment of a patient (undergoing surgery for FAI) in a left hip (femoral head to the right). Below is the anterior femoral neck, in the center of the picture is the medial synovial fold, and at the top is the zona orbicularis. (*B*) Another patient (undergoing surgery for synovial chondromatosis and FAI) showing the zona orbicularis (bottom of the picture going up and to the right) oriented posteriorly (femoral neck above) in a right hip (femoral head on the left). (*Courtesy of* Marc R. Safran, MD.)

although it requires several millimeters before it becomes taut. The iliopsoas, whose bursa communicates with the hip joint in 20% of adults, and rectus femoris, whose reflected head inserts on the anterior capsule, run in front of the hip joint and are dynamic stabilizers of the hip in extension.

Normal acetabular anteversion is 15 to 20 degrees, whereas coronal abduction is 45 degrees. The femoral head can be considered as two-thirds of a sphere, with an average head-neck anteversion of 5 to 15 degrees and neck-shaft angle of 130 degrees. However, great variability exists particularly in the female population with femoral neck anteversion.[21]

The 3 main hip capsular ligaments cannot be seen arthroscopically from within the joint. However, hip capsular ligament anatomy from the perspective of the arthroscope has recently been described in a cadaveric study by our group, and the margins defined by the portals and arthroscopic landmarks (**Fig. 5**). Using the clock face system, with lateral/superior being 12 o'clock, anterior being 3 o'clock, posterior 9 o'clock and inferior being 6 o'clock for all hips, we defined the arthroscopic locations of the hip capsular ligaments. The ILFL ran from 12:45 to 3:00 o'clock. The ILFL was pierced by the anterolateral and anterior portals just within its lateral and medial borders, respectively. The pubofemoral ligament (PFL) was located from 3:30 to 5:30 o'clock; the lateral border was at the recess of the acetabulum anteriorly that accommodates the iliopsoas tendon, and the medial border was at the junction of the anteroinferior acetabulum and the cotyloid fossa. The ISFL ran from 7:45 to 10:30 o'clock. The posterolateral portal pierced the ISFL just inside its superior/lateral border and the inferior/lateral border was located at the posteroinferior acetabulum. In the peripheral compartment, the lateral ILFL and superior/lateral ISFL borders were in proximity to the lateral synovial fold. The medial ILFL and lateral PFL borders were closely approximated to the medial synovial fold.

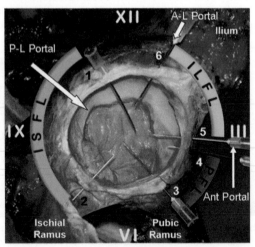

Fig. 5. A right acetabulum in situ from a cadaveric specimen. The needles demarcate the borders of the hip capsular ligaments. The locations of the standard central compartment arthroscopic portals are noted. The roman numerals represent hours on a clockface: III, anterior; VI, inferior; IX, posterior; XII, lateral. (A-L Portal, anterolateral portal; Ant Portal, anterior portal; P-L Portal, posterolateral portal; PFL, pubofemoral ligament; 1, ISFL superior/lateral border; 2, ISFL inferior/medial border; 3, PFL medial border; 4, PFL lateral border; 5, ILFL medial border; 6, ILFL lateral border). (*Courtesy of* Marc R. Safran, MD.)

The named ligaments reinforce 60% of the hip capsule that can be visualized during arthroscopy, leaving 3 sections of the capsule uncovered (see **Fig. 3**). The first large unreinforced interval is adjacent to the transverse acetabular ligament from 5:30 to 7:45 o'clock. A second interval is lateral, 10:30 to 12:45 o'clock. The third interval was smaller, from 3:00 to 3:30 o'clock, and lay just under the iliopsoas muscle, which may serve to support this exposed capsular region.

TRAUMATIC INSTABILITY

Traumatic instability occurs when frank dislocation or subluxation of the hip secondary to an event, such as motor vehicle accident, sports injury, or iatrogenic large capsulectomy, damages the osseous or capsuloligamentous structures about the hip. This damage can result in recurrent instability that generally responds favorably to surgical treatment of the underlying cause.[22] The most common mechanism of dislocation is posterior, caused by a posteriorly directed force transmitted through a bent knee, such as landing on a bent knee or being tackled with the hip and knee flexed. The spectrum of injury ranges from subluxation to dislocation with or without concomitant injuries. Contact from behind with the hip in extension and external rotation can cause anterior subluxation or dislocation. Sports that are linked to traumatic instability include football, skiing, gymnastics, rugby, biking, and soccer.[23,24] Most athletic-related dislocations are posterior, and the classification is the same as with trauma, whether there is an associated fracture or not. Iatrogenic anterior dislocation after arthroscopic capsulotomy has been reported.[14,25]

Most hip dislocations sustained during athletics are pure posterior dislocations and, because of the low-energy mechanism, usually have no associated fractures or small acetabular rim fractures. Hip subluxation may be more subtle in its presentation, and has been described with both contact injuries (fall on a flexed knee) as well as noncontact injuries while running with sudden changes in direction.

Evaluation of the individual with a hip dislocation includes the position of the extremity. In a posterior dislocation, the hip is slightly flexed, adducted and internally rotated, as well as a little shortened. In an anterior dislocation, the hip is extended, abducted, and externally rotated, and may not be shortened. A neurovascular examination is to be performed, paying special attention to sciatic nerve function. Because of the force being applied through the knee, it is important to also examination the ipsilateral knee.

Hip dislocations are treated with prompt reduction with sedation or general anesthesia, to reduce the risk of avascular necrosis (AVN). The risk of AVN increases with time following hip dislocation, with 6 hours being a critical threshold. Following reduction, imaging of the hip is important, preferably anteroposterior (AP) pelvis and cross-table lateral hip radiographs, to confirm concentric reduction and to evaluate for fractures and intra-articular loose bodies. If suspicion for fracture or incarcerated fragments is raised, perhaps because of widened joint space compared with the contralateral hip, computed tomography (CT) should be obtained (**Fig. 6**). After reduction, the hip is assessed for stability and smoothness of motion. Dislocations without fracture are inherently stable. Because the hip is inherently stable, if there is no associated fracture, surgical stabilization is often not warranted.

Although posterior wall acetabular fractures involving less than 20% based on CT measurement are generally believed to be stable,[26] a substantial portion have been shown to be unstable under dynamic fluoroscopy in small trauma series. Stress fluoroscopy under anesthesia may be considered early to evaluate for unstable fracture.[27] Intra-articular fragments or subluxed labrum should be addressed acutely to allow for

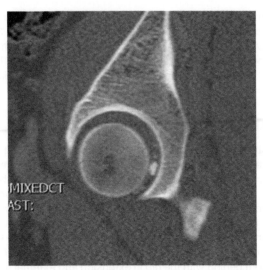

Fig. 6. Postreduction CT following a hip dislocation showing incarcerated bony fragment within the joint necessitating arthroscopic removal. (*Courtesy of* Marc R. Safran, MD.)

concentric reduction and early passive range of motion, and this can be done arthroscopically or open.

Some clinicians advocate magnetic resonance imaging (MRI) in addition to plain radiographs. MRI in the setting of an acute hip dislocation may show a characteristic triad of findings of hemarthrosis, a posterior acetabular lip fracture or posterior labral tear, and an ILFL disruption.[24] Anterior labral abnormalities are often present as well, and may represent a traumatic avulsion of the labrum or indicate the presence of some underlying bony impingement. Chondral injury to the femoral head may also be present, in addition to chondral loose bodies (**Fig. 7**).

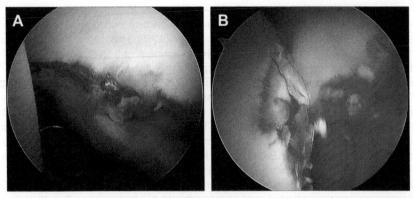

Fig. 7. Arthroscopic view of the left hip of a 24-year-old competitive athlete who sustained a hip subluxation playing field hockey. (*A*) A posterior labral injury, separation from the posterior acetabular rim. (*B*) A chondral injury to her medial femoral head as a result of the subluxation. (*Courtesy of* Marc R. Safran, MD.)

Hip arthroscopy may play a role after both dislocation and subluxation to address femoral head disorders, loose bodies, chondral injuries, and associated labral disorders. The optimal timing of the procedure is debatable because of the concern of placing a hip in traction and capsular distention for hip arthroscopy in the acute phase of injury. AVN is the feared complication of hip dislocation, and the management of acute hemarthrosis that could congest blood flow to the femoral head is debated. Reducing intracapsular pressure via hip aspiration and open capsulotomy have been described. Controversy exists with regard to management after reduction. Rest up to 48 hours is often recommended, with a knee immobilizer, hip abduction pillow, or brace to prevent going into a position of possible redislocation, although active and passive range of motion can begin as soon as tolerated by the patient. Frequently, hip motion precautions are recommended in the direction of dislocation (posterior shall refrain from flexion >90 degrees, internal rotation >10 degrees; anterior shall refrain from extension past neutral and external rotation). Controversy also exists regarding weight bearing after dislocation, although most recommend protected weight bearing for 2 to 6 weeks after reduction of dislocation. With significant bony injury, or if concern for AVN arises, limited weight bearing for even longer than 6 weeks may be recommended.[23,28] MRI is the most sensitive study for osteonecrosis and has been advocated as early as 6 weeks after trauma, although most clinicians wait 4 to 6 months for a repeat MRI to rule out avascular necrosis.[20] If no complications arise, the athlete may begin return to sports training in a progressive fashion when asymptomatic, with return to sports for an uncomplicated dislocation without fracture at about 3 months. The late sequelae of traumatic dislocation or subluxation is recurrent instability and pain, which can be managed similarly to atraumatic instability.[20]

ATRAUMATIC INSTABILITY

Atraumatic hip instability is an evolving concept and can be divided into those of dysplastic and idiopathic origin. Management of a patient with dysplasia stemming from bony deficiency (developmental dysplasia of the hip, Perthes, acetabular retroversion) should include discussion of corrective osteotomy and joint arthroplasty, based on the age and presence of degenerative changes. Patients with dysplasia caused by connective tissue disorders (Ehlers Danlos, Marfan) may present initially to Orthopaedics, and require additional work-up for diagnosis and proper referral to Genetics and Medicine to manage his or her syndrome. Because of abnormal collagen biology, these patients may be ideal for an extended strengthening program and activity modification counseling rather than surgical intervention.

Patients with idiopathic hip instability may have any or several of the following associated factors: generalized laxity (or subclinical connective tissue disorder), mild osseous hip dysplasia not meeting radiographic diagnosis, or history consistent with focal capsular redundancy and laxity caused by repetitive microtrauma. Overuse/microtraumatic injuries are common in athletes who participate in sports involving repetitive hip rotation with axial loading (eg, golf, figure skating, football, tennis, baseball, ballet, martial arts, gymnastics). Normally the femoral head moves within the acetabulum. The labrum or ILFL may be damaged from these repetitive forces, increasing the translation of the femoral head relative to the acetabulum, stressing these structures (the labrum and capsular ligaments) even further. These abnormal forces cause increased tension in the joint capsule that can lead to painful labral injury, capsular redundancy, and subsequent microinstability. The hip must rely more on the dynamic stabilizers for stability once the static stabilizers of the hip, such as the ILFL or labrum, are injured.

The history should be carefully reviewed for location and provocative maneuvers that reproduce the pain, and mechanical symptoms such as clicking, snapping, popping, and catching. The athlete may complain of hip instability or a feeling the hip is coming out of its socket. Hip impingement symptoms (pain with extended sitting or high flexion) are also common. A thorough physical examination, particularly including the low back and knee, should aid by focusing on the hip as the culprit. Specific clinical tests include posterior and anterior apprehension tests; a lateral decubitus apprehension test has also been described (**Box 1**). Generalized laxity can be noted by using the Beighton criteria for benign joint hypermobility (**Box 2**), although this diagnosis is still controversial in the rheumatology literature.[29–31] In addition to the apprehension tests, the log roll test (externally rotating the lower extremity in a supine patient) may provide a clue to ILFL insufficiency, particularly if asymmetric. Laying the patient in a figure-of-4 position, supine with the ipsilateral foot placed on the contralateral knee, and measuring the distance between the examination table and lateral knee, may also provide a clue, especially if asymmetric (**Fig. 8**). If radiographs do not suggest femoroacetabular impingement but examinations such as labral stress test and impingement test with flexion to 90 degrees and internal rotation are positive, hip instability should be in the differential diagnosis. Femoroacetabular impingement can present with generalized ligamentous laxity concomitantly and may raise a red flag to the surgeon if central compartment capsulotomy is performed.[14] Reproducing internal snapping hip with flexion abduction to extension adduction, or extension abduction to adduction can be a clue.[32] Alternately, the Thomas test for hip flexion iliopsoas contracture and the Ober test for iliotibial band tightness can be positive as the muscles try to stabilize an unstable hip. Rarely, hip subluxation may be demonstrable by the patient in clinic.

Plain films should initially include high quality AP pelvis and cross-table lateral views of the hips. Radiographs should be assessed for appropriate acetabular coverage of the femoral head, assessment for femoroacetabular impingement (FAI) anatomy, and retroversion of the acetabulum. Radiographic anterolateral dysplasia can be defined by a lateral center-edge angle of Wiberg less than 20 to 25 degrees on AP pelvis, and Lequesne vertical-center-anterior angle of less than 24 degrees on false profile view.[33,34] Radiographic retroversion may be suggested by the posterior wall sign and/or the ischial spine sign (**Fig. 9**). It has been suggested that the projection of the ischial spines into the pelvis on the AP pelvis radiograph indicates retroversion.[35] A posterior wall sign is present when the rim of the posterior wall is medial to the center of the femoral head. This condition suggests posterior wall insufficiency, which may be a result of retroversion of the acetabulum. There is some discussion that FAI may predispose athletes to hip dislocations. Particularly with the contracoup mechanism of joint injury in pincer impingement, the extreme of the levering of the anterior femoral

---

Box 1
Apprehension testing in hip instability

Anterior apprehension: patient lies at end of bed with hip almost off table; examiner extends hip and leg past neutral and the hip is externally rotated

Posterior apprehension: examiner flexes, adducts and internally rotates the hip and knee and applies force posteriorly

Lateral apprehension: patient lies in lateral decubitus position with affected leg suspended in adduction

Box 2
Physical examination findings in patients with generalized ligamentous laxity

Extreme skin extensibility on the dorsum of the hand

Thumb touches forearm in flexion

Small finger or all 4 fingers hyperextension at metacarpophalangeal past 90 degrees

Elbows and knees hyperextend past −10 degrees

Palms touch floor on forward bend (without dance/yoga training)

Foot excessive dorsiflexion, eversion

Marfanoid body habitus

History of genitourinary prolapse

Data from Beighton P. Hypermobility scoring. Br J Rheumatol 1988;27:163.

head-neck region against the acetabulum may result in dislocation (**Fig. 10**). This situation would be even easier in the case of acetabular retroversion or posterior wall insufficiency.

Beyond inspecting plain radiographs for dysplasia, FAI, old trauma, and other osseous abnormality, advanced imaging can be helpful. MRI, particularly with arthrogram, can aid in assessing chondral labral disorders, presence of effusion, and, if distended by fluid or contrast, capsular redundancy, as noted earlier.[9] CT may be helpful in mild dysplasia or if fracture is suspected. Traction/axial distraction dynamic fluoroscopy has also been described but requires general anesthesia and paralysis.[23,36] Dynamic fluoroscopy evaluation of hip stability in positions of apprehension may also be diagnostic.[20]

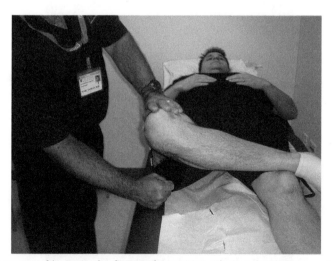

Fig. 8. Assessment of laxity in the figure-of-4 position. Placing the patient supine with the ipsilateral foot placed on the contralateral knee, and measuring the distance between the examination table and lateral knee, may also provide a clue to laxity. (*Courtesy of* Marc R. Safran, MD.)

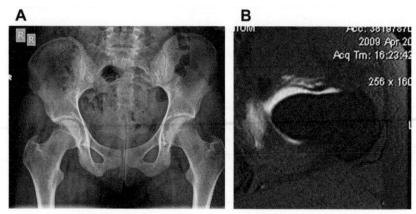

Fig. 9. AP pelvis radiographs of a Division 1 female collegiate volleyball player who sustained a hip dislocation playing volleyball. (*A*) AP pelvis radiograph showing the ischial spine sign (seeing the ischial spines on the AP pelvis) and posterior wall sign (posterior wall of the acetabulum medial to the center of the femoral head). (*B*) MRI showing injury to the ILFL as a result of the dislocation. (*Courtesy of* Marc R. Safran, MD.)

TREATMENT

As with most orthopaedic issues, the algorithm for treating hip stability depends on the severity and frequency of the problem as well as the underlying cause. A concentrated physical therapy program, focusing on strengthening of the hip and trunk,[37] should generally be the first line of treatment, particularly for patients with connective tissue disorders or generalized ligamentous laxity. Activity modification counseling may also

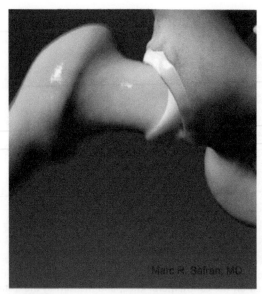

Fig. 10. The femoral head being levered out by the acetabular rim as a proposed mechanism for hip dislocation in the setting of FAI. (*Courtesy of* Marc R. Safran, MD.)

be considered. Evidence of frank subluxation of the hip would favor early operative intervention because longitudinal studies of patients with developmental dysplasia whose hips sublux suggest fairly rapid degenerative changes in the joint.[38] Dysplastic patients with primarily osseous abnormality benefit from corrective redirecting osteotomies of the acetabulum and/or proximal femur.[20] Instability following hip arthroplasty successfully treated with arthroscopic suture capsulorrhaphy has also been reported.[39] In addition, recurrent hip dislocation following hip arthroplasty has been treated with open ILFL reconstruction.[40]

In caring for the nondysplastic patient with hip instability who has failed nonoperative modalities, surgical soft tissue balancing via capsular plication/capsulorrhaphy and/or thermal capsulorrhaphy are options. In the presence of avulsion or acetabular wall fractures, fixation and augmentation of the deficit wall along with capsulorrhaphy is recommended.[22,41,42] Recently, the importance of the labrum in hip stability, pain, and cartilage protection has gained attention.[12,43] The labrum should be debrided and repaired if possible, although entry into the central compartment is then necessary.[28,44] Labral repair techniques have been discussed elsewhere and may be performed with the arthroscope. Capsulotomies created to enter the central and peripheral compartments, such as standard anterolateral and anterior portals piercing the ILFL should be made as small as possible for all patients with capsular laxity, and closure may be considered.[14]

There are 2 recently published reports of iatrogenic hip dislocation following arthroscopic capsulotomy/capsulectomy without closure, and more cases have been discussed at meetings. As a result, it is recommended that any patient undergoing hip arthroscopy with a large capsular defect or ligamentous laxity should be considered for capsule repair and/or plication. For those who perform routine capsulotomies with hip arthroscopies, it is prudent to create as small a capsulotomy as possible to perform the procedure.[14,25] Also, being aware of ligamentously lax patients with intra-articular disorders (labral tear, pincer FAI) should be considered for closure of the capsulotomy and may influence a surgeon's decision to perform the procedure arthroscopically. A torn capsule can be approached solely from outside of the peripheral compartment; however, labral repair will require entry into the joint, thus violating the capsule further for access to the joint to repair the labrum.[14]

Because of the rarity of symptomatic hip instability for which surgical remedy is sought, all case reports and sequential series have been single-surgeon, small numbered series to date. Further complicating the picture is the lack of a good, validated, nonarthritic hip outcomes assessment tool. Recently the MAHORN hip outcomes tool has been introduced.[45]

Open capsulorrhaphy, before the advent of accessible hip arthroscopy, has been performed with success.[32,41,42,46,47] The primary benefit is enhanced visualization and access, and there may always be a role for open procedures because of the limitations of arthroscopic entry.[14] Arthroscopic techniques for addressing soft tissue disorders in patients with hip instability have been described.[43] Although there are no direct comparisons in the literature of open and arthroscopic procedures, the minimally invasive advantage of arthroscopy is clear and should be considered as first-line treatment when capsular redundancy, labral tear, and/or bony defect are within the working arena of the arthroscope. Limitations of an arthroscopic approach are the steep learning curve and technically demanding nature of these new procedures, access limitations based on nearby neurovascular structures, and limitations when bony deformity or bony insufficiency are the cause of instability.

Thermal capsulorrhaphy for the hip was first reported by Philippon[9] and continues to be used. Thermal energy by laser or radiofrequency causes collagen denaturation and tissue shrinkage. The quantity of tissue contraction is directly related to the temperature or heat energy transferred, with 65 to 75°C advocated.[23] Concerns of thermal capsulorrhaphy certainly exist. In the shoulder, thermal necrosis of the capsule and chondrolysis are known complications, as well as gradual stretching of the capsule with recurrent instability.[48,49] However, none of these complications have been reported in the hip. The potential reasons why these have not been seen in the hip could be surgeons performing this procedure more carefully in the hip, based on the shoulder experience; the hip capsule is much thicker; and greater contribution to stability via the bony architecture. It is possible that it is not performed as frequently as it has been in the shoulder and is just a matter of time before these complications surface. Using even, nonrepeating parallel passes with several millimeters of space left between each stripe, allowing the heated arthroscopy fluid to exit the joint, and applying the thermal wand intermittently may help prevent overheating or necrosis of the tissue (**Fig. 11**). Because of the inherent stability provided by the bony architecture of the hip, delayed recurrence of laxity has not been seen by the senior author, nor reported. If adequate capsular tightening does not occur, suture plication is recommended.[20]

Plication and suture capsulorrhaphy is technically demanding arthroscopically, but remains the mainstay of repair when the capsule is torn or cut via planned capsulotomy.

Suture shuttling techniques adapted from shoulder arthroscopy with a curved hook or bird beak can be used to perform mechanical capsulorrhaphy from the central and peripheral compartments as well as just outside the peripheral compartment (**Fig. 12**). Most reports discuss anterior and anterolateral plication, with instruments in the anterior portal and a 30 degree arthroscopic lens in the anterolateral portal.[20,23,43] Roughening of the capsule before suture plication helps in the healing of the plication. Capsular tears or capsulotomy sites are closed first, then, if additional tightening is necessary, iliofemoral-to-ISFL plication is suggested next, or, in essence, closure of 1 of the ligament bare areas.[43] It is possible that closure of these ligament bare intervals as described earlier may tighten the hip capsule without direct plication of the ligaments (**Fig. 13**). Posterior and superior plication has also been advocated.[20] Lateral and posterior capsular redundancy in a patient with hip arthroplasty has been approached with instrumentation through a posterolateral portal and the

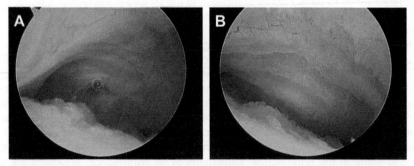

Fig. 11. Thermal capsulorrhaphy. A 24-year-old woman presented with a several-year history of hip instability and instability of other joints. She was sent for evaluation and diagnosis of Ehlers-Danlos syndrome was confirmed. After failed rehabilitation, she underwent thermal capsulorrhaphy. (*A*) The patulous capsule in the peripheral compartment. (*B*) Similar view after thermal capsulorrhaphy with parallel stripping every few millimeters. At 5-year follow-up, she continues to be asymptomatic in this hip. (*Courtesy of* Marc R. Safran, MD.)

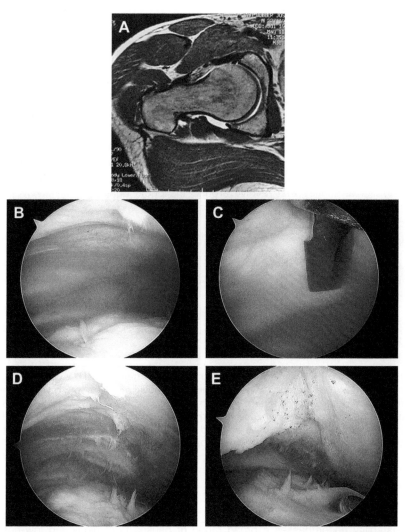

Fig. 12. 22-year-old student dislocated his right hip while playing soccer 6 years before being evaluated by the senior author. The hip was reduced on the field; however, despite physical therapy, he continued to have pain deep in the hip that prevented him from participation in sports. (*A*) Chronic ILFL changes. (*B*) A patulous anterior capsule in the peripheral compartment consistent with ILFL insufficiency. (*C*) The rasping of the anterior capsule and ILFL, causing irritation to help with the scarring or healing from the suture plication of the ligament. (*D*) The patulous anterior capsule after rasping. (*E*) The same view after capsular plication with 3 sutures in the ILFL. This patient returned to sports and continues to be asymptomatic 3 years after the plication. (*Courtesy of* Marc R. Safran, MD.)

arthroscope in an anterolateral portal. Parallel incisions in the capsule posterolaterally with a single, looping, knotting suture pulls the capsule taut.[39] Most investigators agree that protected weight bearing with or without bracing and specific hip precautions for up to 8 weeks will allow a capsuloligamentous and/or labral repair to heal adequately before increasing hip range of motion.

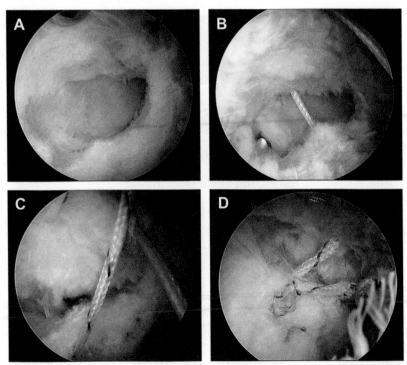

Fig. 13. Closure of capsulotomy. This patient underwent surgery for FAI but was noted to be ligamentously lax. Her hip capsule was tightened by removal of a 1-cm by 2-cm area of non-ligamentous capsule anterolaterally (*A*). Two nonabsorbable sutures were passes using a suture relay (*B, C*) and tied (*D*). Closure of the capsule results in tightening. This patient had no problems with hip instability and had a complete recovery following her surgery, with return to sports at 4 months. (*Courtesy of* Marc R. Safran, MD.)

SUMMARY

Hip instability encompasses a broad range of causes from high- and low-energy trauma to repetitive microtrauma, generalized ligamentous laxity, and bony and soft tissue dysplasia. Evaluation requires careful history, physical examination, and plain radiographs and advanced imaging studies are essential adjuncts. Physical therapy and activity modification play important roles in initial management and should be particularly considered in patients with connective tissue disorders. However, for a patient with a chronically subluxating hip or grossly unstable hip after dislocation, surgery is indicated. Surgery is also indicated for those with a traumatic dislocation with fragments within the joint preventing concentric reduction to remove or repair the fragments. Patients with osseous dysplasia may benefit from corrective osteotomy. In the nondysplastic patient, arthroscopic thermal or suture capsulorrhaphy and plication may be options rather than open approaches, but should take into consideration the technical and anatomic demands of the problem. The surgical treatment must address the underlying cause and consider associated disorders such as acetabular rim fracture, injury to the labrum and/or capsuloligamentous envelope, and hip impingement. A skilled hip arthroscopist familiar with this emerging concept can aid in the diagnosis and management of the patient with symptoms of pain and hip instability.

REFERENCES

1. Cereatti A, Margheritini F, Donati M, et al. Is the human acetabulofemoral joint spherical? J Bone Joint Surg Br 2010;92(2):311–4.
2. Menschik F. The hip joint as a conchoid shape. J Biomech 1997;30(9):971–3.
3. Afoke NY, Byers PD, Hutton WC. The incongruous hip joint. A casting study. J Bone Joint Surg Br 1980;62(4):511–4.
4. Gilles B, Christophe FK, Magnenat-Thalmann N, et al. MRI-based assessment of hip joint translations. J Biomech 2009;42(9):1201–5.
5. Dy CJ, Thompson MT, Crawford MJ, et al. Tensile strain in the anterior part of the acetabular labrum during provocative maneuvering of the normal hip. J Bone Joint Surg Am 2008;90(7):1464–72.
6. Safran MR, Zaffagnini S, Lopomo N, et al. The influence of soft tissues on hip joint kinematics: an in vitro computer assisted analysis. Orthopaedic Research Society 55th Annual Meeting. Las Vegas (NV), February 22–25, 2009.
7. Gray H, Clemente CD. Anatomy of the human body. 30th American edition. Philadelphia: Lea & Febiger; 1985.
8. Konishi N, Mieno T. Determination of acetabular coverage of the femoral head with use of a single anteroposterior radiograph. A new computerized technique. J Bone Joint Surg Am 1993;75(9):1318–33.
9. Philippon MJ. The role of arthroscopic thermal capsulorrhaphy in the hip. Clin Sports Med 2001;20(4):817–29.
10. Tan V, Seldes RM, Katz MA, et al. Contribution of acetabular labrum to articulating surface area and femoral head coverage in adult hip joints: an anatomic study in cadavera. Am J Orthop (Belle Mead NJ) 2001;30(11):809–12.
11. Ferguson SJ, Bryant JT, Ganz R, et al. An in vitro investigation of the acetabular labral seal in hip joint mechanics. J Biomech 2003;36(2):171–8.
12. Crawford MJ, Dy CJ, Alexander JW, et al. The 2007 Frank Stinchfield Award. The biomechanics of the hip labrum and the stability of the hip. Clin Orthop Relat Res 2007;465:16–22.
13. Greaves LL, Gilbart MK, Yung AC, et al. Effect of acetabular labral tears, repair and resection on hip cartilage strain: a 7T MR study. J Biomech 2010;43(5): 858–63.
14. Ranawat AS, McClincy M, Sekiya JK. Anterior dislocation of the hip after arthroscopy in a patient with capsular laxity of the hip. A case report. J Bone Joint Surg Am 2009;91(1):192–7.
15. Telleria JJM, Lindsey DP, Giori NJ, et al. An anatomic arthroscopic description of the hip capsular ligaments for the hip arthroscopist. Arthroscopy 2011 [Epub ahead of print].
16. Martin HD, Savage A, Braly BA, et al. The function of the hip capsular ligaments: a quantitative report. Arthroscopy 2008;24(2):188–95.
17. Harty M. The anatomy of the hip joint. Surgery of the hip joint. 2nd edition. New York: Springer-Verlag; 1984. p. 49–74.
18. Drake RLV, Vogl AW, Mitchell AW, et al. Gray's atlas of anatomy. 1st edition. Philadelphia: Churchill Livingstone, Elsevier; 2008.
19. Ito H, Song Y, Lindsey DP, et al. The proximal hip joint capsule and the zona orbicularis contribute to hip joint stability in distraction. J Orthop Res 2009;27(8): 989–95.

20. Shindle MK, Ranawat AS, Kelly BT. Diagnosis and management of traumatic and atraumatic hip instability in the athletic patient. Clin Sports Med 2006;25(2): 309–26, ix–x.
21. Yoshioka Y, Cooke TD. Femoral anteversion: assessment based on function axes. J Orthop Res 1987;5(1):86–91.
22. Nelson CL. Traumatic recurrent dislocation of the hip. Report of a case. J Bone Joint Surg Am 1970;52(1):128–30.
23. Smith MV, Sekiya JK. Hip instability. Sports Med Arthrosc 2010;18(2):108–12.
24. Moorman CT 3rd, Warren RF, Hershman EB, et al. Traumatic posterior hip subluxation in American football. J Bone Joint Surg Am 2003;85(7):1190–6.
25. Matsuda DK. Acute iatrogenic dislocation following hip impingement arthroscopic surgery. Arthroscopy 2009;25(4):400–4.
26. Vailas JC, Hurwitz S, Wiesel SW. Posterior acetabular fracture-dislocations: fragment size, joint capsule, and stability. J Trauma 1989;29(11):1494–6.
27. Moed BR, Ajibade DA, Israel H. Computed tomography as a predictor of hip stability status in posterior wall fractures of the acetabulum. J Orthop Trauma 2009;23(1):7–15.
28. Kelly BT, Weiland DE, Schenker ML, et al. Arthroscopic labral repair in the hip: surgical technique and review of the literature. Arthroscopy 2005;21(12): 1496–504.
29. Beighton P. Hypermobility scoring. Br J Rheumatol 1988;27(2):163.
30. Grahame R, Bird HA, Child A. The revised (Brighton 1998) criteria for the diagnosis of benign joint hypermobility syndrome (BJHS). J Rheumatol 2000;27(7):1777–9.
31. Remvig L, Jensen DV, Ward RC. Epidemiology of general joint hypermobility and basis for the proposed criteria for benign joint hypermobility syndrome: review of the literature. J Rheumatol 2007;34(4):804–9.
32. Bellabarba C, Sheinkop MB, Kuo KN. Idiopathic hip instability. An unrecognized cause of coxa saltans in the adult. Clin Orthop Relat Res 1998;355:261–71.
33. Wiberg G. Studies on dysplastic acetabula and congenital subluxation of the hip joint with special reference to the complication of osteoarthritis. Acta Chir Scand 1939;83:1–130.
34. Lequesne M, de S. False profile of the pelvis. A new radiographic incidence for the study of the hip. Its use in dysplasias and different coxopathies. Rev Rhum Mal Osteoartic 1961;28:643–52 [in French].
35. Kalberer F, Sierra RJ, Madan SS, et al. Ischial spine projection into the pelvis: a new sign for acetabular retroversion. Clin Orthop Relat Res 2008;466(3): 677–83.
36. Arvidsson I. The hip joint: forces needed for distraction and appearance of the vacuum phenomenon. Scand J Rehabil Med 1990;22(3):157–61.
37. Guanche CA. Hip & pelvis injuries in sports medicine. Philadelphia: Wolters Kluwer Health/Lippincott Williams & Wilkins; 2010.
38. Lovell WW, Winter RB, Morrissy RT, et al. Lovell and Winter's pediatric orthopaedics. 4th edition. Philadelphia: Lippincott-Raven; 1996.
39. Cuellar R, Aguinaga I, Corcuera I, et al. Arthroscopic treatment of unstable total hip replacement. Arthroscopy 2010;26(6):861–5.
40. Fujishiro T, Nishikawa T, Takikawa S, et al. Reconstruction of the iliofemoral ligament with an artificial ligament for recurrent anterior dislocation of total hip arthroplasty. J Arthroplasty 2003;18(4):524–7.
41. Lieberman JR, Altchek DW, Salvati EA. Recurrent dislocation of a hip with a labral lesion: treatment with a modified Bankart-type repair. Case report. J Bone Joint Surg Am 1993;75(10):1524–7.

42. Rashleigh-Belcher HJ, Cannon SR. Recurrent dislocation of the hip with a "Bankart-type" lesion. J Bone Joint Surg Br 1986;68(3):398–9.
43. Philippon MJ. New frontiers in hip arthroscopy: the role of arthroscopic hip labral repair and capsulorrhaphy in the treatment of hip disorders. Instr Course Lect 2006;55:309–16.
44. Safran MR. The acetabular labrum: anatomic and functional characteristics and rationale for surgical intervention. J Am Acad Orthop Surg 2010;18(6):338–45.
45. Safran MR, Hariri S. Hip arthroscopy assessment: tools and outcomes. Op Techn Orthop 2010;20(4):264–77.
46. Dall D, Macnab I, Gross A. Recurrent anterior dislocation of the hip. J Bone Joint Surg Am 1970;52(3):574–6.
47. Liebenberg F, Dommisse GF. Recurrent post-traumatic dislocation of the hip. J Bone Joint Surg Br 1969;51(4):632–7.
48. Good CR, Shindle MK, Kelly BT, et al. Glenohumeral chondrolysis after shoulder arthroscopy with thermal capsulorrhaphy. Arthroscopy 2007;23(7):797, e791–5.
49. Wong KL, Williams GR. Complications of thermal capsulorrhaphy of the shoulder. J Bone Joint Surg Am 2001;83(Suppl 2; Pt 2):151–5.

Femoroacetabular Impingement: The Femoral Side

Leandro Ejnisman, MD[a], Marc J. Philippon, MD[a,b,c,*],
Pisit Lertwanich, MD[a]

KEYWORDS

• FAI • CAM • Femoral osteoplasty • Impingement

Femoroacetabular impingement (FAI) has been recognized as a cause of hip pain, chondrolabral damage, and developing osteoarthritis of the hip.[1–3] This impingement results from abnormal femoral head-neck offset (cam) and excessive coverage of the acetabular rim (pincer). However, the combined pathology is the most common pattern found in patients with FAI.[1,4]

Smith-Petersen was the first to describe FAI in 1936, when he stated "The impingement of the femoral neck on the anterior acetabular margin... would result in traumatic arthritis."[5] In this article, a surgical technique was also described, which resembles the technique still used today for FAI treatment. After this description, FAI was mentioned in sparse publications,[6,7] until the 1990s when investigators started to recognize fragments of the syndrome, such as the impingement sign,[8] retroversion, as a cause of hip pain[9] and overcorrection of a acetabular osteotomy leading to impingement.[10] In 2003, Ganz and colleagues[2] established the modern concept of FAI and proposed the types of impingement. They also described open surgical treatment and demonstrated the association of impingement with acetabular labral tears and early osteoarthritis of the hip. Since then, the literature regarding FAI has grown immensely. Arthroscopic treatment is recognized as an alternative to the open technique with excellent results in a less-invasive approach.[11,12] Moreover, hip arthroscopy has

Grants: In 2010/2011 Leandro Ejnisman was a Visiting Scholar in Hip Arthroscopy and Biomechanics. Scholarship provided with grants from the Instituto Brasil de Tecnologias da Saúde. Financial disclosures: Board member/owner/officer/committee appointments: Arthrocare (MJP). Royalties: Smith & Nephew, Arthrocare, DonJoy, Bledsoe (MJP). Paid consultant or employee: Smith & Nephew (MJP). Research or institutional support from companies or suppliers: Smith & Nephew, Ossur, Arthrex, Siemens (MJP, LE).
[a] Steadman Philippon Research Institute, 181 West Meadow Drive, Suite 1000, Vail, CO 81657, USA
[b] The Steadman Clinic, Vail, CO, USA
[c] Department of Surgery, McMaster University, Hamilton, Ontario, Canada
* Corresponding author. Steadman Philippon Research Institute, 181 West Meadow Drive, Suite 1000, Vail, CO 81657.
E-mail address: karen.briggs@sprivail.org

Clin Sports Med 30 (2011) 369–377
doi:10.1016/j.csm.2010.12.007
0278-5919/11/$ – see front matter © 2011 Published by Elsevier Inc.

sportsmed.theclinics.com

shown good results in the athletic population, with the majority of patients returning to their previous sport.[13,14] One cannot overemphasize the importance of correction of bony abnormality because it is critical for good surgical outcome.[15,16] The aim of this article is to describe the diagnosis and treatment of the cam lesion.

ETIOLOGY AND PATHOMECHANICS OF CAM IMPINGEMENT

Cam impingement is characterized by a nonspherical head with abnormal head-neck offset of the proximal femur (**Fig. 1**). The causes of this bony abnormality remain unclear. Siebenrock and colleagues[17] used MRI to measure epiphyseal extension of the proximal femur comparing subjects with FAI and control subjects. Their findings demonstrated that an abnormal epiphyseal extension correlates with a nonspherical femoral head and a decreased femoral head-neck offset. Several developmental disorders can be the cause of cam-type deformity, such as slipped capital femoral epiphysis[18] and Legg-Calvé-Perthes disease.[19] Malunion of the femoral neck fracture in retroversion and varus position also results in cam impingement.[20]

Abnormal morphologic features in cam and pincer impingement create pathologic contact between the femoral head-neck junction and the acetabular rim at certain positions of hip motion. However, the patterns of articular and labral damages found in the cam impingement are different from the pincer type.[1] A nonspherical femoral head sliding into the anterosuperior labrum during hip flexion produces compression and shear stresses at the chondrolabral junction resulting in a separation between the labrum and the articular cartilage (**Fig. 2**). Avulsion of cartilage from the labrum and the subchondral bone can be seen as a wave sign[21] when the cartilage is probed during arthroscopy or as a frank cartilage delamination.

Beck and colleagues[1] compared intraoperative findings from surgical dislocation of the hip for the treatment of FAI between subjects with isolated cam lesions and those with isolated pincer lesions. All hips with isolated cam impingement had articular damage in the anterosuperior part of the acetabulum with a mean depth of cartilage damage of 11 mm, which was approximately one-third of the total cartilage depth

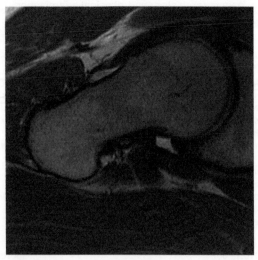

Fig. 1. A nonspherical femoral head as seen on MRI.

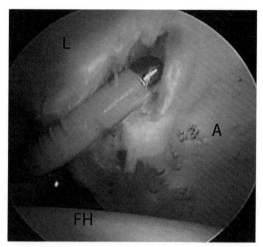

Fig. 2. Injury to the labrum and the adjacent cartilage as commonly seen with cam impingement. A, acetabulum; FH, femoral head; L, labrum.

at this location. A separation of the acetabular cartilage from the labrum was observed in all hips of this group. Cartilage and labral damages in hips with isolated pincer impingement were more circumferential. Chondral lesions found in pincer type were less severe compared with cam type and often limited to a small rim area (mean depth of 4 mm). In pincer and mixed-type impingement, repeated abutment between the femoral neck and the acetabular rim causes degeneration of the labrum. The labrum may be bruised and flattened, and intrasubstance ganglion formation may be found in more severe cases.

CLINICAL PRESENTATION

The majority of patients (50%–65%) with FAI have insidious onset of symptoms.[4,22] Pain onset following traumatic episode and acute symptoms without a traumatic event are also reported by some patients. Pain is the most common complaint, with moderate or marked severity.[4] The groin area is the most common location of pain (81%–83%) reported by patients with FAI.[4,22] Nonetheless, some patients also report pain at their lateral hip, buttock, thigh, and low-back area. Mechanical symptoms and feeling of instability are also reported. These symptoms usually worsen with particular daily activities and sports.

The anterior impingement test is a provocative test that is commonly used and is nearly always positive in patients with FAI.[2,4] In the supine position, the hip is passively flexed to 90°, followed by forced adduction and internal rotation. The presence of hip pain during this maneuver is considered a positive test. The flexion/abduction/external rotation test is also a useful test for diagnosis of FAI. While the patient is lying supine, the affected leg is brought to the figure-four position of flexion, abduction, and external rotation, so that the ankle is placed proximal to the contralateral knee. Gentle downward force is applied to the knee of the affected extremity while the contralateral side of the pelvis is stabilized. A positive test is demonstrated by an increased distance between the lateral aspect of the knee and the examination table, compared with the contralateral side.

RADIOGRAPHIC EXAMINATION

Abnormal morphology of the proximal femur and the acetabulum can be confirmed with radiographs. The senior author (MJP) uses an anteroposterior (AP)-pelvis, a cross-table lateral, and a false profile as the radiograph work-up[23]; however, many other views have been described and can also be used to better evaluate the bony morphology.[24] An AP-pelvis radiograph is generally used to demonstrate pincer-type deformity but some features of cam impingement can be shown, such as pistol-grip deformity, head tilt deformity, a lateral bump, and a herniation pit. A herniation pit is a juxta-articular change that can be seen as a radiolucency area at the anterosuperior femoral neck with a surrounding sclerotic margin. Leunig and colleagues[25] demonstrated an association between the presence of this lesion and FAI. It is also important to measure the minimum joint space in the AP radiograph, because patients with a joint space of less than 2 mm are more likely to have a lower postoperative modified Harris hip score and are 39 times more likely to progress to a total hip replacement.[12]

Because the nonspherical part of the femoral head is usually located at the anterosuperior part of the head-neck junction, this can be demonstrated in a lateral view of the femur (**Fig. 3**). The femoral head-neck offset can be assessed by measuring the alpha angle as described by Nötzli and colleagues (see **Fig. 3**).[26] In the original description, the alpha angle was measured in magnetic resonance (MR) scans, but several recent studies used plain radiographs to determine the alpha-angle.[23,27–29] Values of more than 50° are suggestive of abnormal femoral head-neck offset. Dunn view and the cross-table lateral seem to be the best radiographic views for alpha angle evaluation.[30] Several parameters can be used as alternative measurements, such as the head-neck offset ratio[31] and the triangular index.[32]

MRI provides details of soft-tissue disorders related to FAI. This imaging modality also reveals other causes of hip pain, which can be found concomitant with FAI, such as trochanteric bursitis and hip abductors tears. Moreover, viability of the femoral head is confirmed preoperatively. It is essential to have a study dedicated to the hip because a single-hip MRI has a better resolution than a pelvic MRI. MR arthrography may be used to better demonstrate labral and chondral damages.[33] Three-dimensional reconstructed CT scans can be used to delineate the bony abnormality[34] but it is not used routinely at the authors' institution.

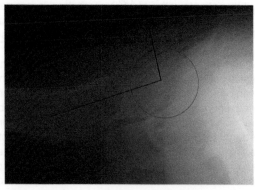

Fig. 3. Alpha angle as measured on cross-table lateral radiograph for the diagnosis of cam impingement.

SURGICAL TECHNIQUE

Arthroscopic treatment of FAI aims to improve the clearance for hip motion and diminish abutment between the proximal femur and acetabular rim. A normal femoral head-neck offset is created by femoral osteoplasty while normal labral seal is maintained. This can be performed either in supine or lateral position depending on surgeon preference. The senior author (MJP) uses the modified supine position (**Fig. 4**) (the affected leg is placed in a position of 10° flexion, 15° internal rotation, 10° lateral tilt, and neutral abduction) with 2 arthroscopic portals (anterolateral and midanterior portals).

After patients are properly positioned and traction is applied, the anterolateral portal is established at 1 cm proximal and 1 cm anterior to the tip of the greater trochanter. Then, the midanterior portal is made 6 to 7 cm from the anterolateral portal at a 45° to 60° angle with respect to the longitudinal line passing through the anterolateral portal. This location is the middle between the longitudinal lines passing through the anterior superior iliac spine and the anterolateral portal. The midanterior portal has a greater distance from the lateral femoral cutaneous nerve compared with the anterior portal.[35] Interportal capsulotomy connecting both portals is performed using an arthroscopic blade to allow better mobility of arthroscopic instruments. The central compartment now can be inspected to identify and treat all concomitant pathologies, such as labral tears, chondral lesions, ligamentum teres tears, and a pincer lesion of the acetabular rim.

For femoral osteoplasty, traction is then released and the peripheral compartment is approached. The cam lesion can be usually identified as a bump on the femoral head-neck junction with changes in color (gray, purplish) and texture (fibrillation, fissure, flap) of the cartilage over this area (**Fig. 5**). While the hip is placed in 45° of flexion, femoral osteoplasty can be performed proximally at 1 cm from the peripheral edge of the labrum with the burr introduced through the anterolateral portal. The resection should taper distally along the femoral neck for 1.5 to 2.0 cm. The medial synovial fold and the lateral epiphyseal vessels should be observed and protected during the procedure and these can be used as the inferior and superior boundaries of osteoplasty.

Positioning of the hip is important for accessing different parts of the femoral head-neck junction in the peripheral compartment. The anteroinferior part of the femoral

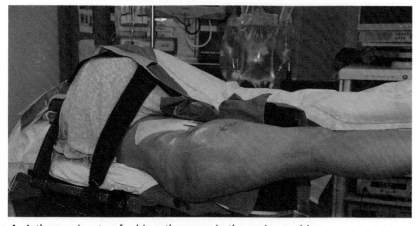

Fig. 4. Arthroscopic setup for hip arthroscopy in the supine position.

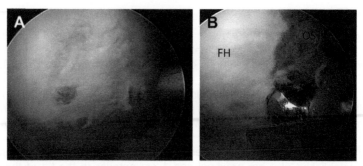

Fig. 5. (*A*) Femoral head neck bump as seen arthroscopically. (*B*) Burr shown performing osteoplasty of the area of impingement. FH, femoral head; OST, osteoplasty.

neck can be better visualized by increasing the amount of flexion of the hip. Moving the hip to a lesser degree of flexion and changing the arthroscope to the anterolateral portal facilitates burring at the superolateral part of the femoral neck. The arthroscope can be used as a capsular retractor by a levering maneuver during the procedure.

During femoral osteoplasty, the cam lesion should be adequately removed while a smooth and concave head-neck transition is created. Over-resection can increase the risk of femoral neck fracture and also has a negative effect on the labral seal. A herniation pit, which can be found in some patients, should be evacuated and usually becomes a shallow defect after finishing the femoral osteoplasty. For a large herniation pit, the senior author (MJP) prefers to fill the bony void with a bone-graft substitute plug. Periodic examination by moving the hip in all impinging motions is crucial to ensure that adequate bony resection is achieved while good labral seal is well maintained (**Fig. 6**). Capsular closure is performed using an absorbable suture. Platelet-rich plasma is injected for homeostasis purpose.

POSTOPERATIVE REHABILITATION

Postoperative protocol after hip arthroscopic treatment of FAI involves restriction of weight bearing, rotation, and motion.[36] Patients are kept at 20 lb of flat-foot weight

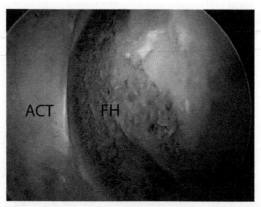

Fig. 6. Femoral head (FH) articulating in acetabulum (ACT) verifying adequate decompression and labral seal.

bearing for 2 to 3 weeks to protect the femoral neck after osteoplasty. Four hours of continuous passive motion machine is used for 2 weeks combined with use of a stationary bike at 0 resistance for 20 minutes. A modified hip brace and an antirotational bolster are used for 2 to 3 weeks to limit hip external rotation and extension, which will protect the early phase of capsular healing.

Physiotherapy should start with restoration of passive motion, followed by active motion and then strength. Passive circumduction movements are recommended to prevent adhesion. Active flexion of the hip should be gradually progressed to avoid flexor tendonitis.

COMPLICATIONS

Complications related to femoral osteoplasty have been reported and should be prevented, such as residual cam lesion, over-resection of the femoral neck, femoral neck fracture, avascular necrosis of the femoral head, and capsular adhesion.

A residual cam lesion is one of common causes of revision surgery after arthroscopic FAI treatment.[15] This lesion can be prevented by carefully identifying the cam deformity and performing periodic dynamic examination during femoral osteoplasty. On the other hand, over-resection of the femoral neck can increase the risk of femoral neck fracture and has an adverse effect on the labral seal. Aggressive osteoplasty should be avoided. A smooth contour of the bony resection can be achieved by switching the arthroscopic portals to appreciate the 3-dimensional geometry of the femoral neck.

Femoral neck fractures have been reported as complications of arthroscopic femoral osteoplasty[37] and of combined arthroscopical and limited anterior approach.[38] Mardones and colleagues[39] performed a cadaveric study showing that resections up to 30% of the anterolateral head-neck junction of a morphologically normal femur did not significantly alter the load-bearing capacity of the proximal femur bone, and advised that 30% should be the greatest resection performed. Nonetheless, this amount of resection is seldom necessary. Weight-bearing restriction after femoral osteoplasty is emphasized to prevent this complication and the duration should be prolonged for patients with lower bone quality.

Avascular necrosis of the femoral head is a rare complication.[40] Both the medial synovial fold and the lateral epiphyseal vessels should be well visualized and protected during osteoplasty. Capsular adhesion is another common cause for revision surgery.[15] Progressive range-of-motion exercise, both passive and active motions, is used to prevent this problem.

SUMMARY

Femoroacetabular impingement is an abnormal conflict of the acetabular rim and the femoral head-neck junction. This condition causes labral and cartilage damage and leads to early osteoarthritis of the hip. After clinical evaluation and radiographic examination, hip arthroscopy is one of the treatment options for FAI. During hip arthroscopy, the bony abnormalities can be corrected. Femoral osteoplasty is performed to restore normal femoral head-neck offset while the amount of bony resection is monitored by periodic examination. Postoperatively, patients are kept at partial weight bearing and rehabilitation focuses on range of motion. Complications related to this procedure are not common.

REFERENCES

1. Beck M, Kalhor M, Leunig M, et al. Hip morphology influences the pattern of damage to the acetabular cartilage: femoroacetabular impingement as a cause of early osteoarthritis of the hip. J Bone Joint Surg Br 2005;87:1012–8.
2. Ganz R, Parvizi J, Beck M, et al. Femoroacetabular impingement: a cause for osteoarthritis of the hip. Clin Orthop Relat Res 2003;417:112–20.
3. Ganz R, Leunig M, Leunig-Ganz K, et al. The etiology of osteoarthritis of the hip: an integrated mechanical concept. Clin Orthop Relat Res 2008;466:264–72.
4. Philippon MJ, Maxwell RB, Johnston TL, et al. Clinical presentation of femoroacetabular impingement. Knee Surg Sports Traumatol Arthrosc 2007;15: 1041–7.
5. Smith-Petersen MN. Treatment of malum coxae senilis, old slipped upper femoral epiphysis, intrapelvic protrusion of the acetabulum, and coxa plana by means of acetabuloplasty. J Bone Joint Surg Am 1936;18:869–80.
6. Carlioz H, Pous JG, Rey JC. Upper femoral epiphysiolysis. Rev Chir Orthop Reparatrice Appar Mot 1968;54:387–491.
7. Murray RO, Duncan C. Athletic activity in adolescence as an etiological factor in degenerative hip disease. J Bone Joint Surg Br 1971;53:406–19.
8. Klaue K, Durnin CW, Ganz R. The acetabular rim syndrome. A clinical presentation of dysplasia of the hip. J Bone Joint Surg Br 1991;73:423–9.
9. Reynolds D, Lucas J, Klaue K. Retroversion of the acetabulum. A cause of hip pain. J Bone Joint Surg Br 1999;81:281–8.
10. Myers SR, Eijer H, Ganz R. Anterior femoroacetabular impingement after periacetabular osteotomy. Clin Orthop Relat Res 1999;363:93–9.
11. Byrd J, Jones K. Prospective analysis of hip arthroscopy with 10-year follow-up. Clin Orthop Relat Res 2010;468:741–6.
12. Philippon MJ, Briggs KK, Yen YM, et al. Outcomes following hip arthroscopy for femoroacetabular impingement with associated chondrolabral dysfunction: minimum two-year follow-up. J Bone Joint Surg Br 2009;91:16–23.
13. Philippon M, Weiss D, Kuppersmith D, et al. Arthroscopic labral repair and treatment of femoroacetabular impingement in professional hockey players. Am J Sports Med 2010;38:99–104.
14. Brunner A, Horisberger M, Herzog RF. Sports and recreation activity of patients with femoroacetabular impingement before and after arthroscopic osteoplasty. Am J Sports Med 2009;37:917–22.
15. Philippon MJ, Schenker ML, Briggs KK, et al. Revision hip arthroscopy. Am J Sports Med 2007;35:1918–21.
16. Shindle MK, Voos JE, Nho SJ, et al. Arthroscopic management of labral tears in the hip. J Bone Joint Surg Am 2008;90:2–19.
17. Siebenrock KA, Wahab KH, Werlen S, et al. Abnormal extension of the femoral head epiphysis as a cause of cam impingement. Clin Orthop Relat Res 2004; 418:54–60.
18. Leunig M, Casillas MM, Hamlet M, et al. Slipped capital femoral epiphysis: early mechanical damage to the acetabular cartilage by a prominent femoral metaphysis. Acta Orthop Scand 2000;71:370–5.
19. Eijer H, Podeszwa DA, Ganz R, et al. Evaluation and treatment of young adults with femoro-acetabular impingement secondary to Perthes' disease. Hip Int 2006;16:273–80.
20. Eijer H, Myers SR, Ganz R. Anterior femoroacetabular impingement after femoral neck fractures. J Orthop Trauma 2001;15:475–81.

21. Philippon MJ, Schenker ML. Arthroscopy for the treatment of femoroacetabular impingement in the athlete. Clin Sports Med 2006;25:299–308, ix.
22. Clohisy JC, Knaus ER, Hunt DM, et al. Clinical presentation of patients with symptomatic anterior hip impingement. Clin Orthop Relat Res 2009;467:638–44.
23. Johnston TL, Schenker ML, Briggs KK, et al. Relationship between offset angle alpha and hip chondral injury in femoroacetabular impingement. Arthroscopy 2008;24:669–75.
24. Clohisy J, Carlisle J, Beaule P, et al. A systematic approach to the plain radiographic evaluation of the young adult hip. J Bone Joint Surg Am 2008;90:47–66.
25. Leunig M, Beck M, Kalhor M, et al. Fibrocystic changes at anterosuperior femoral neck: prevalence in hips with femoroacetabular impingement. Radiology 2005; 236:237–46.
26. Nötzli HP, Wyss TF, Stoecklin CH, et al. The contour of the femoral head-neck junction as a predictor for the risk of anterior impingement. J Bone Joint Surg Br 2002;84:556–60.
27. Neumann M, Cui Q, Siebenrock KA, et al. Impingement-free hip motion: the 'normal' angle alpha after osteochondroplasty. Clin Orthop Relat Res 2009;467:699–703.
28. Ochoa LM, Dawson L, Patzkowski JC, et al. Radiographic prevalence of femoroacetabular impingement in a young population with hip complaints is high. Clin Orthop Relat Res 2010;468:2710–4.
29. Allen D, Beaulé PE, Ramadan O, et al. Prevalence of associated deformities and hip pain in patients with cam-type femoroacetabular impingement. J Bone Joint Surg Br 2009;91:589–94.
30. Meyer DC, Beck M, Ellis T, et al. Comparison of six radiographic projections to assess femoral head/neck asphericity. Clin Orthop Relat Res 2006;445:181–5.
31. Peelle MW, Della Rocca GJ, Maloney WJ, et al. Acetabular and femoral radiographic abnormalities associated with labral tears. Clin Orthop Relat Res 2005; 441:327–33.
32. Gosvig KK, Jacobsen S, Palm H, et al. A new radiological index for assessing asphericity of the femoral head in cam impingement. J Bone Joint Surg Br 2007;89:1309–16.
33. Czerny C, Hofmann S, Neuhold A, et al. Lesions of the acetabular labrum: accuracy of MR imaging and MR arthrography in detection and staging. Radiology 1996;200:225–30.
34. Beaulé PE, Zaragoza E, Motamedi K, et al. Three-dimensional computed tomography of the hip in the assessment of femoroacetabular impingement. J Orthop Res 2005;23:1286–92.
35. Robertson WJ, Kelly BT. The safe zone for hip arthroscopy: a cadaveric assessment of central, peripheral, and lateral compartment portal placement. Arthroscopy 2008;24:1019–26.
36. Philippon MJ, Christensen JC, Wahoff MS. Rehabilitation after arthroscopic repair of intra-articular disorders of the hip in a professional football athlete. J Sport Rehabil 2009;18:118–34.
37. Sampson TG. Complications of hip arthroscopy. Tech Orthop 2005;20:63–6.
38. Laude F, Sariali E, Nogier A. Femoroacetabular impingement treatment using arthroscopy and anterior approach. Clin Orthop Relat Res 2009;467:747–52.
39. Mardones RM, Gonzalez C, Chen Q, et al. Surgical treatment of femoroacetabular impingement: evaluation of the effect of the size of the resection. J Bone Joint Surg Am 2005;87:273–9.
40. Scher DL, Belmont PJ, Owens BD. Case report: osteonecrosis of the femoral head after hip arthroscopy. Clin Orthop Relat Res 2010;468:3121–5.

Impingement (Acetabular Side)

Michael B. Cross, MD*, Peter D. Fabricant, MD,
Travis G. Maak, MD, Bryan T. Kelly, MD

KEYWORDS

- Femoroacetabular impingement • Hip arthroscopy
- Labral detachment • Labral refixation • Rim impingement

Femoroacetabular impingement (FAI), popularized by Ganz and colleagues,[1] is now recognized as a major cause of hip pain and is a predictor of early-onset osteoarthritis of the hip.[1–9] At present, there are two distinct types of FAI: cam and rim impingement.[10–12] Cam impingement occurs with loss of the anterior offset on the femoral head and neck, resulting in an abnormally shaped femoral head contacting a normal acetabulum.[13] Rim impingement, on the other hand, occurs with increased coverage of the femoral head by the anterior portion of the acetabulum.[13,14] Isolated rim impingement lesions are found most commonly in females, but combined cam and rim impingement lesions are common in both sexes.[15] Both types of FAI result in very distinct patterns of labral injury. A cam lesion will cause a detachment of the labrum from the articular cartilage at the transition zone secondary to the shear force created by the "bump" at the head-neck junction, whereas a rim lesion will cause one or more cleavage planes of variable depths within the labrum itself as a result of a crushing type injury seen with rim impingement.[13,14] Seldes and colleagues[16] have termed the pattern of labral injury associated with rim impingement a "type II tear," which consists of intrasubstance delamination, cystic degeneration, and tears involving the anterosuperior portion of the labrum. This situation occurs as a result of repetitive crushing injury, leaving the labrum bruised and flattened.[14] Over time, repetitive injury to the labrum results in pathologic ossification of the labrum, leaving the rim even more prominent. Further, there can be an associated injury of the posterior inferior acetabular chondral surfaces or the posteromedial femoral head, termed a "contracoup" injury," which is thought to be caused by subtle posterior subluxation of the femoral head.[11,13–15] Given the recent knowledge of the important functions of the labrum, including absorbing shock, distributing force across the hip joint, and joint lubrication, recent efforts in the arthroscopic treatment of FAI lesions have stressed labral repair/refixation rather than debridement alone, if at all possible.[17–22] Also, Philippon and

Department of Orthopaedic Surgery, Hospital for Special Surgery, 535 East 70th Street, New York, NY 10021, USA
* Corresponding author.
E-mail address: crossm@hss.edu

Clin Sports Med 30 (2011) 379–390
doi:10.1016/j.csm.2011.01.002
0278-5919/11/$ – see front matter © 2011 Elsevier Inc. All rights reserved.

sportsmed.theclinics.com

colleagues[23] have shown histologic evidence of labral healing in the ovine model with labral repair, further strengthening the argument for labral repair/refixation during arthroscopic management of FAI.

Rim impingement can be subclassified by the type of pathologic morphology of the acetabulum causing the rim lesion, which includes anterosuperior overhang (also known as cephalad retroversion), coxa profunda, acetabular protrusio, and acetabular retroversion.[13,24,25] With anterosuperior acetabular overhang, there is linear overhang proximally, but a normal relationship between the anterior and posterior walls further distally.[13] Radiographically one may see a "cross-over sign," demonstrating that proximally, the posterior wall is medial to the anterior wall, or a "posterior wall sign," in which the posterior wall is medial to the center of femoral head.[13,26] The result of anterosuperior acetabular overhang is focal damage of the anterosuperior labrum.[13] Radiographic interpretation of the cross-over sign is highly dependent on appropriate positioning of the beam to normalize pelvic tilt and rotation. Distalization or elongation of the anterior inferior iliac spine (AIIS) can sometimes be misinterpreted as a cross-over sign that clinically is associated with "subspine" impingement rather than "rim" impingement.

Coxa profunda and acetabular protrusion both define a pathologic condition of global overcoverage of the femoral head. In coxa profunda, there is medialization of the femoral head, but the femoral head still remains lateral to the ilioischial line.[13,15] However, protrusio is defined as a center-edge angle greater than 40°, whereby the femoral head lies medial to the ilioischial line.[13,15] In this situation, there is acetabular remodeling such that the medial wall of the acetabulum is medial to the ilioischial line.[13,27,28] In both cases, as a result of global overcoverage there is extensive, circumferential damage of the labrum caused by repetitive crushing injury by the femoral head and neck.[13] Finally, acetabular retroversion is a complex situation in which there is anterior overcoverage and posterior acetabular deficiency.[13] A "posterior wall sign" (posterior wall of acetabulum lies medial to center for femoral head) is highly suggestive of acetabular retroversion.

CLINICAL PRESENTATION OF FAI

A complete history should be performed on all patients. Most patients with FAI will present with complaints of anterior groin pain that is exacerbated by hip flexion.[14] Other common complaints include pain with prolonged sitting, getting in and out of a chair, and putting on socks and shoes.[14] In the athletic population, patients will often complain of pain during cutting exercises.[15] In addition to gait analysis, motor strength testing, and range of motion, one should examine the patient for the presence of an "impingement sign." The impingement sign is pain with internal rotation of the hip when the hip is flexed at 90°.[14] Range of motion may be limited with hip flexion and internal rotation.[15] Another common finding is an increased distance from the lateral genicular line to the examination table when the patient's leg is placed in flexion, abduction, and external rotation (FABER). Lateral hip pain may also be reported in this position. The "SCOUR" test may also elicit groin pain in patients with rim-type impingement, and is performed by circumducting the hip from a position of flexion, internal rotation, adduction to extension, and then circumducting the hip from flexion, external rotation, abduction to extension.[15,29]

PREOPERATIVE PLANNING

Preoperative planning is essential for treating rim (and cam) impingement lesions. Routine radiographs of the hip, including an anteroposterior (AP) view of the pelvis, a false profile lateral, and a cross-table lateral radiograph are performed to diagnose coxa profunda, protrusio acetabuli, acetabular retroversion, or acetabular dysplasia (often diagnosed by an upsloping sourcil), as well as cam impingement.[19] A true AP pelvis must have 0 to 3 cm between the coccyx and pubis symphysis, to minimize any error when determining actabular coverage.[15,30] A cross-over sign, indicating actabular retroversion, or a posterior wall sign, indicating global overcoverage, may be present on the AP pelvis radiograph.[24,31] A center edge angle (CE angle), or the angle formed by a vertical line drawn from the center of the femoral head and a line drawn from the center of the femoral head to the most lateral aspect of the acetabulum, can be measured on an AP radiograph to assess for acetabular undercoverage (CE <25°) or global overcoverage (CE >30°).[19] Wolff and colleagues[32] have recently described a method for templating the amount of rim trimming that needs to be performed during surgery to adequately resect a rim impingement lesion.

Magnetic resonance imaging (MRI) is used to evaluate the extent and location of the labral degeneration, as well as to assess the quality of the remaining labral tissue and the chondrolabral junction. Some investigators also recommend obtaining a 3-dimensional computed tomography scan to obtain a better appreciation of the bony anatomy.[15] By using these methods, one can adequately plan for arthroscopic management of rim (and cam) impingement lesions, as well as their associated labral injuries.[19]

INDICATIONS/CONTRAINDICATIONS

In general, the indication for surgical intervention in a patient with FAI is intermittent groin pain that has failed conservative management for 6 weeks to 3 months, and has minimal to no osteoarthritis on plain radiographs. Conservative management includes core strengthening, range of motion exercises, and activity modification. Patients with any radiographic joint space narrowing have predominately achy pain at rest, and bipolar grade 4 lesions seen on MRI have been found by some investigators to have poor outcomes following surgical management of FAI.[15]

SURGICAL MANAGEMENT

FAI lesions have traditionally been managed by open surgical procedures (ie, open surgical dislocation). Ganz and others[33] have supported open treatment of these lesions using a surgical hip dislocation, due to the fact that one can obtain an unobstructed 360° view of the acetabulum.[11,14] Good mid-term results have been recently published on surgical dislocation for FAI.[34] Hip arthroscopy is increasingly being used to surgically manage specific types of rim impingement lesions.[35,36] However, these are often challenging cases, and arthroscopic management should only be performed in situations where the anatomy of the acetabulum does not require major bony correction. For example, in cases with severe acetabular retroversion and posterior undercoverage, alternative procedures may be more appropriate than arthroscopy.[13] The main goal of surgery is to eliminate the impingement lesion without altering the physiologic function of the labrum.[13] In general terms, this is accomplished by careful surgical release of the labrum, osseus correction, and refixation of the labrum to the bony rim of the acetabulum.[13]

Positioning

In general, hip arthroscopy can be performed in the supine or lateral decubitus positions on either a fracture table or a hip distractor.[37] A modified supine position has been described, with the operative hip in 10° of hip flexion (to relax the anterior hip capsule), 15° of internal rotation, 30° of abduction, and the operative table in 10° of lateral tilt toward the nonoperative side.[19,38–40] Both general and epidural anesthesia can be used; however, a muscle relaxant (ie, paralytic) must be given to all patients undergoing general anesthesia to allow adequate distraction of the hip joint.[37,39–41] The perineum is positioned around a well-padded post to decrease the risk of pudendal nerve palsy, and the foot is well padded and secured in a boot with tape, to avoid injury to the superficial peroneal nerve.[13,37] The nonoperative leg is placed in 60° of abduction, 20° of flexion, and neutral rotation.[19] Under fluoroscopy, approximately 25 to 50 pounds of traction is applied to the operative leg, to achieve at least 8 to 10 mm of joint distraction, which is required prior to portal placement to break the normal seal of the hip joint. Fluoroscopically this is seen as the "vacuum sign."[13,19,37] A small amount of traction can be applied to the nonoperative leg as well, to hold the pelvis against the peroneal post. The operative leg is then slightly adducted to enhance the bony landmarks, and to create a lateral force vector against the peroneal post for distraction.[37]

Portals

Once the patient has been positioned, and before portal placement, the anterior superior iliac spine (ASIS) and greater trochanter are marked using a surgical marking pen. A line is then drawn from the ASIS down the anterior thigh, to mark the course of the lateral femoral cutaneous nerve (LFCN) of the thigh. Placement of portals lateral to this line will minimize injury to the LFCN.[42,43] A variety of portals have been described in the literature, including the anterior, anterolateral, mid-anterior, posterolateral, and proximal mid-anterior; however, the anterolateral and mid-anterior portals are usually sufficient to address both the rim lesion and the labral pathology.[13] The anterolateral portal is 1 cm superior and 1 cm anterior to the greater trochanter.[13,42] The authors' preferred anterior portal is 1 cm lateral to the ASIS in line with the tip of the greater trochanter.[13] This position is slightly different to that of the standard anterior portal, which is in line with the ASIS, and is used to minimize risk to the LFCN. Finally, the mid-anterior portal is 2 to 3 cm distal and between the anterior and anterolateral portals. In cases of significant retroversion or overhang, portal placement may need to be placed 1 to 2 cm distal to the standard positions to allow easier access into the hip joint.[13]

Diagnostic Arthroscopy

The location of lesions in the acetabulum traditionally has been described by using a clock-face method, whereby 12 o'clock corresponds to superior, 3 o'clock is anterior, and 9 o'clock is posterior.[44] However, some prefer to describe the acetabulum in 1 of 6 zones, defined by a vertical line drawn at the anterior and posterior aspects of the acetabular fossa and a horizontal line drawn at the superior limit of the fossa.[44,45] Furthermore, most investigators define the hip joint in 1 of 3 compartments: central, peripheral, and peritrochanteric space. The central compartment refers to the capsule (anterior and posterior triangles), acetabular zones, the anterior/posterior/superior labrum, the ligamentum teres, the acetabular cartilage, the transverse ligaments, and the femoral head cartilage.

As part of the standard diagnostic arthroscopy, using a 70° scope viewing through the anterolateral portal, one should be able to obtain a 360° view of the acetabulum to confirm the presence of the rim impingement lesion.[13] Starting with the scope in the anterior aspect of the acetabulum and the light source pointed inferior, the entire rim of the acetabulum can be seen by withdrawing the scope and rotating the light source counterclockwise.[13] In this same position, one can evaluate the medial and lateral portions of the femoral head and the central/parafoveal region.[43,45]

Portal Use Based on Pathology

For lesions, up to the 12 o'clock position on the acetabular rim or more posterior, the working portal should be the anterolateral portal, while viewing through the anterior portal (or modified anterior as described above).[13] In coxa profunda or protrusio, where the lesion is far posterior, a separate posterolateral portal may be necessary for bony work, while viewing through the anterolateral portal.[13] For anterior and anterosuperior (3 to 1 o'clock) lesions, the anterolateral portal is often used for viewing, while the anterior portal is the working portal.[13]

Findings

Rim impingement classically leads to a type II labral injury, with local crushing of the labrum, capsular edema, and erythema associated with repetitive impaction (**Fig. 1**).[13] There is often a contracoup injury in the posterior aspect of the joint, which can consist of an injury to the cartilage, labrum, or synovium.[13] This lesion is most commonly caused by posterior shear or overload forces in the posterior aspect of the joint.[13] A probe can be used to assess the labral injury, the extent of the bony impingement lesion, and calcifications within the substance of the labrum.[13]

SURGICAL TECHNIQUES

In general, there are 3 different techniques to manage rim impingement lesions: (1) labral debridement and rim resection, (2) capsular elevation, rim resection, and labral advancement, and (3) labral detachment, rim resection, and labral refixation.[13] Which

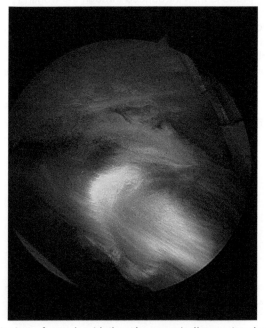

Fig. 1. Arthroscopic view of capsular sided erythema typically associated with a type II crushing injury to the labrum as a result of primary rim impingement.

procedure to perform is based on location of the rim lesion, the degree of labral injury, and surgeon's preference.[13] In each of these techniques, the same overlying principles exist: (1) a generous capsular cut using a beaver blade between the anterolateral and anterior portals to allow adequate visualization, (2) finding the exact location of the impingement lesion, (3) adequately clearing of the soft tissue (eg, capsule) off the lesion, (4) protecting the uninjured labral tissue, (5) adequate resection of the bony impingement lesion using a 5.5-mm burr (or smaller, based on surgeon preference), (6) reattachment of the uninjured labrum to the bony rim of the acetabulum (if possible), and (7) addressing any cam lesion that is present. Combined rim and cam lesions are common, and the best outcomes occur by addressing both sources of pathology.[14] The specific steps of each treatment option are discussed.

Labral Debridement and Rim Resection

In cases where there is severe crush injury to the labrum (eg, with global overcoverage), or extensive intrasubstance calcification, the labrum may not be amenable to refixation. In these cases, the labrum has a decreased ability to heal, therefore partial labral debridement using an arthroscopic shaver is advised. Debridement should occur at the exact location of the bony impingement lesion, as confirmed by intraoperative probing and by fluoroscopic assessment (**Fig. 2**). The working and viewing portals are dependent on the location of the lesion, as described earlier. Once the injured labrum at the area of the bony impingement lesion has been adequately debrided, debridement should be tapered to the viable labral tissue around the periphery. In cases where there is no viable labral tissue, Philippon and colleagues[46] have described a technique for reconstructing the labrum using the iliotibial (IT) band as autograft, while Sierra and Trousdale[47] have described a technique to reconstruct the labrum using the ligamentum teres capitis.

A radiofrequency probe is then introduced through the working portal to ablate the tissue, and further expose the bony impingement lesion. Radiofrequency ablation is also helpful in removing any unstable tissue adjacent to healthy labral tissue.[48] Location of the lesion is again confirmed by fluoroscopy and intraoperative probing. While protecting the viable labral tissue, a high-speed burr is used to resect the bony impingement lesion, which usually is about 5 to 8 mm. One should also be careful

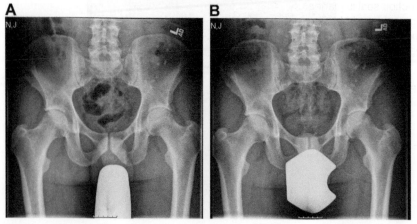

Fig. 2. Pre- and postoperative radiographs showing prominent rim ossification (*A*) and arthroscopic removal of rim ossification (*B*).

not to overresect the rim lesion, as postoperative instability may develop in these cases. If the lesion extends into the superolateral aspect of the acetabulum, then the reflected head of the rectus femorus must be indentified and protected. If a cam lesion is identified, it should be addressed at this time. Fluoroscopy is used to confirm that reestablishment of the normal anatomic relationship in the acetabulum has been achieved; specifically, that the anterior wall is medial to the posterior wall. Dynamic arthroscopy is also used to confirm that there is no impingement throughout range of motion under direct visualization.

Capsular Elevation, Rim Resection, and Labral Advancement

In situations where there is an extensive bony rim lesion that extends past the labral tissue, the rim can be resected by elevating the capsular tissue off the lesion, and resecting the rim lesion without taking down the labrum. This technique is a controlled method of preserving of a large amount of labral tissue.[38,49] After the cut in capsule to connect the anterolateral and anterior portals, one should debride the inflamed capsular tissue with an arthroscopic shaver and then elevate the capsule off the rim lesion using a radiofrequency ablator (**Fig. 3**). At this point, the labrum is peeled off the rim to the level of the transition zone, thus fully exposing the rim impingement lesion. Any nonviable labral tissue that is seen should be debrided at this point. Using a 5.5-mm burr (or smaller based on surgeon preference), the bony rim lesion is removed. Labral tissue can be protected by placing the burr in a position that allows the smooth backside of the burr sheath faces the labrum. As described for the first technique, resection should be continued until the normal relationship of the acetabulum is established (ie, the anterior wall of the acetabulum lies medial to the posterior

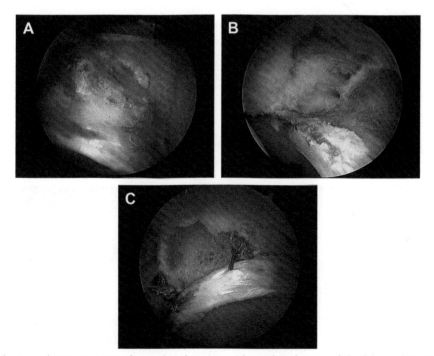

Fig. 3. Arthroscopic view of capsular elevation without detachment of the labrum (*A*), rim decompression (*B*), and labral refixation (*C*).

wall). Again, as already described, one should be careful not to overresect the rim impingement lesion, to prevent postoperative instability.

If the labrum destabilizes from the transition zone, then refixation is required. However, often the majority of the labrum stays attached to the transition zone of the cartilage, therefore 1 to 4 suture anchors, placed as close to the transition zone as possible, should be adequate. The labral tissue is advanced to the new bony rim of the acetabulum after adequate removal of the rim lesion. Sutures should be passed through the capsular side of the labrum, from the base of the labrum to the tip, so as to prevent suture from being in hip joint itself and to minimize the chance of everting the labrum when it is tied down (**Fig. 4**). Furthermore, when the labrum is tensioned, the femoral head should be in the reduced position, so as to recreate the anatomic suction seal of the labrum.[20–22] The sutures are tied using a standard arthroscopic knot-tying technique. As with the previous technique, if a cam lesion is present it should also be addressed, and dynamic arthroscopy should be performed at the completion of surgery to ensure there is no remaining impingement (**Fig. 5**).

Labral Detachment, Rim Resection, and Labral Refixation

Labral detachment, rim resection, and labral refixation is often used in situations where the labrum is healthy, and rim impingement lesion does not significantly overhang the labrum. After a capsular cut is made, and after diagnostic arthroscopy is performed to locate the lesion, an arthroscopic beaver blade can be used to primarily release the labrum from the acetabulum. This step is best performed by viewing from an intra-articular position, and freeing the labrum from the peripheral space from the outside in.[19] In addition to performing the resection holding the burr so

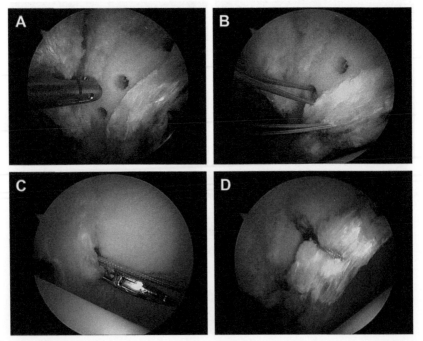

Fig. 4. Arthroscopic view of suture anchor placement (*A*), intrasubstance suture passage (*B, C*), and labral refixation (*D*).

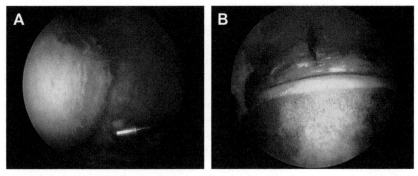

Fig. 5. Arthroscopic view of refixed labrum after the hip joint has been reduced before (*A*) and after (*B*) resection of the cam lesion.

that the smooth portion of the burr sheath is pointing toward the labrum, the labrum can be retracted by placing stay sutures in the labrum to hold traction. Using a radio-frequency ablator, the remaining soft tissues are removed from the rim lesion, and resection is performed as described in the previous 2 techniques. After adequate resection, the labrum is reattached to the bony rim of the acetabulum using suture anchors placed as close to the transition zone of the articular cartilage as possible. As already described, sutures should be passed through the capsular side of the labrum, from the base of the labrum to the tip; this prevents suture from being in the hip joint itself and also minimizes the chance of everting the labrum when it is tied/tensioned down. Again, when the labrum is tensioned, the femoral head should be reduced to recreate the fluid seal of the labrum.[20–22] As in both of the previous techniques, if a cam lesion is present it should also be addressed, followed by dynamic arthroscopy at the completion of surgery to ensure there is no remaining impingement.

POSTOPERATIVE REHABILITATION

Early range of motion is encouraged as soon as 4 hours postoperatively to prevent adhesions from forming. The patient is allowed to toe-touch weight bear (TTWB), applying 20 pounds of foot flat weight bearing, using crutches, for at least 4 weeks, and up to 8 weeks depending on the surgical procedure. If chondral work was performed, then restricted weight bearing should be used up to 8 weeks postoperatively. A continuous passive motion (CPM) machine is used for up to 4 to 8 weeks based on surgeon preference, for up to 8 hours per day.

RESULTS

If patient selection is appropriate, most investigators have published good short- to medium-term results following arthroscopic management of FAI.[14,15,18,50–57] Furthermore, studies comparing labral debridement and labral refixation in the treatment of these disorders have demonstrated improved results and less osteoarthritis in the hip with labral refixation at 1 and 2 years postoperatively.[15,18,50,51] However, long-term results following arthroscopic management of cam and/or rim type FAI are lacking in the literature.

DISCUSSION AND SUMMARY

Rim impingement lesions vary based on the underlying pathology. In general, rim impingement occurs with anterosuperior overhang, coxa profunda, protrusio acetabuli, and acetabular retroversion. The method for addressing these pathologic lesions depends on location and size of the impingement lesion, the underlying pathology, and the degree of labral damage. The ultimate goals of surgical management include accurate localization of the rim impingement lesion, adequate removal of the bony impingement lesion, and preservation and refixation of the viable labral tissue. However, if the surgeon feels that these goals cannot be accomplished safely and effectively by arthroscopic methods, then alternative procedures should be considered.

REFERENCES

1. Ganz R, Parvizi J, Beck M, et al. Femoroacetabular impingement: a cause of osteoarthritis of the hip. Clin Orthop Relat Res 2003;417:112–20.
2. Tonnis D, Heinecke A. Acetabular and femoral anteversion: relationship with osteoarthritis of the hip. J Bone Joint Surg Am 1999;81(12):1747–70.
3. Wenger DR, Bomar JD. Human hip dysplasia: evolution of current treatment concepts. J Orthop Sci 2003;8(2):264–71.
4. Delaunay S, Dussault RG, Kaplan PA, et al. Radiographic measurements of dysplastic adult hips. Skeletal Radiol 1997;26(2):75–81.
5. Giori NJ, Trousdale RT. Acetabular retroversion is associated with osteoarthritis of the hip. Clin Orthop Relat Res 2003;417:263–9.
6. Beck M, Kalhor M, Leunig M, et al. Hip morphology influences the pattern of damage to the acetabular cartilage. J Bone Joint Surg Br 2005;87(7):1012–8.
7. Wagner S, Hofstetter W, Chiquet, et al. Early osteoarthritic changes of human femoral head cartilage subsequent to femoro-acetabular impingement. Osteoarthritis Cartilage 2003;11(7):508–18.
8. Goodman DA, Feighan JE, Smith AD, et al. Subclinical slipped capital femoral epiphysis: relationship to osteoarthritis of the hip. J Bone Joint Surg Am 1997; 79:1489–97.
9. Leunig M, Casillas MM, Hamlet M, et al. Slipped capital femoral epiphysis: early mechanical damage to the acetabular cartilage by a prominent femoral metaphysis. Acta Orthop Scand 2000;71(4):370–5.
10. Ito K, Minka MA, Leunig M, et al. Femoroacetabular impingement and the cam-effect: a MRI-based quantitative anatomical study of the femoral head-neck offset. J Bone Joint Surg Br 2001;83(2):171–6.
11. Lavigne M, Parvizi J, Beck M, et al. Anterior femoroacetabular impingement: part I: techniques of joint preserving surgery. Clin Orthop Relat Res 2004;418:61–6.
12. Notzli HP, Wyss TF, Steocklin CH, et al. The contour of the femoral head-neck junction as a predictor for the risk of anterior impingement. J Bone Joint Surg Br 2002;84(4):556–60.
13. Ayeni OR, Pruett A, Kelly BT. Arthroscopic management of pincer impingement. In: Kelly BT, Philippon MJ, editors. Arthroscopic techniques in the hip. Thorofare (NJ): SLACK Incorporated; 2010. p. 69–88.
14. Philippon MJ, Schenker ML. Arthroscopy for the treatment of femoroacetabular impingement in the athlete. Clin Sports Med 2006;25(2):299–308.
15. Larson CM. Arthroscopic management of pincer-type impingement. Sports Med Arthrosc 2010;18(2):100–7.

16. Seldes RM, Tan V, Hunt J, et al. Anatomy, histologic features, and vascularity of the adult acetabular labrum. Clin Orthop Relat Res 2001;382:232–40.
17. Ferguson SJ, Bryant JT, Ganz R, et al. The acetabular labrum seal: a poroelastic finite element model. Clin Biomech 2000;15(6):463–8.
18. Espinosa N, Rothenfluh DA, Beck M, et al. Treatment of femoro-acetabular impingement: preliminary results for labral refixation. J Bone Joint Surg Am 2006;88(5):925–35.
19. Philippon MJ, Dewing CB, Briggs KK. Arthroscopic acetabular labral repair with rim trimming and femoral head-neck osteoplasty. In: Kelly BT, Philippon MJ, editors. Arthroscopic techniques in the hip. Thorofare (NJ): SLACK Incorporated; 2010. p. 15–26.
20. Ferguson SJ, Bryant R, Ganz R, et al. The influence of the acetabular labrum on hip joint cartilage consolidation: a poroelastic finite element model. J Biomech 2000;33:953–60.
21. Ferguson SJ, Bryant JT, Ganz R, et al. An in vitro investigation of the acetabular labral seal in hip joint mechanics. J Biomech 2003;36:171–8.
22. Ferguson SJ, Bryant JT, Ito K. The material properties of the bovine acetabular labrum. J Orthop Res 2001;19:887–96.
23. Philippon MF, Arnocsky SP, Torrie A. Arthroscopic repair of the actabular labrum: a histologic assessment of healing in an ovine model. Arthroscopy 2007;23(4):376–80.
24. Reynolds D, Lucas J, Klaue K. Retroversion of the acetabulum: a cause of hip pain. J Bone Joint Surg Br 1999;81(2):281–8.
25. Seibenrock KA, Schoeniger R, Ganz R. Anterior femoroacetabular impingement due to acetabular retroversion: treatment with periacetabular osteotomy. J Bone Joint Surg Am 2003;85(2):278–86.
26. Maheshwari A, Malik A, Dorr L. Impingement of the native hip joint. J Bone Joint Surg Am 2007;89:2508–18.
27. Leunig M, Nho SJ, Turchetto L, et al. Protrusio acetabuli: new insights and experience with joint preservation. Clin Orthop Relat Res 2009;467(9):2241–50.
28. McBride MT, Muldoon MP, Santore RF, et al. Protrusio acetabuli: diagnosis and treatment. J Am Acad Orthop Surg 2001;9(2):79–88.
29. Martin RL, Ensek KR, Draovitch P, et al. Acetabular labral tears of the hip: examination and diagnostic challenges. J Orthop Sports Phys Ther 2006;35:503–15.
30. Clohisy JC, Carlisle JC, Beaule PE, et al. A systematic approach to the plain radiographic evaluation of the young adult hip. J Bone Joint Surg Am 2008;90:47–65.
31. Siebenrock KA, Kalbermatten DF, Ganz R. Effect of pelvic tilt on acetabular retroversion: a study of pelves from cadavers. Clin Orthop Relat Res 2003;407:241–8.
32. Wolff AB, Philippon MJ, Briggs KK, et al. Acetabular rim reduction for the treatment of femoroacetabular impingement correlates with pre- and post-operative center edge angle. American Academy of Orthopaedic Surgeons Annual Meeting 2009. Las Vegas (NV), February 27, 2009.
33. Ganz R, Gill TJ, Gautier E, et al. Surgical dislocation of the adult hip a technique with full access to the femoral head and acetabulum without the risk of avascular necrosis. J Bone Joint Surg Br 2001;83(8):1119–24.
34. Beck M, Leunig M, Parvizi J, et al. Anterior femoroacetabular impingement: part II: midterm results of surgical treatment. Clin Orthop Relat Res 2004;418:67–73.
35. Byrd JW. Hip arthroscopy: evolving frontiers. Opin Tech Orthop 2004;14(2):58–67.
36. Sampson T. Hip morphology and its relationship to pathology: dysplasia to impingement. Opin Tech Sports Med 2005;13(1):37–45.
37. Bharam S, Tong A. Positioning and set-up. In: Kelly BT, Philippon MJ, editors. Arthroscopic techniques in the hip. Thorofare (NJ): SLACK Incorporated; 2010. p. 1–12.

38. Kelly BT, Williams RJ, Philippon MJ. Hip arthroscopy: current indications, treatment options, and management issues. Am J Sports Med 2003;31:1020–37.
39. Schenker ML, Martin RR, Weiland DE, et al. Current trends in hip arthroscopy: a review of injury diagnosis, techniques, and outcome scoring. Curr Opin Orthop 2005;16:89–94.
40. Bharam S. Labral tears, extra-articular injuries, and hip arthroscopy in the athlete. Clin Sports Med 2006;25(2):279–92.
41. Kelly BT, Weiland DF, Schenker ML, et al. Arthroscopic labral repair in the hip: surgical technique and review of the literature. Arthroscopy 2005;21(12):1496–504.
42. Robertson WJ, Kelly BT. Portals. In: Kelly BT, Philippon MJ, editors. Arthroscopic techniques in the hip. Thorofare (NJ): SLACK Incorporated; 2010. p. 15–26.
43. Robertson WJ, Kelly BT. The safe zone for hip arthroscopy: a cadaveric assessment of central, peripheral, and lateral compartment portal placement. Arthroscopy 2008;24(9):1019–26.
44. Martin H. Diagnostic arthroscopy. In: Kelly BT, Philippon MJ, editors. Arthroscopic techniques in the hip. Thorofare (NJ): SLACK Incorporated; 2010. p. 15–26.
45. Ilizaliturri VM Jr, Byrd JW, Sampson TG, et al. A geographic zone method to describe intra-articular pathology in hip arthroscopy: cadaveric study and preliminary report. Arthroscopy 2008;24:534–9.
46. Philippon M, Stubbs AJ, Schenker ML, et al. Arthroscopic management of femoroacetabular impingement: osteoplasty technique and literature review. Am J Sports Med 2007;35:1571–80.
47. Sierra RJ, Trousdale RT. Labral reconstruction using the ligamentum teres capitis: report of a new technique. Clin Orthop Relat Res 2009;467(3):753–9.
48. Byrd JWT. The role of hip arthroscopy in the athletic hip. Clin Sports Med 2006;25:255–78.
49. Kelly BT. Arthroscopy of the hip. In: Kibler WB, editor. Orthopaedic knowledge update: sports medicine. 4th edition. Rosemont (IL): American Academy of Orthopaedic Surgeons; 2009. p. 101–8.
50. Larson CM, Giveans MR. Arthroscopic management of femoro-acetabular impingement: early outcomes measures. Arthroscopy 2008;24:540–6.
51. Larson CM, Giveans RM. Arthroscopic debridement versus refixation of the acetabular labrum associated with femoroacetabular impingement. Arthroscopy 2009;25:369–76.
52. Philippon M, Briggs K, Yen Y, et al. Outcomes following hip arthroscopy for femoroacetabular impingement with associated chondrolabral dysfunction minimum two-year follow-up. J Bone Joint Surg Br 2009;91:16–23.
53. Byrd JW, Jones KS. Arthroscopic femoroplasty in the management of cam-type femoroacetabular impingement. Clin Orthop Relat Res 2009;467:739–46.
54. Bedi A, Chen N, Robertson W, et al. The management of labral tears and femoroacetabular impingement of the hip in the young, active hip. Arthroscopy 2008;24:1135–45.
55. Ilizaliturri VM Jr, Orozco-Rodriguez L, Acosta-Rodriguez E, et al. Arthroscopic treatment of cam-type femoroacetabular impingement: preliminary report at 2 years minimum follow-up. J Arthroplasty 2008;23:226–34.
56. Guanche CA, Bare AA. Arthroscopic treatment of femoroacetabular impingement. Arthroscopy 2006;22:95–106.
57. Philippon M, Schenker M, Briggs K, et al. Femoroacetabular impingement in 45 professional athletes: associated pathologies and return to sport following arthroscopic decompression. Knee Surg Sports Traumatol Arthrosc 2007;15:908–14.

Soft Tissue Pathology Around the Hip

Victor M. Ilizaliturri Jr, MD[a],*, Javier Camacho-Galindo, MD[a],
Alberto Nayib Evia Ramirez, MD[a], Yari Lizette Gonzalez Ibarra, MD[a],
Sean Mc Millan, DO[b], Brian D. Busconi, MD[c]

KEYWORDS

- Peritrochanteric space • Snapping hips • Endoscopy

Hip arthroscopy is used increasingly to treat early hip disease in cases where nonarthroplasty hip-preserving techniques are indicated. This technique is ideal for the younger patients experiencing hip problems. More recently, endoscopic access to the periarticular areas of the hip has allowed endoscopic forms of treatment for soft tissue pathology.

There are several different pathologic conditions produced by soft tissue around the hip joint that may be adequate for endoscopic treatment. Found in current medical literature are (1) the greater trochanteric pain syndrome (and associated pathology), (2) snapping hip syndromes, and more infrequently, (3) piriformis syndrome. Other soft tissue conditions that may require open surgical treatment that involves other muscles around the hip include avulsion injuries of the anterior iliac spines, hamstring injuries, and sports hernias or athletic pubalgia.

GREATER TROCHANTERIC PAIN SYNDROME

It has been traditionally described that the etiology of the greater trochanteric pain syndrome is related to a single traumatic episode or multiple microtraumas resulting in chronic inflammation of the greater trochanteric bursa.

The use of the term "greater trochanteric bursitis" erroneously implies that there is inflammation of the greater trochanteric bursa involved in the etiology of painful symptoms in the peritrochanteric region. The "bursitis idea" has been reinforced by the significant relief of symptoms obtained after injections containing glucocorticoids and local anesthetics in the area around the greater trochanter. However, there is a recent tendency in the literature to refer to this condition as the greater trochanteric

[a] National Rehabilitation Institute of Mexico, Universidad Nacional Autónoma de México, Avenue México Xochimilco 289, Col. Arenal de Guadalupe, Mexico City 14389, Mexico
[b] Division of Sports Medicine, Department of Orthopedics, University of Massachusetts Memorial Medical Center, 281 Lincoln Street, Worcester, MA 01605, USA
[c] Department of Orthopedics and Physical Rehabilitation, University of Massachusetts Medical School, 281 Lincoln Street, Worcester, MA 01605-2192, USA
* Corresponding author.
E-mail address: vichip2002@yahoo.com.mx

Clin Sports Med 30 (2011) 391–415
doi:10.1016/j.csm.2010.12.009
0278-5919/11/$ – see front matter © 2011 Elsevier Inc. All rights reserved.

pain syndrome, arising from the paucity of histologic evidence supporting inflammation of the bursal tissue around the greater trochanter in cases diagnosed with trochanteric bursitis.[1,2]

The term "greater trochanteric hip syndrome" implies that there is a group of signs and symptoms related to pain in the trochanteric region. This condition is usually more complex than a simple bursal inflammation, and is frequently related to other pathologic conditions or is associated with other lesions within the peritrochanteric space.[3]

Epidemiology

Pain localized around the greater trochanter is a common affliction seen by the orthopedic surgeon. In a large multicenter observational study of 3026 patients the prevalence of greater trochanteric pain syndrome in the age group between 50 and 79 years was 15% for women and 6.6% for men in unilateral presentation, and 8.5% for women and 1.9% for men in bilateral presentation.[4]

Diagnostic Criteria

Attempts to make clinical diagnostic criteria have been made. Krout and Anderson proposed a set of diagnostic criteria that were later modified by Rasmussen and Fano.[5] These criteria required at least 2 criteria from the following be present: lateral hip pain, tenderness about the greater trochanter, and one of the following: pain at the extremes of rotation, abduction, or adduction; pain on strong contraction of hip abductors; or pseudoradiculopathy (pain radiating down the lateral aspect of the thigh).

Imaging

Imaging studies are usually done to rule out evidence of hip osteoarthritis, bony hip deformities, or the presence of bone pathology at the greater trochanter. An anteroposterior (AP) pelvis radiograph, as well as an AP and lateral hip series, are standard initial images. Further imaging, such as magnetic resonance imaging (MRI), can be pursued to evaluate for muscle tears and strains in the hip abductor region. More recently, hip abductor muscle pathology has been described in relation to greater trochanteric pain syndrome; this is discussed later in this article.

Treatment Options

Many of the patients suffering greater trochanteric pain syndrome are frequently seen by 2 or more orthopedic surgeons, and receive multiple modes of treatment ranging from oral anti-inflammatory nonsteroidal drugs (NSAIDs) to multiple local infiltrations and physical therapy. In many cases there is very little or no improvement.[5,6]

Surgical Considerations

Failure of conservative treatment is the indication for surgical treatment. In this situation, associated pathology such as abductor tendon muscle tears and compression from a tight iliotibial band should be investigated. Different open surgical techniques have been described for the treatment of the greater trochanteric pain syndrome, ranging from iliotibial band release and bursectomy, to iliotibial band lengthening and bursectomy and trochanteric reduction osteotomies.[7–13] This condition has been treated endoscopically with greater trochanteric bursectomy and bursectomy combined with iliotibial band release or iliotibial band partial resection. **Table 1** compares the results of open and endoscopic procedures. Results between open and endoscopic techniques are comparable, but articles of a higher level of evidence and longer follow-up are needed for better evaluation of the results of both open and endoscopic techniques.

Table 1
Results of surgical treatment for greater trochanteric pain syndrome

First Author, Year[Ref.]	Number of Hips	Technique	Follow-Up (Months)	Pain
Slawski, 1997[7]	6	Open Iliotibial band decompression and bursectomy	20 (2 lost to follow-up)	3 patients with occasional pain
Craig, 2007[8]	17	Open Iliotibial band Z-plasty leaving 5 cm posterior defect and bursectomy	47	1 poor result 1 Further surgery for gluteus medius repair
Govaert, 2003[9]	12 5 had previous open iliotibial band decompression and bursectomy	Open trochanteric reduction osteotomy and bursectomy	23.5	2 mild pain 1 pain related to screws that required removal 1 postoperative hematoma drained surgically in a subsequent procedure developed heterotopic ossification requiring removal with removal of screws
Bradley, 1998[10] (Case report)	2 (bilateral case)	Endoscopic removal of fibrotic bands from iliotibial band and bursectomy	7	None
Fox, 2007[11] (Technical note)	27	Endoscopic bursectomy	None reported	Not reported
Farr, 2007[12]	2	Endoscopic bursectomy and longitudinal iliotibial band release	40	None
Baker[13]	30	Endoscopic iliotibial band release (cross-cut and flap resection) and bursectomy	26 (5 patients lost to follow-up)	1 seroma requiring further surgery 1 failed procedure requiring open revision

GREATER TROCHANTERIC PAIN SYNDROME (ASSOCIATED LESIONS)
Abductor Muscle Tears

The cause for tendinosis, and eventually rupture, of the gluteus medius and minimus is still uncertain. Local anatomic and/or traumatic conditions may be involved, just as systemic conditions may predispose certain individuals for spontaneous rupture (**Fig. 1**).

Epidemiology
In a study by Bunker and colleagues,[14] the prevalence of such lesions was initially estimated to be 22% in a series of patients with surgical treatment for femoral neck fractures. In their study, tears were frequently observed at the anterior third of the gluteus medius and the gluteus minimus tendon. The term rotator cuff of the hip was adopted because of the similarities of these tears with tears occurring on the rotator cuff of the shoulder. Howell and colleagues[15] found degenerative tears in the gluteus medius and minimus in 20% of 176 patients undergoing total hip arthroplasty.

Anatomic and physiologic considerations
The mechanical or local components postulated as causes for this pathology may consist of pelvic morphology, a high valgus angle of the knee, and/or leg-length discrepancy. All of these alterations surmount to a tense iliotibial band, which in turn would cause mechanical abrasion on the gluteal muscles as the greater trochanter impinges against it. Predisposing conditions that have been described as possible causes in hip rotator cuff tears are anabolic steroid use, chondrocalcinosis, diabetes mellitus, dystrophic calcification, gout, hyperparathyroidism, myofascial pain syndrome, obesity, Paget disease, rheumatoid arthritis, and systemic lupus erythematosus.[16–20]

Presentation
Hip rotator-cuff tears or tendinitis may present with buttock, lateral hip, or groin pain. History of trauma is frequently absent. Patients may describe a grinding sensation and difficulty climbing stairs. Pain will be elicited on palpation of the gluteus medius

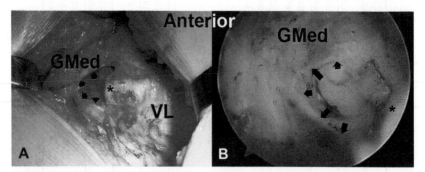

Fig. 1. (A) Clinical photograph taken during total hip replacement in a right hip. A gluteus medius (GMed) tear was found. The vastus lateralis (VL) is to the right; asterisk indicates the tip of the greater trochanter. The black arrows indicate the limits of the tear on the gluteus medius. The gluteus minimus is observed through the tear. (B) Endoscopic image demonstrating a similar tear (different patient) to the one shown A. The photograph shows the peritrochanteric space in a right hip. The tip of the greater trochanter (asterisk) is to the right. The black arrows indicate the limits of the gluteus medius tear. A calcification is observed through the tear.

insertion, or directly over the greater trochanter. The patients may present a positive "fatigue" Trendelenburg test.[21]

Imaging

Plain radiographs are usually the first imaging examination obtained in patients with greater trochanteric pain syndrome. In the case of gluteal tendinopathy it may show avulsion fractures of the greater trochanter or calcification within the tendon substance. Plain radiographs are very important in evaluating the anatomy of the hip joint. An anteroposterior pelvis radiograph should always be obtained for comparative purposes, as well as a lateral view of both hips.

MRI and ultrasonography have been considered more accurate in diagnosing this pathology. Direct signs of injury of the gluteus medius and/or minimus on the MRI include surrounding soft tissue edema, tendon thickening, intrasubstance signal abnormality, focal discontinuity, or absence of tendon fibers (**Fig. 2**). Indirect signs include subminimus or submedius bursitis, enthesopathic changes along the great trochanteric insertion, and fatty atrophy. Ultrasonography may detect tendinopathy by decreased and often heterogeneous echogenicity and tendon thickening. Kingzett-Taylor and colleagues[22] presented a series of 35 MRI studies of patients with buttock, lateral hip, or groin pain. Twenty-two patients had a gluteus medius tear (14 complete tears and 8 partial tears). Five of these 22 patients had a partial tear of the gluteus minimus, and one had an additional partial tear of the gluteus maximus. Thirteen patients had signs of tendinosis of the gluteus medius, and 5 of those also had tendinitis of the gluteus minimus. Cvitanic and colleagues[23] presented a more recent series of MRI and gluteus medius and minimus tears. These investigators studied 74 hips in 45 patients. Fifteen hips had surgically proven abductor tendon tears, while the other 59 were either asymptomatic or had surgically confirmed intact tendons. T2 hypersensitivity superior to the greater trochanter had the highest sensitivity and specificity for tears among other signs (73% and 95%, respectively). The authors' preference is MRI.

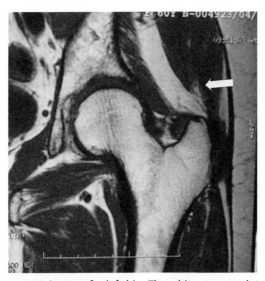

Fig. 2. Magnetic resonance image of a left hip. The white arrow points to a hyperintense signal in the substance of the muscle-tendon junction in the gluteus medius. This was reported as gluteus medius tendinosis.

Treatment options

Gluteus tendon ruptures may be treated nonoperatively if they are diagnosed early. Treatment involves unloading of the affected hip, NSAIDs, and physical therapy once the patients symptoms have subsided. Conservative treatment is similar to that commonly applied to patients who are diagnosed with greater trochanteric pain syndrome.

Patients presenting more advanced lesions, or chronic pain, may be subject to operative treatment. Fisher and colleagues[20] describe an open operative technique employed in a case of bilateral spontaneous hip rotator cuff tears. The patient had no predisposing condition that could be identified, and presented with spontaneous ruptures of the gluteus medius and minimus with a 5-year period between each hip. Diagnosis was clinical, and included MRI showing edema and rupture of the gluteus minimus and partial tearing of the gluteus medius. A direct lateral approach was performed through the tensor fasciae latae, and in both hips the trochanteric bursa appeared normal. The tears were compatible with the images seen in the MRI. Repair of the gluteus minimus was performed with several intraosseous sutures with an orthobiologic patch as augmentation. Postoperative management began with protected weight bearing using 2 crutches for the first 2 weeks. Resistance-free abduction exercises were begun at the third week along with the use of one crutch. At 5 weeks the investigators reported remission of the pain and the limp, with full abduction and flexion strength. Four months postoperatively the patient was asymptomatic and able to walk 3 km.

Five years later, similar findings led to a repeat operation on the contralateral hip. Results and management were similar, obtaining pain-free asymptomatic walking within 6 months. More recently, endoscopic access to the peritrochanteric space and endoscopic repair of gluteus medius tears have been described,[3] but this is only a technical description and no results are reported.

In a recent publication, Voos and colleagues[24] presented a consecutive series of 10 patients treated with endoscopic repair of gluteus medius tears, who all presented with chronic multitreated greater trochanteric pain. Diagnosis was made by clinical examination and MRI and was confirmed during endoscopy. All patients in the series were free of pain and had a full recovery of motor strength at 25 months. Seven patients described their hip as normal and 3 as nearly normal. Domb and colleagues[25] recently presented a technique for partial thickness gluteus medius tears; however, no results or follow-up were data were given.

Even though greater trochanteric pain syndrome, described as trochanteric bursitis, is a frequent condition in general orthopedics practice; associated lesions such as abductor tendon tears have only recently been described. Long-term follow-up studies of larger series of patients are needed to understand the value of surgical treatment of this condition. The current available evidence of both open and endoscopic repair is anecdotal.

Snapping Hip Syndromes

Three different types of snapping hip syndrome have traditionally been described[26]: (1) external snapping hip syndrome, produced by the iliotibial band snapping over the posterior edge of the greater trochanter; (2) internal snapping hip syndrome, produced by the iliopsoas tendon snapping over the iliopectineal eminence of the femoral head; AND (3) the intra-articular snapping hip syndrome, which was originally attributed to diverse intra-articular pathology (loose bodies, labral tears, and so forth). We no longer refer to the intra-articular snapping hip because today there is more accuracy in the description and diagnosis of intra-articular hip pathology.

EXTERNAL SNAPPING HIP SYNDROME

External snapping hip syndrome[27] originates through the iliotibial band snapping over the prominence of the greater trochanter. This condition is caused by a thickening of the posterior part of the iliotibial band, which is positioned posterior to the posterior edge of the greater trochanter. Flexion of the hip causes the iliotibial band to slide anteriorly over the greater trochanter. When the posterior thickened part of the iliotibial band passes over the greater trochanter it snaps to an anterior position, and extension brings the thickened part of the iliotibial band back to the posterior position, repeating the snapping phenomenon (**Fig. 3**). The greater trochanteric bursa lies between the iliotibial and the greater trochanter, over the tendinous insertion of the gluteus medius and the origin of vastus lateralis muscles. It may become inflamed with the snapping, causing pain. Tendinopathy, degeneration, and tears of the gluteus medius tendon are also likely to develop because of this constant rubbing.

Presentation

Diagnosis is evident when patients are able to reproduce the snapping.

Clinical presentation of this phenomenon is typical in 2 different forms. The first clinical form is the "hip dislocator." The patient usually refers the ability to dislocate the hip joint without a correlating pain elicitation. This action is usually reproducible, and the patients often volunteer to demonstrate it by standing with bilateral weight bearing while doing a tilting and rotating motion of the pelvis with lateral displacement of the affected side. The snapping phenomenon can be visible or palpable around the area of the greater trochanter. As mentioned, this phenomenon occurs without pain and usually represents no problems in performing sporting activity or activities of daily living. Stretching exercises of the iliotibial band may be indicated to treat this condition.

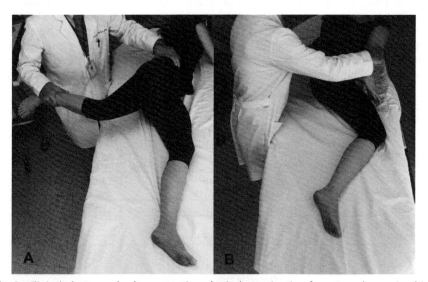

Fig. 3. Clinical photographs demonstrating physical examination for external snapping hip. The patient is in left lateral decubitus as the right hip is examined. (*A*) The hip is in extension. (*B*) The hip is brought to flexion; the examiner should look for the snapping phenomenon on the greater trochanteric region.

The second clinical form is a "true" external snapping hip, characterized by a snapping phenomenon at the area of the greater trochanter that occurs while flexing and extending the hip. The patients often complain of the snapping occurring during stair climbing, exercising, or while sitting down on or standing up from a chair. The phenomenon is frequently associated with pain and tenderness around the greater trochanter.

Treatment Options

Asymptomatic snapping should be considered a normal occurrence. Stretching exercises of the iliotibial band should be indicated in asymptomatic snappers to prevent the condition from becoming symptomatic. Most of the symptomatic cases improve with stretching physical therapy, NSAID therapy, and corticosteroid infiltration of the greater trochanteric bursa. If there is failure of a positive response to conservative treatment of the external snapping hip syndrome, surgical release is indicated.

Surgical Considerations

Open surgical release and lengthening techniques[28–31] have been described in the literature. More recently, endoscopic techniques have been introduced. To date the only results that have been published of endoscopic treatment of the external snapping hip is the authors' own series.[27] The original report included 11 hips treated for external snapping hip syndrome using an endoscopic technique in which a diamond-shaped window on the iliotibial band is created, allowing the greater trochanter to freely rotate within the window. At an average follow-up of 25 months, all of the patients were free of pain. One patient presented with mild resnapping that was treated successfully with further physical therapy. These results compare well with those of open surgical techniques used for this pathology (**Table 2**).

The diamond-shape release of the iliotibial band was initially used to treat the external snapping hip syndrome (**Fig. 4**). More recently, the authors have used the technique to provide access to the peritrochanteric space. The release itself is used to relieve pressure from the iliotibial band over the area of the greater trochanter. The resulting defect on the iliotibial band provides access to the greater traochanteric bursa. After resection of the bursa, the gluteus medius tendon is accessible for inspection. Internal rotation provides access to the area of the short external rotators.

Table 2
Results of surgical treatment of external snapping hip syndrome (open and endoscopic)

First Author, Year[Ref.]	Number of Hips	Technique	Follow-Up	Pain	Resnapping
Fery, 1988[28]	35	Open cross-cut, and inverted flap suture	7 y	21 cases	10 cases
Faraj, 2001[29]	11	Open Z-plasty	12 mo	3 cases	0
Provencher, 2004[30]	9	Open Z-Plasty	22 mo	1	0
White, 2004[31]	17	Open vertical incision and multiple transverse cuts	32.5 mo	0	2 cases (reoperated)
Ilizaliturri, 2006[33]	11	Diamond-shape defect	25 mo	0	1 case, improved with physical therapy

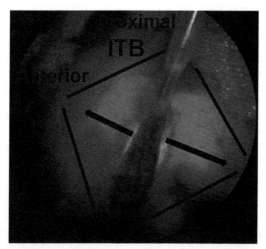

Fig. 4. Endoscopic photograph of a left hip. The view is from the subcutaneous space lateral to the iliotibial band (ITB); a radiofrequency hook probe is used to perform a vertical release of the iliotibial band over the prominence of the greater trochanter. The black arrows indicate the direction of subsequent releases done at the mid-portion of the vertical release anteriorly and posteriorly. The black lines indicate the "diamond" shape defect on the iliotibial band that will result after the flaps are resected.

Surgical Technique

The patient is positioned in the lateral decubitus position. Next, the patient is draped with care taken to ensure for free range of motion of the lower extremity, enabling reproduction of the snapping phenomenon during surgery. Traction is not necessary to access the greater trochanteric bursa and the iliotibial band. The greater trochanter is marked on the skin using a skin marker. The greater trochanter is the main landmark for portal establishment. The authors use 2 portals, a proximal trochanteric and distal trochanteric. The area of snapping should be between both portals and is also marked on the skin (**Fig. 5**). The authors start by infiltrating the space under the iliotibial band

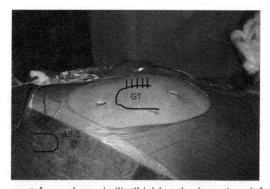

Fig. 5. Portal placement for endoscopic iliotibial band release in a left hip. The anterior superior iliac spine (ASIS) and the greater trochanter (GT) are outlined. The area of snapping is indicated by the horizontal lines. The proximal trochanteric portal is to the left of the tip of the greater trochanter and the distal trochanteric portal to the right.

with 40 to 50 mL of saline. Next, the inferior trochanteric portal is established using a standard arthroscopic cannula that is introduced under the skin and directed proximally to the site of the superior trochanteric portal, using the blunt obturator to develop a working space above the iliotibial band. The site of the proximal trochanteric portal is identified arthroscopically using a needle inserted at the portal landmark. The skin incision is made next, and a shaver is introduced to dissect subcutaneous tissue from the iliotibial band situated between the portals. Hemostasis is performed in this step to allow clear visualization of the iliotibial band. Then a radiofrequency hook probe is introduced from the proximal trochanteric portal and a 4- to 5-cm vertical retrograde cut is made on the iliotibial band starting at the level of the inferior trochanteric portal, which is the viewing portal. The pump pressure should be kept low while working on the subcutaneous space to avoid complications with the skin. Once the vertical cut on the iliotibial band is complete, the pump pressure can be increased and a transverse anterior cut of 2 cm length is performed, starting at the middle of the vertical cut. The resulting superior and inferior anterior flaps are resected using a shaver to develop a triangular defect on the anterior iliotibial band; this will provide access to the posterior iliotibial band. Next, a transverse posterior cut is started at the same level of the transverse anterior cut. This release is the most important, and should be performed until the snapping phenomenon is solved. Finally the superior and inferior posterior flaps are resected, which results in a diamond shape defect on the iliotibial band (**Figs. 6** and **7**). The greater trochanter will rotate freely within the defect without snapping. The greater trochanteric bursa should be removed through the defect on the iliotibial band and the abductor tendons inspected for tears. When central or peripheral compartment hip arthroscopy is also necessary, the authors begin with those compartments before addressing the peritrochanteric region.

INTERNAL SNAPPING HIP SYNDROME

Internal snapping hip syndrome is produced by the iliopsoas tendon over the iliopectineal eminence or the femoral head. The iliopsoas tendon is located lateral to the iliopectineal eminence when the hip is in full flexion; with hip extension the tendon is displaced medially until it positions medial to the iliopectineal eminence when the hip is in neutral position.[26]

Epidemiology

The snapping phenomenon can occur without pain in up to 10% of the general population, and should be considered a normal occurrence.[32]

Presentation

The symptomatic internal snapping hip syndrome always presents with pain in the groin associated with the snapping phenomenon. The snapping phenomenon is reproduced when bringing the hip to extension from a flexed position. Patients will report snapping while climbing stairs or rising from a chair. The snapping phenomenon is usually voluntary and reproducible.[33]

Physical examination of the internal snapping phenomenon is done with the patient supine by flexing the affected hip more than 90° and extending to neutral position. This movement may be accentuated with abduction and external rotation in flexion and adducting and internally rotating while extending. The snapping phenomenon is not visible at the groin. It may be audible or may be palpated by placing the hand over

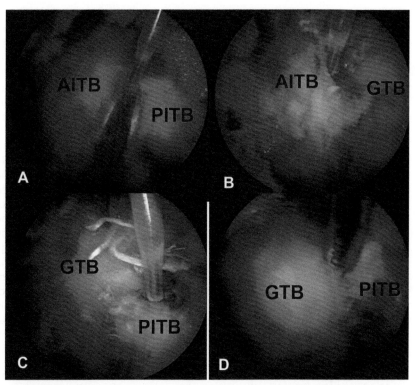

Fig. 6. The sequence illustrates an endoscopic release of the iliotibial band in a left hip. (*A*) The first cut is a vertical release, which is performed in a retrograde fashion using a radiofrequency hook probe; the arthroscope is in the distal trochanteric portal and the radiofrequency hook in the proximal trochanteric portal. The iliotibial band is divided by this cut in 2 portions: anterior iliotibial band (AITB) and posterior iliotibial band (PITB). (*B*) At the mid-portion of the AITB cut, an anterior transverse release is performed, usually 2 cm in length. The greater trochanteric bursa (GTB) is to the right. (*C*) The PITB is released at the mid-portion of the vertical cut. The GTB can be observed at the left. (*D*) The diamond-shape defect is complete; the GTB is observed through the defect.

the affected groin. There is always an apprehension response from the patient when the snapping occurs.

Imaging

Plain radiographs consist of an AP pelvis, AP hip, and lateral radiographs. These films are usually normal; however, in some cases a cam femoroacetabular impingement deformity may be documented. Psoas bursography may outline the tendon and, if combined with fluoroscopy, may document the snapping phenomenon dynamically. The limiting factor with this examination is the technical proficiency of the test performer related to his or her ability to reproduce the snapping while examining hip motion within the range of view of the C-arm.[34] Ultrasonography of the iliopsoas tendon is a dynamic noninvasive study that may document the snapping phenomenon as well as pathologic changes of the iliopsoas tendon and its bursa. Psoas ultrasonography also depends on the ability and experience of the examiner.[35] More recently, ultrasonography has also been used to describe new mechanisms of iliopsoas

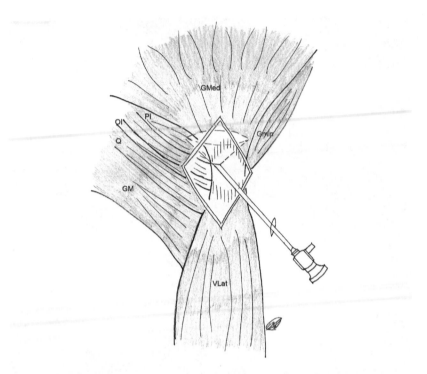

Fig. 7. Endoscopic examination of the peritrochanteric space in a right hip. The arthroscope is introduced though a distal trochanteric portal and onto the peritrochanteric space through a diamond-shape defect on the iliotibial band. The insertion of the gluteus medius (GMed) at the greater trochanter is examined. Behind the greater trochanter the tendons of the piriformis muscle (PI), obturator internus (OI), quadratus femoris (Q), and gluteum maximus (GM) are presented. Anterior to the gluteus medius is the gluteus minimus (Gmin).

snapping, including snapping of bifid iliopsoas tendons, snapping of the iliopsoas over the iliacus muscle, and snapping of the iliopsoas tendon over paralabral cysts.[36]

Because almost half of the patients with internal snapping hip syndrome have associated intra-articular hip parthology,[32,33,37] magnetic resonance arthrography (MRA) is the diagnostic study preferred by the authors. MRA may demonstrate intra-articular pathology and report changes related to the iliopsoas tendon and bursa. The snapping phenomenon cannot be documented using MRA.

Treatment Options

Treatment is initially conservative with trial of physical therapy, NSAID therapy, and corticosteroid injections used. If there is a failure of a positive response to conservative treatment, surgical treatment is indicated.[26]

Surgical Considerations

Open surgical release or lengthening has traditionally been the standard procedure for symptomatic internal snapping hip syndrome.[38–41] Recently, successful endoscopic iliopsoas tendon release has been reported in the literature.[32,33,37,42] Results of endoscopic release of the iliopsoas tendon for internal snapping hip syndrome compare well with results reported for open release or open lengthening techniques (**Table 3**).

Table 3
Results of surgical treatment of internal snapping hip syndrome (open and endoscopic)

First Author, Year[Ref.]	Number of Hips	Technique	Follow-Up	Pain	Resnapping
Taylor, 1995[39]	17	Open release	17 mo	0	5
Jacobson, 1990[38]	20	Open Z-plasty	20 mo	2 (reoperated)	6
Dobbs, 2002[40]	11	Open Z-plasty	4 y	0	1
Gruen, 2002[41]	11	Open Z-plasty	3 y	0	0
Byrd, 2005[32]	9	Endoscopic release at lesser trochanter	20 mo	0	0
Ilizaliturri, 2005[33]	7	Endoscopic release at the lesser trochanter	21 mo	0	0
Wettstein, 2006[42]	9	Endoscopic release (preserving iliacus muscle) transcapsular	3 mo (Technique report)	0	0
Flanum, 2007[37]	6	Endoscopic release at the lesser trochanter	12 mo	0	0
Contreras, 2010[43]	7	Endoscopic release, capsulotomy from central compartment (hip with traction)	24 mo	0	0

Endoscopic iliopsoas release is always performed in conjunction with hip arthroscopy. The rationale for this derives from studies having demonstrated that almost half of the patients with internal snapping hip syndrome present with associated intra-articular pathology.[32,33,37] Endoscopic release can be performed from the hip periphery. This procedure is performed without traction, and the authors prefer accessory portals to access the hip periphery (**Fig. 8**). A communication between the hip capsule and the iliopsoas bursa is established by carrying out an anterior hip capsulotomy between the anterior labrum and zona orbicularis, which provides access from the hip capsule into the psoas bursa (**Fig. 9**). The iliopsoas tendon is identified at this level and released (a radiofrequency hook is frequently used), leaving the iliacus muscle intact behind it (**Fig. 10**).[42] An alternative technique is to release the tendon from its insertion at the level of the lesser trochanter. Only the tendinous portion is released, leaving some muscle fibers intact. Access is gained through accessory portals, which are directed to the psoas bursa by aiming toward the area above the lesser trochanter. The procedure is done without traction and with hip external rotation to further expose the lesser trochanter. A radiofrequency hook is frequently used to perform the release (**Fig. 11**).[32,33,37]

Release at the central compartment with traction has been recently reported.[43] A capsulotomy is performed anteriorly between the anterior labrum and anterior femoral

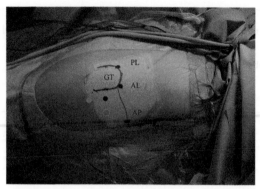

Fig. 8. Positioning of a patient for hip arthroscopy in lateral position. The greater trochanter (GT) and the anterior superior iliac spine (ASIS) are outlined. Portals for central compartment arthroscopy are the anterolateral portal (AL), direct anterior portal (AP), and posterolateral portal (PL). The black dot illustrates the position of the viewing accessory portal for both the anteroinferior hip periphery and the iliopsoas bursa at the level of the lesser trochanter. The red dot illustrates the authors' preference for the working portal for the anterior inferior hip periphery. Note that it is lateral to the position of the ASIS. The green dot illustrates the position of the working portal for the iliopsoas bursa at the level of the lesser trochanter.

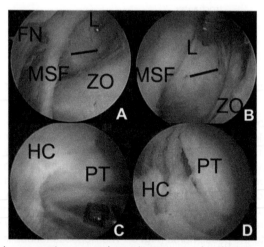

Fig. 9. Sequence demonstrating an endoscopic transcapsular iliopsoas tendon release in a right hip. (*A*) View of the hip periphery; the patient is without traction. The femoral neck (FN) is to the left and next to it is the medial synovial fold (MSF); in close relationship to the MSF, the inferior portion of the zona orbicularis (ZO) is observed. The labrum (L) is at the top, with a probe at the perilabral sulcus. The arrow indicates a thin portion of the anterior-inferior hip capsule. The iliopsoas tendon is behind this area. (*B*) An arthroscopic knife is used to open a "window" at the anterior inferior hip capsule between the anterior labrum and zona orbicularis. The MSF is to the left. (*C*) Once the "window" at the anterior inferior hip capsule (HC) has been established, a shaver is used to further expose the iliopsoas tendon (PT). (*D*) The iliopsoas tendon is completely exposed through the defect at the anterior inferior HC.

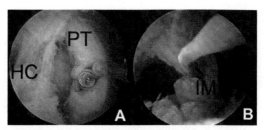

Fig. 10. Sequence demonstrating an endoscopic transcapsular iliopsoas tendon release in a right hip, following the sequence presented in **Fig. 4**. (*A*) The iliopsoas tendon (PT) is accessed though a "window" at the anterior inferior hip capsule (HC). A radiofrequency hook probe is used to release the tendinous portion in retrograde fashion. (*B*) After release of the iliopsoas tendon the iliacus muscle (IM) is left intact.

head. The iliopsoas tendon is exposed through this capsulotomy and is released at that level (**Fig. 12**).

Surgical Complications

Heterotopic ossification requiring further surgical intervention has been reported after open iliopsoas lengthening at the iliopsoas bursa for internal snapping hip syndrome.[44] Byrd has observed 3 cases of heterotopic ossification requiring further surgical intervention after endoscopic release of the iliopsoas tendon internal snapping hip syndrome (Byrd JWT, personal communication, 2005).

The authors performed a prospective randomized study evaluating 19 patients with internal snapping hip syndrome using endoscopic release at the lesser trochanter in comparison with transcapsular release. The results and complications of both techniques were examined and compared.[45] No difference was found in the clinical outcome and an absence of heterotopic ossification was noted. Prophylaxis against heterotopic ossification was used in every patient in the series with Celebrex (200 mg twice a day for 21 days).

PIRIFORMIS SYNDROME
Epidemiology

Piriformis syndrome is an etiologic entity that is difficult to diagnose. It is estimated that it may be responsible for 0.33% to 6% of all cases of low back pain and/or sciatica.

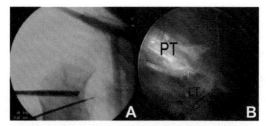

Fig. 11. Release of the iliopsoas tendon at its insertion on the lesser trochanter in a right hip. (*A*) Fluoroscopy image that demonstrates a 30° arthroscope viewing over the iliopsoas insertion. A hook radiofrequency probe is used to release the iliopsoas tendon in retrograde fashion. (*B*) Endoscopic image at the iliopsoas bursa. The iliopsoas tendon (PT) is released with a radiofrequency hook probe close to its insertion on the lesser trochanter (LT).

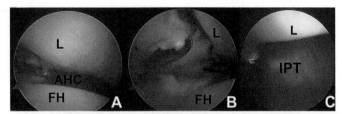

Fig. 12. Arthroscopic series of photographs demonstrating transcapsular release of the iliopsoas tendon from the central compartment in a left hip (the hip is with traction). (*A*) A radiofrequency hook is used to perform a cut on the anterior hip capsule (AHC), parallel to the free margin of the anterior labrum (L). The femoral head (FH) is at the bottom. (*B*) A shaver is used to remove capsular tissue from around the iliopsoas tendon (*black arrow*). The anterior labrum is at the top, the femoral head is at the bottom. (*C*) Once the capsule has been removed, the iliopsoas tendon (IPT) is clearly visible and ready for release with a radiofrequency hook. The labrum is at the top.

Anatomic Considerations

The piriformis muscle has a flat pyramidal shape. Its origin is the anterior surface of the second, third, and fourth sacral vertebrae, the sacrotuberous ligament, and the superior margin of the sciatic notch. It exits the pelvis through the sciatic notch and inserts into the superior aspect of the greater trochanter in the posteromedial corner. Numerous anatomic variations have been described as to the relation of this muscle and the sciatic nerve. Most commonly, the undivided nerve exits the greater sciatic notch below the piriformis muscle (84.2%). Less commonly, divisions of the sciatic nerve pass between and below the bifid muscle belly of the piriformis (11.7%). Rarely, divisions of the nerve pass above and below an undivided muscle (3.3%). Finally, an undivided nerve passing between the bifid muscle bellies of the piriformis has been reported (0.8%) **(Fig. 13)**.[46]

Presentation

Symptoms associated with piriformis syndrome occur from compression of the sciatic nerve by the piriformis muscle, which may be the result of overuse or repetitive trauma. The piriformis muscle may be more prone to hypertrophy than other muscles in the region. Gait abnormalities may influence this hypertrophy, thus facilitating the muscle to become inflamed and subsequently irritating the sciatic nerve. Acute trauma may also be responsible for piriformis muscle inflammation. A blunt blow to the buttock is believed to result in hematoma formation and subsequent scarring between the piriformis muscle and the sciatic nerve. Anatomic variations in the relationship of the piriformis muscle and the sciatic nerve may also be implicated in the development of piriformis syndrome. Variations that have the sciatic nerve or bifurcations of it going through the muscle belly of the piriformis may be more prone to piriformis syndrome.[46]

Diagnostic Criteria

Attempts to define clinical criteria for the diagnosis of piriformis syndrome have been made. In 1937 Freiberg[47] proposed 3 signs: (1) positive Lasegue sign, (2) tenderness at the sciatic notch, and (3) relief of symptoms with traction. Robinson[48] proposed 6 cardinal features in 1947: (1) history of trauma to sacroiliac and gluteal region, (2) pain in the sacroiliac joint, greater sciatic notch, and the piriformis muscle extending down the leg and causing difficulty walking, (3) acute exacerbations brought on by stooping or lifting and relieved by traction on the affected leg, (4) presence of a tender,

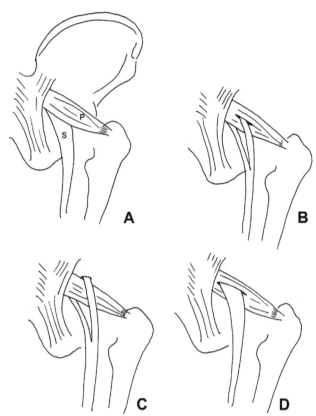

Fig. 13. Relationship between the sciatic nerve and the piriformis muscle belly with anatomic variations. (*A*) The sciatic nerve (*S*) passes under the muscle belly of the piriformis (*P*). (*B*) A bifurcated sciatic nerve with its proximal trunk through the muscle belly of the piriformis. (*C*) A bifurcated sciatic nerve with its trunks going superior and inferior to the muscle belly of the piriformis. (*D*) The sciatic nerve going through the muscle belly of the piriformis.

palpable, sausage-shaped mass over the piriformis muscle, (5) a positive Lasegue sign, and (6) gluteal atrophy.

Physical Examination

There is no single reliable finding for the diagnosis of piriformis syndrome. Posterior pain is nonspecific and may originate from the gluteus maximus or irradiate from the lumbar spine. Palpation of the piriformis muscle is performed directly posterior to the hip joint, close to the sciatic notch. It is relatively easy to differentiate this site from the posterior greater trochanter, the sacroiliac joint, or the ischium. Palpation may produce tenderness, pain, or irradiated sciatic nerve pain. The straight leg raise may be positive in piriformis syndrome, but it is difficult to differentiate from pain of radicular origin at the lumbar spine. Passive external rotation with the hip extended produces tension on the piriformis muscle, which may increase pain by compression of the sciatic nerve. Resisted external rotation of the leg may produce pain around the piriformis area for the same reason. In flexion the piriformis tendon becomes an abductor. As such, resisted abduction may produce symptoms. Passive adduction and internal rotation with the hip in flexion will also produces tension on the piriformis tendon, which may produce symptoms.[46]

Imaging

Imaging studies are usually addressed to establish a differential diagnosis. Plain AP radiographs of the pelvis and lateral projections of both hips are always evaluated. MRI of the pelvis is necessary to discard the possibility of intrapelvic masses producing sciatic nerve or nerve root compressions. Electromyographic studies complement evaluation of possible root compressions but are unspecific for piriformis syndrome.

Treatment Options

Conservative treatment is initially established with lifestyle modifications to avoid offending activities. NSAIDs are often successfully used. Physical therapy with piriformis stretching and correction of gait abnormalities, as well as compensation of leg length discrepancies, is necessary. Local injections with corticosteroids and local anesthetics are used both therapeutically and as a diagnostic test, as improvement of the symptoms after injection is evaluated. Accuracy of piriformis injections may be increased by ultrasound guidance.[49]

Low-dose botulinum toxin type A has been recently used for the treatment of chronic piriformis syndrome. This procedure has demonstrated an improvement in the quality of life of patients suffering from piriformis syndrome when compared with patients receiving dexamethasone.[50]

Failure of conservative treatment is the indication for surgery.

Surgical Considerations

Open surgical release of the piriformis tendon and decompression of the sciatic nerve through a standard posterior approach is the traditional form of treatment for this condition. Most of the evidence on the results of open surgical release of the piriformis tendon for the treatment of piriformis syndrome is anecdotal. The largest cohorts were published by Fishman and colleagues[51] in 2002, with 43 patients showing 68.8% of good results, and Indrekvam and Sudmann[52] in 2002 with a series of 19 patients. At an average follow-up of 8 years (range 1–16), two-thirds of the patients evaluated their clinical state as being better.

Evidence on endoscopic release of the piriformis tendon for piriformis syndrome is anecdotal. Dezawa and colleagues[53] published a technical note in 2003 describing an endoscopic release technique under local anesthesia, which was used with good results in 6 patients. The procedure was described as a combination of palpation to localize the piriformis muscle through a 2-cm incision and endoscopic release at the muscle-tendon junction. Local anesthesia was used so that the symptoms could be reproduced by palpating the piriformis muscle during surgery. The investigators describe pain control as difficult during the operation.

Using newer access techniques to the peritrochanteric space[3,27] and modern hip arthroscopy instruments, it is possible to visualize the area of the piriformis tendon. No other reports are available in the literature regarding endoscopic release of the piriformis muscle.

The first and most important aspect of surgical treatment of the piriformis syndrome is patient selection. Diagnosis has to be precise, and if associated pathologies are present this should be understood by both the surgeon and the patient. Today, evidence supports a limited open release as the technique of choice. An understanding of the anatomic relationship of the piriformis tendon and the sciatic nerve is very important when attempting surgical release. If the sciatic nerve or a bifurcation of it go through the belly of the piriformis muscle, a selective release from the muscle may be necessary.

HAMSTRING INJURIES
Epidemiology

Hamstring injuries are common in the athletic population. Most of these injuries are strains, which occur more frequently at the musculotendinous junction and are more frequently treated with nonoperative measures consisting in rest, ice, NSAIDs, and ambulatory aids.[54] Avulsions of the proximal insertion of the hamstring tendons from the ischium are much less common, but result in significant disability and are a separate topic of this review.[55] Apophyseal ischial avulsions occur between the ages of 11 and 15 years and are also related to sporting activity.

Presentation

The most common mechanism of injury is an acute forced hip flexion with the knee in extension. This mechanism may occur in different sporting activities that require rapid acceleration and deceleration and occur more frequently in water skiing.[54] Proximal hamstring avulsions are classified as acute or chronic (acute when seen within 1 month of injury). These injuries can be subcategorized as partial or complete avulsions, apophyseal avulsions, or degenerative avulsions (tendinosis). Degenerative tears of hamstring origin are more insidious in onset and are more commonly seen as an overuse injury.[56] Diagnosis is most commonly made by clinical history and physical examination. Sudden onset of pain in the posterior thigh during physical activity with painful weight bearing and sometimes related to an audible "pop" is typically described.

Physical Examination

Physical examination is performed with the patient prone and with slight knee flexion. Palpation of the posterior thigh may reveal muscle spasm. A very painful area may be identified at the site of proximal hamstring insertion. Ecchymosis is observed is the fascia is disrupted. When the injury is chronic, symptoms may be less clear and gait problems may be identified along with giving way.[55,56]

Imaging

Standard radiographs, including an AP pelvis, AP hip, and lateral hip are the initial step in imaging pelvis injuries. Hamstring avulsion injuries may be visible on radiographs by demonstrating a "floating fleck" of bone attached to the avulsed tendon.

MRI is the most common imaging technique in the diagnosis of proximal hamstring avulsion. The typical finding is an increased signal on T2-weighted MRI, which represents edema and hemorrhages at the site of proximal insertion of the hamstring tendons.

Treatment Options

Nonoperative treatment is initially similar to the treatment for strains, with gentle stretching exercises, normalization of gait, and slow return to sporting activity. Muscle weakness may result after conservative treatment. Nonoperative treatment of complete hamstring avulsions has resulted in unsatisfactory results in the athletic population.[57,58] For injuries recalcitrant to nonoperative management, or those falling outside the nonsurgical criteria; surgical intervention should be pursued.

Surgical Considerations

Surgical treatment is indicated if fragment displacement is more than 1.5 to 2 cm.[59,60] Overall, surgical intervention of hamstring avulsion injuries has produced mixed results. Reports in the literature have yielded good to excellent results in athletes with surgical correction of acute proximal hamstring avulsion.[54,56,57] The technique consists of reattachment of the avulsed hamstring origin to the ischial tuberosity using metallic anchors. Reports of poor to fair outcomes cite persistent pain, weakness, and limitation in functional performance as common findings.[61,62]

APOPHYSEAL AVULSION INJURIES OF THE ANTERIOR SUPERIOR AND ANTERIOR INFERIOR ILIAC SPINES
Epidemiology

Apophyseal injuries of the anterior superior iliac spine (ASIS) and the anterior inferior iliac spine (AIIS) are typically observed in the immature athlete population between the ages of 10 and 15 years.[63]

Anatomic Considerations

The mechanism of injury is usually a powerful muscle contracture or a forceful stretch during physical or sporting activity. The ASIS is avulsed from traction from the sartorius muscle and the AIIS from the direct head of the rectus femoris muscle.

Presentation

Diagnosis is based in clinical history and physical examination. Pain is usually found at the site of the avulsion, and reproduced with active hip flexion against gravity and against resistance.

Imaging

Plain radiographs in different projections may demonstrate avulsion injuries of both the ASIS and AIIS. Nondisplaced avulsions may not be apparent in plain radiographs and may be identified with MRI.[64]

Treatment Options

AIIS and ASIS avulsions injuries can be treated conservatively if there is no displacement or minimal displacement of the fragment. Nonoperative treatment consists in rest, ice, NSAIDs, ambulatory aids, and physical therapy.[65] When there is fragment displacement of 1 cm or more, surgical intervention consisting of internal fixation of the fragment is indicated.[66] Pincer-type femoroacetabular impingement may result from an inferiorly displaced AIIS avulsion.[67]

Surgical Considerations

Repair of avulsed AIIS and ASIS fragments can be treated in multiple ways. The use of anchor fixation has been employed for true tendon avulsion. Transosseous fixation is also a viable option for repair of an avulsed tendon from its bony insertion. For avulsions with a substantial bony component, repair via screw and washer fixation may be performed.

SPORTS HERNIAS AND ATHLETIC PUBALGIA
Epidemiology

Estimates suggest that 5% of all sports injuries occur in the groin. This figure may be an underestimation of their frequency because of inaccurate diagnosis of hip or groin pathology. In general terms, a sports hernia may be described as incompetence of the abdominal wall musculature in the absence of a clinically detectable hernia bulge. The prevalence of such hernias found at surgical exploration in athletes with chronic groin pain is reported to be in the region of 80%.[68,69]

Anatomic Considerations

The pathoanatomy of sports hernias and athletic pubalgia is complex. The site of injury includes the extent of the inguinal canal with the transversalis fascia posteriorly, the tendinous rectus abdominis and conjoined tendon anteriorly, and the bony pubic symphysis medially. The adductor tendons and their proximal attachment define the distal extent. The various nerves of the inguinal region are commonly involved, thus explaining the cutaneous pain.[70]

The rectus insertion on the pubis has been cited as the primary site of pathology in athletic pubalgia. This syndrome has been described primarily in high-level athletes and is almost exclusive to males.

Mechanism

The typical mechanism of injury involves repetitive hyperextension of the trunk in association with hyperabduction of the thigh pivoting on the anterior pelvis. Shearing forces generated across the pubic symphysis during adductor contraction may stress the posterior inguinal wall. In addition, repetitive forces or a sudden severe force may lead to separation of the internal oblique and or the transversalis fascia from the inguinal ligament. This mechanism may also account for the possible coexistent findings in osteitis pubis and adductor tendinitis.[70]

Treatment Options

Nonoperative therapy consisting of anti-inflammatory medications, physical therapy, heat/ice therapies, steroid injections, and activity restriction may be used in the face of an athletic pubalgia diagnosis. Unfortunately, nonsurgical modalities have had limited success in this condition. Core strengthening and corticosteroid injections have been described as bridge therapy for athletes attempting to finish their season until definitive surgical intervention can be performed.

Surgical Considerations

Surgical intervention for athletic pubalgia is best performed in an open fashion. Repair is performed via reattachment of the rectus abdominis muscle to the pubis. Anterior and lateral release of the epimysium of the adductor fascia may be performed if secondary chronic inflammatory symptoms are present in the adductor compartment. Laparoscopic surgery for athletic pubalgia has demonstrated suboptimal results to date.[68–70]

SUMMARY

The peritrochanteric space and the pathology within is a new field of research in the area of endoscopic hip surgery. Treatment of snapping hip syndromes has offered a gateway to this compartment and has helped in the development of access and visualization techniques, which has stimulated further interest for the pathology in this area. The high prevalence of the greater trochanteric pain syndrome and failure of conservative treatment in many cases opens the door to endoscopic surgery as an option for effective and minimally invasive treatment. Further development of the techniques and understanding of the pathology will contribute to placing endoscopic surgery of the peritrochanteric space in its right dimension. Medical literature of higher level of evidence is necessary, but this is sure to appear in the near future. Muscle injury around the hip joint is complex, and requires a dedicated clinical history and detailed physical examination. Avulsion tendon injuries around the hip joint usually occur in the sports-active population, and in some cases almost exclusively in high-level athletes. Success in treatment depends on adequate patient selection, an understanding of the pathology, and surgical techniques.

REFERENCES

1. Alvarez-Nemegyei J, Canoso JJ. Evidence-based soft tissue rheumatology III: trochanteric bursitis. J Clin Rheumatol 2004;10:123–4.
2. Silva F, Adams T, Feinstein J, et al. Trochanteric bursitis. Refuting the myth of inflammation. J Clin Rheumatol 2008;14:82–6.
3. Voos JE, Rudzki JR, Shindle MK, et al. Arthroscopic anatomy and surgical techniques for peritrochanteric space disorders in the hip. Technical note. Arthroscopy 2007;23:1246,e1–5.
4. Segal NA, Felson DT, Torner JC, et al. Greater trochanteric pain syndrome: epidemiology and associated factors. Arch Phys Med Rehabil 2007;88:988–92.
5. Rasmussen KJ, Fano N. Trochanteric bursitis. Treatment by corticosteroid injection. Scand J Rheumatol 1985;14:417–20.
6. Gordon EJ. Trochanteric bursitis and tendonitis. Clin Orthop 1961;20:193–202.
7. Slawski DP, Howard RF. Surgical management of refractory trochanteric bursitis. Am J Sports Med 1997;25:86–9.
8. Craig RA, Gwynne Jones DP, Oakley AP, et al. Iliotibial band z-lengthening for refractory trochanteric bursitis (greater trochanteric pain syndrome). ANZ J Surg 2007;77:996–8.
9. Govaert LH, van der Vis HM, Marti RK, et al. Trochanteric reduction osteotomy as a treatment for refractory trochanteric bursitis. J Bone Joint Surg Br 2003;85: 199–203.
10. Bradley DM, Dillingham MF. Bursoscopy of the trochanteric bursa. Case report. Arthroscopy 1998;14:884–7.
11. Fox JL. The role of arthroscopic bursectomy in the treatment of trochanteric bursitis. Technical note. Arthroscopy 2002;18:E34.
12. Farr D, Selesnick H, Janecki C, et al. Arthroscopic bursectomy with concomitant iliotibial band release for the treatment of recalcitrant trochanteric bursitis. Technical note. Arthroscopy 2007;23:905,e1–5.
13. Baker CL, Massie V, Hurt G, et al. Arthroscopic bursectomy for recalcitrant trochanteric bursitis. Arthroscopy 2007;23:827–32.
14. Bunker TD, Esler CN, Leach WJ. Rotator-cuff tear of the hip. J Bone Joint Surg Br 1997;79:618–20.
15. Howell GE, Biggs RE, Bourne RB. Prevalence of abductor mechanism tears of the hips in patients with osteoarthritis. J Arthroplasty 2001;16:121–3.
16. Karpinski MR, Piggott H. Greater trochanteric pain syndrome. A report of 15 cases. J Bone Joint Surg Br 1985;67:762–3.
17. Traycoff RB. "Pseudotrochanteric bursitis": the differential diagnosis of lateral hip pain. J Rheumatol 1991;18:1810–2.
18. Lonner JH, Van Kleunen JP. Spontaneous rupture of the gluteus medius and minimus tendons. Am J Orthop 2002;31:579–81.
19. LaBan MM, Weir SK, Taylor RS. 'Bald trochanter' spontaneous rupture of the conjoined tendons of the gluteus medius and minimus presenting as a trochanteric bursitis. Am J Phys Med Rehabil 2004;83:806–9.

20. Fisher DA, Almand JD, Watts MR. Operative repair of bilateral spontaneous gluteus medius and minimus tendon ruptures a case report. J Bone Joint Surg Am 2007;89:1103–7.
21. Lequesne M, Mathieu P, Vuillemin-Bodaghi V, et al. Gluteal tendinopathy in refractory greater trochanter pain syndrome: diagnostic value of two clinical tests. Arthritis Rheum 2008;59:241–6.
22. Kingzett-Taylor A, Tirman PF, Feller J, et al. Tendinosis and tears of gluteus medius and minimus muscles as a cause of hip pain: MR imaging findings. AJR Am J Roentgenol 1999;173:1123–6.
23. Cvitanic O, Henzie G, Skezas N, et al. MRI Diagnosis of tears of the hip abductor tendons (gluteus medius and gluteus minimus). AJR Am J Roentgenol 2004;182: 137–43.
24. Voos JE, Shindle MK, Pruett A, et al. Endoscopic repair of gluteus medius tendon tears of the hip. Am J Sports Med 2009;37(4):743–7.
25. Domb BG, Nasser RM, Boster IB. Partial-thickness tears of the gluteus medius: rationale and technique for transtendinous endoscopic repair. Arthroscopy 2010;26(12):1697–705.
26. Allen WC, Cope R. Coxa saltans: the snapping hip revisited. J Am Acad Orthop Surg 1995;3:303–8.
27. Ilizaliturri VM Jr, Martinez-Escalante FA, Chaidez PA, et al. Endoscopic iliotibial band release for external snapping hip syndrome. Arthroscopy 2006;22:505–10.
28. Fery A, Sommelet J. The snapping hip. Late results of 24 surgical cases. Int Orthop 1988;12:277–82.
29. Faraj AA, Moulton A, Sirivastava VM. Snapping iliotibial band. Report of ten cases and review of the literature. Acta Orthop Belg 2001;67:19–23.
30. Provencher MT, Hofmeister EP, Muldoon MP. The surgical treatment of external coxa saltans (the snapping hip) by Z-plasty of the iliotibial band. Am J Sports Med 2004;32:470–6.
31. White RA, Hughes MS, Burd T. A new operative approach in the correction of external coxa saltans. Am J Sports Med 2004;32:1504–8.
32. Byrd JW. Evaluation and management of the snapping iliopsoas tendon. Tech Orthop 2005;20:45–51.
33. Ilizaliturri VM Jr, Villalobos FE, Chaidez PA, et al. Internal snapping hip syndrome: treatment by endoscopic release of the iliopsoas tendon. Arthroscopy 2005;21: 1375–80.
34. Harper MC, Schaberg JE, Allen WC. Primary iliopsoas bursography in the diagnosis of disorders of the hip. Clin Orthop Relat Res 1987;221:238–41.
35. Cardinal E, Buckwalter KA, Capello WN, et al. US of the snapping iliopsoas tendon. Radiology 1996;198:521–2.
36. Deslandes M, Guillin R, Cardinal E, et al. The snapping iliopsoas tendon: new mechanisms using dynamic sonography. AJR Am J Roentgenol 2008;190(3): 576–81.
37. Flanum ME, Keene JS, Blankenbaker DG, et al. Arthroscopic treatment of the painful "internal" snapping hip: results of a new endoscopic technique and imaging protocol. Am J Sports Med 2007;35:770–9.
38. Jacobson T, Allen WC. Surgical correction of the snapping iliopsoas tendon. Am J Sports Med 1990;18:470–4.
39. Taylor GR, Clarke NM. Surgical release of the "snapping iliopsoas tendon". J Bone Joint Surg Br 1995;77:881–3.
40. Dobbs MB, Gordon JE, Luhmann SJ, et al. Surgical correction of the snapping iliopsoas tendon in adolescents. J Bone Joint Surg Am 2002;84:420–4.

41. Gruen GS, Scioscia TN, Lowenstein JE. The surgical treatment of internal snapping hip. Am J Sports Med 2002;30:607–13.
42. Wettstein M, Jung J, Dienst M. Arthroscopic psoas tenotomy. Arthroscopy 2006; 22:907,e1–4.
43. Contreras ME, Dani WS, Endges WK, et al. Arthroscopic treatment of the snapping iliopsoas tendon trough the central compartment of the hip. A pilot study. J Bone Joint Surg Br 2010;92:777–80.
44. McCulloch PC, Bush-Joseph CA. Massive heterotopic ossification complicating iliopsoas tendon lengthening. A case report. Am J Sports Med 2006;31:2022–5.
45. Ilizaliturri VM Jr, Chaidez C, Villegas P, et al. Prospective randomized study of 2 different techniques for endoscopic iliopsoas tendon release in the treatment of internal snapping hip syndrome. Arthroscopy 2009;25:159–63.
46. Byrd JW. Piriformis syndrome. Oper Tech Sports Med 2005;13:71–9.
47. Freiberg AH. Sciatic pain and its relief by operations on the muscle and fascia. Arch Surg 1937;34:337–50.
48. Robinson DR. Piriformis syndrome in relation to sciatic pain. Am J Surg 1947;73: 355–8.
49. Peng PW, Tumber PS. Ultrasound guided interventional procedures for patients with chronic pelvic pain-a description of techniques and review of the literature. Pain Physician 2008;11:215–24.
50. Yoon SJ, Ho J, Kang HY, et al. Low-dose botulinum toxin type A for the treatment of refractory piriformis syndrome. Pharmacotherapy 2007;27:657–65.
51. Fishman LM, Dombi GW, Michaelsen C, et al. Piriformis syndrome: diagnosis treatment and outcome a 10-year study. Arch Phys Med Rehabil 2002;83: 295–301.
52. Indrekvam K, Sudmann E. Piriformis muscle syndrome in 19 patients treated by tenotomy a 1 to 16-year follow-up study. Int Orthop 2002;26:101–3.
53. Dezawa A, Kusano S, Miki H. Arthroscopic release of the piriformis muscle under local anesthesia for piriformis syndrome. Arthroscopy 2003;19:554–7.
54. Clanton TO, Coupe KJ. Hamstring strains in athletes: diagnosis and treatment. J Am Acad Orthop Surg 1998;6:237–48.
55. Ishikawa K, Kai K, Mizuta H. Avulsion of the hamstring muscles from the ischial tuberosity: a report of two cases. Clin Orthop Relat Res 1988;232:153–5.
56. Klingele KE, Sallay PI. Surgical repair of complete proximal hamstring tendon rupture. Am J Sports Med 2002;30:742–7.
57. Sallay PI, Friedman RL, Coogan PG, et al. Hamstring muscle injuries among water skiers: functional outcome and prevention. Am J Sports Med 1996;24: 130–6.
58. Cohen S, Bradley J. Acute proximal hamstring rupture. J Am Acad Orthop Surg 2007;15:350–5.
59. Servant CT, Jones CB. Displaced avulsion of the ischial apophysis: a hamstring injury requiring internal fixation. Br J Sports Med 1998;32:255–7.
60. Gill DR, Clark WB. Avulsion of the ischial apophysis. Aust N Z J Surg 1996;66: 564–5.
61. Wootton JR, Cross MJ, Holt KW. Avulsion of the ischial apophysis: the case for open reduction and internal fixation. J Bone Joint Surg Br 1990;72:625–7.
62. Schlonsky J, Olix ML. Functional disability following avulsion fracture of the ischial epiphysis. Report of two cases. J Bone Joint Surg Am 1972;54:641–4.
63. Waters PM, Millis MB. Hip and pelvic injuries in the young athlete. Clin Sports Med 1988;7:513–26.

64. Ouellette H, Thomas BJ, Nelson E, et al. MR imaging of rectus femoris origin injuries. Skeletal Radiol 2006;35:665–72.
65. Metzemaker JN, Pappas AN. Avulsion fractures of the pelvis. Am J Sports Med 1985;13:349–58.
66. Kocher MS, Tucker R. Pediatric athlete hip disorders. Clin Sports Med 2006;25: 241–53.
67. Ilizaliturri VM Jr, Nossa-Barrera JM, Acosta-Rodríguez E, et al. Arthroscopic treatment of femoroacetabular impingement secondary to pediatric hip disorders. J Bone Joint Surg Br 2007;89:1025–30.
68. Azurin DJ, Go LS, Schuricht A, et al. Endoscopic preperitoneal herniorrhaphy in professional athletes with groin pain. J Laparoendosc Adv Surg Tech A 1997;7: 7–12.
69. Akita K, Niga S, Yamato Y, et al. Anatomic basis of chronic groin pain with special reference to sports hernia. Surg Radiol Anat 1992;21:1–5.
70. Smedberg SG, Broome AE, Gullmo A, et al. Herniography in athletes with groin pain. Am J Surg 1985;149:378–82.

Athletic Pubalgia (Sports Hernia)

Demetrius E.M. Litwin, MD[a],*, Erica B. Sneider, MD[a],
Patrick M. McEnaney, MD[b], Brian D. Busconi, MD[c]

KEYWORDS
- Sports hernia • Athletic pubalgia
- Lower abdomen and groin pain • Hernia
- Inguinal canal • Laparoscopic

Athletic pubalgia or sports hernia is a syndrome of chronic lower abdomen and groin pain that may occur in both athletes and nonathletes. It is defined as weakness or tearing of the rectus abdominus insertion to the superior pubic ramus. Activity restricting lower abdomen and groin pain is a frequent occurrence in some sports, such as soccer, accounting for 10% to 13% of all injuries per year.[1,2] However, most lower abdomen and groin injuries are self-limited and only a small percentage cause symptoms for greater than 3 weeks.[2] There are several causes of chronic lower abdomen and groin pain that may be related to disorders of the hip joint, injury to muscles of the thigh or abdominal wall, and even genitourinary or intraabdominal disease.[3,4] Because the differential diagnosis of chronic lower abdomen and groin pain is so broad, only a small number of patients with chronic lower abdomen and groin pain fulfill the diagnostic criteria of athletic pubalgia (sports hernia).

Over the years, many different names have been associated with this injury, such as athletic pubalgia, sports hernia, Gilmore's groin, pubic inguinal pain syndrome, sportsmen's groin, footballers groin injury complex, hockey player's syndrome, and athletic hernia.[3,5–9] None of the terms listed earlier is perfect, but they all seek to describe a poorly understood disease complex that is generally not well accepted by general surgeons as a real syndrome warranting surgical therapy, and for which there is a paucity of good clinical studies. However, sports hernia is becoming more widely diagnosed and more frequently operated on in part because of a greater awareness generated by the media on high-profile athletes.

The literature published to date regarding the cause, pathogenesis, diagnosis, and treatment of sports hernias is confusing. The goal of this article is to summarize the

[a] Department of Surgery, UMass Memorial Medical Center, University of Massachusetts Medical School, 55 Lake Avenue North, Worcester, MA 01655, USA
[b] Department of Surgery, Milford Hospital, University of Massachusetts Medical School, Worcester, MA, USA
[c] Department of Orthopedics and Physical Rehabilitation, University of Massachusetts Medical School, 281 Lincoln Street, Worcester, MA 01605-2192, USA
* Corresponding author.
E-mail address: litwind@ummhc.org

Clin Sports Med 30 (2011) 417–434
doi:10.1016/j.csm.2010.12.010
0278-5919/11/$ – see front matter © 2011 Elsevier Inc. All rights reserved.

sportsmed.theclinics.com

current information and our present approach to this chronic lower abdomen and groin pain syndrome.

HISTORICAL CONTEXT

In 1980, Gilmore[10] recognized and undertook to surgically repair groin disruption in a group of athletes who presented with a syndrome of chronic lower abdomen and groin pain. In 1992, he reported his experience in a large series of 313 athletes, most of whom were soccer players, who presented with groin pain and underwent surgery.[10,11] This entity of groin disruption that he identified associated with groin pain in athletes was subsequently called Gilmore's groin.[10] At that same time, there were other reports emanating from Europe,[12–15] usually involving soccer players, also identifying a similar chronic lower abdomen and groin pain syndrome in athletes. This disorder was called pubalgia by Taylor and colleagues[16] in 1991, who reported their own series of athletes with chronic pain who were unable to compete, and in which they found "abnormalities of the abdominal wall in the groin region, including palpable hernias, nonpalpable hernias, and microscopic tears or avulsions of the internal oblique muscles."[16]

However, whereas some investigators were describing a chronic pain syndrome related to muscular injury in athletes, there were others who felt that chronic lower abdomen and groin pain was secondary to an incipient posterior inguinal wall hernia. This condition was first described by Gullmo[17] in 1980 and Ekberg and colleagues[18] in 1981 in Sweden. By 1991, Polglase and colleagues[19] reported the finding of a substantially deranged posterior wall of the inguinal canal in most (85%) of the 64 Australian Rules football players with chronic lower abdomen and groin pain enrolled in their study. In 1992, Malycha and Lovell[20] reported the detection of a bulge at the time of surgery in the posterior inguinal wall in 80% of athletes with chronic undiagnosed lower abdomen and groin pain, which they felt represented an incipient direct inguinal hernia.

Cause and Pathogenesis

One can see that 2 major schools of thought emerged regarding the cause and pathogenesis of athletic pubalgia or sports hernia. The first is characterized by the concept of muscular injury and disruption that was popularized by Gilmore.[3,11] Athletes in Gilmore's study were found to have "1) a torn external oblique aponeurosis causing dilatation of the superficial inguinal ring; 2) a torn conjoined tendon; and 3) dehiscence between the inguinal ligament and the torn conjoined tendon."[11,21]

The term pubalgia, coined by Taylor and colleagues,[16] also encompassed the notion of muscle injury, which they described as "groin pain ... most commonly caused by musculotendinous strains of the adductors and other muscles crossing the hip joint, but ... also ... related to abdominal wall abnormalities." They went on to state "cases may be termed 'pubalgia' if physical examination does not reveal an inguinal hernia and there is an absence of other etiology for lower abdomen and groin pain."

Meyers and colleagues[22] further characterized the injury leading to chronic lower abdomen and groin pain as a hyperextension injury. They asserted that the pubis serves as a pivot point into which both the rectus abdominis and the adductor longus insert, thereby causing 1 muscle to pull against the other, leading to injury, which usually occurs to the weaker abdominal wall muscles.[22] This concept of a tug-of-war at the pubis is lent credence by the high prevalence of concomitant adductor symptoms.[22–24] It has also led to one of the major strategies of surgery, which is to stabilize the anterior pelvis.[22,25–27] In a recent paper outlining what is now his vast experience with this condition, Meyers enlarged this concept of rectifying the biomechanics of the pubic joint to include not only tightening and broadening the abdominal muscular insertion but also loosening the attachment of muscles on the other side of the symphysis, such as the adductor longus via selective epimysiotomy.[22,28]

The second school of thought focuses on the concept of athletic pubalgia as an occult hernia process, a prehernia condition, or an incipient hernia, with the major abnormality being a defect in the transversalis fascia, which forms the posterior wall of the inguinal canal, and not a muscle tear per se.[19,20,26,29–31] Malycha and Lovell[20] described a series of 50 athletes who underwent inguinal hernia repair after examination; investigation did not reveal a cause of chronic lower abdomen and groin pain, and 40 of the athletes were found to have a bulge in the posterior inguinal wall. In addition, in these investigators' subsequent study of 15 athletes with chronic lower abdomen and groin pain in whom the conjoined tendon was biopsied, they could not find histologic evidence of injury and concluded "injury to the conjoint tendon is not the cause of chronic lower abdomen and groin pain in these athletes."[32] Similarly, Polglase and colleagues[19] discovered as the main finding a substantially deranged posterior wall of the inguinal canal in 61 operations of the groin in 72 athletes (85%), most of whom were Australian Rules football players with debilitating lower abdomen and groin pain. These investigators concluded, "the most common finding in athletes with chronic lower abdomen and groin pain was a deficiency of the posterior wall of the inguinal canal." Furthermore, herniography has long been advocated as a means of detecting nonpalpable hernias in football players with lower abdomen and groin pain. For example, in a study of 60 soccer players with lower abdomen and groin symptoms but no detectable hernia on clinical examination, herniography discovered occult hernias in 51 of the players.[33] In a group of Australian Rules football players with chronic lower abdomen and groin pain, but no clinical signs of hernia, Orchard and colleagues[34] used ultrasound as a tool to show posterior wall deficiency of the inguinal canal. They concluded that dynamic ultrasound (ie, ultrasound performed while the patient strains) was useful in detecting posterior inguinal canal deficiency, and that it was more prevalent in those players with pain. Mushaweck and Berger[7] have recently reported the use of dynamic ultrasound as the diagnostic modality of choice for sports hernia. Using ultrasound to monitor motion of the inguinal canal and its posterior wall during a Valsalva maneuver, these investigators report "sportsmen's groin was diagnosed if a convex anterior bulge of the posterior inguinal wall was observed during stress." In addition, at surgery, the typical finding Mushaweck and Berger[7] describe is "a circumscribed weakness found in the posterior wall, with the tissue around it being firm and intact." Joesting[35] too was emphatic in describing the injury in these patients as a tear of the transversalis fascia, which forms the posterior wall of the inguinal canal.

How do we reconcile these philosophic differences? Are there 2 subgroups of patients, or is it the same entity viewed from different vantage points?
Zimmerman[36] suggested that a tear of the conjoined tendon might be the cause of the bulge in the posterior wall of the inguinal canal seen in these patients. Although Taylor and colleagues[16] postulated that muscle strain was the major cause of pain in these athletes, 7 of the 9 patients operated on had evidence of a bulge in the posterior wall, which the investigators believed represented a direct hernia. Also, even although Meyers and colleagues[22] found a significant incidence of muscular injury in their series of athletic pubalgia (eg, 48% of their patients had obvious tiny defects of the external oblique aponeurosis, 17% had a thin rectus insertion, and 6% had a clear-cut tear in the region of the rectus insertion), these investigators also reported that 57% of the 157 athletes operated on "had subjectively 'loose feeling' inguinal floors

(Hesselbach's triangle)." On the other hand, Polglase and colleagues,[19] who believed that the principle defect seen in athletic pubalgia was of the posterior wall of the inguinal canal, also reported "apparent splitting of the conjoined tendon" in 26% of their cases. Mushaweck and Berger,[7] proponents of the minimal repair technique that Mushaweck has pioneered, which focuses principally on repair of the posterior wall defect that Mushaweck feels is typically present in this disorder, stress that during the repair the rectus abdominis must be, in their words, "lateralized with suture....to counteract the increased tension at the pubic bone, caused by retraction of the rectus muscle in the upward and medial direction." One could postulate that rectus abdominis injury led to the retraction that was noted during surgery.

How does one put this all together? It is likely that several factors contribute to the formation of a sports hernia. However, we believe that a large tear, or multiple small tears (microtears), must be taking place, involving 1 or several muscles in the region, which includes the external oblique aponeurosis, rectus abdominis, conjoined tendon/rectus abdominis interface, or individual muscles that form the conjoined tendon (internal oblique or transversus abdominis). Tears to any of these muscles could lead to the operative findings of attenuation, disruption, or retraction of the muscle, thereby weakening the boundaries of the posterior wall of the inguinal canal (**Figs. 1** and **2**). The repetitive stress of high-level training on the region, the demands of competition that requires explosive muscle contraction, the pulsion effect generated by increases in intraabdominal pressure during sports, and abrupt Valsalva maneuvers that occur during contact may cause failure of the transversalis fascia in the posterior wall of the inguinal canal and lead to the formation of a bulge. The bulge is most likely secondary to other biomechanical issues, specifically muscle injury and weakness. The chronic pain is likely secondary to muscle injury, not the mere presence of a bulge, which is usually minimally symptomatic in patients with conventional groin hernias irrespective of hernia size.

DIFFERENTIAL DIAGNOSIS OF GROIN PAIN IN ATHLETES

Several clinical entities that revolve around the pubic bone and hip joint can be confused with athletic pubalgia (**Box 1**). Before diagnosing a sports hernia, many of

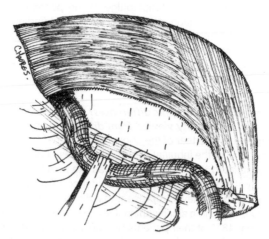

Fig. 1. The inguinal region after the external oblique is opened and reflected both superiorly and inferiorly. The spermatic cord is retracted in a caudad direction. (*Artwork created by* Craig Moores, Medical Student, Albany Medical College, Albany, NY.)

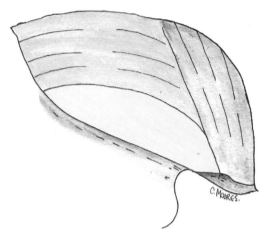

Fig. 2. The main anatomic structures are depicted. The posterior wall of the inguinal canal (*yellow*), also known as the Hesselbach triangle, is covered by the transversalis fascia. It is in the medial aspect of this yellow area that bulges occur in sports hernias. Muscular tears are usually found in the rectus abdominis (*red*) or the conjoined tendon (*green*), or at the interface of the 2 structures. The pubis (*purple*) and the shelving portion of the ilioinguinal ligament (*blue*) participate in the repair. (*Artwork created by* Craig Moores, Medical Student, Albany Medical College, Albany, NY.)

the diseases listed in **Box 1** must be considered, because many of these processes can cause symptoms that are similar to and in the same location as athletic pubalgia.[9,23,24,37–40] However, athletic pubalgia in many cases is a clear and distinct clinical entity with typical history and physical findings, so that many of these other conditions are improbable as the cause of pain.

Disorders of the hip joint, in particular acetabular labral tears, femoroacetabular impingement, and injuries to the adductors can be difficult to distinguish from sports hernia, or may even coexist. Similarly, osteitis pubis or a conventional groin hernia may cause groin symptoms. Genitourinary issues such as epididymitis, prostatitis, or testicular tumors could be a cause of chronic groin pain in men, and a host of intraabdominal conditions in women must be considered before attributing groin pain to athletic pubalgia. This finding was particularly notable in Meyers and colleagues'[22] series, in which laparoscopic evaluation determined that overall 80% of the women in the series had another cause for their pain, such as endometriosis, ovarian cystic disease, PID, Crohn disease, or adhesions.

Magnetic resonance imaging (MRI) is particularly valuable to help rule out other significant musculoskeletal causes for lower abdomen and groin pain and must be obtained before accepting the final diagnosis as athletic pubalgia.[41,42] However, athletes may have several injuries that coexist, such as an acetabular labral tears and a sports hernia.

Because of the wide range of potential disorders and the potential overlap, we have developed a multidisciplinary team approach to assess all patients with possible sports hernia. This approach includes an orthopedic sports medicine specialist and a general surgeon with a special interest in abdominal wall disorders.

IS NERVE ENTRAPMENT A CAUSE FOR PAIN?

There is increasing speculation that nerve entrapment is a reason for chronic pain, and that either nerve release or nerve division should be incorporated into the operative procedure. This observation has been described in the literature as part of both

Box 1
Differential diagnosis of groin pain in athletes

Inflammatory

    Inflammatory bowel disease

    Endometriosis

    Pelvic inflammatory disease (PID)

    Appendicitis

    Osteoarthritis

    Lymphadenopathy

Musculoskeletal

    Stress fracture

    Muscle strain

    Muscle contusion

    Tendon rupture (adductors)

    Adductor tendinitis

    Bursitis

    Avascular necrosis of the femoral head

    Acetabular labral tear

    Adductor longus dysfunction (other adductor injury)

    Osteitis pubis

    Sports hernia

    Femoroacetabular impingement

    Hockey player's syndrome

    Pubic instability

    Conjoined tendon dehiscence

    Herniated nucleus pulposus

    Inguinal or femoral hernia

    Hip flexor/iliopsoas injury (tendinosis)

    Iliac apophysis injury

    Symphyseal instability

    Hip osteoarthritis

Infectious

    Osteomyelitis

    Prostatitis

    Epididymitis

    Septic arthritis

    Urinary tract infections

    Diverticulitis

Neurologic

    Nerve entrapment (ilioinguinal, obturator)

Neoplastic

    Testicular cancer

    Sarcoma

    Bony tumors

Congenital

    Growth plate stress injury or fracture

    Legg-Calvé-Perthes disease

Other

    Ovarian cyst

    Postpartum symphysis separation

    Hydrocele/varicocele

    Testicular torsion

Data from LeBlanc KE, LeBlanc KA. Groin pain in athletes. Hernia 2003;7:68–71; and Caudill P, Nyland J, Smith C, et al. Sports hernias: a systematic literature review. Br J Sports Med 2008;42:954–64.

laparoscopic and open approaches. It has been postulated that injury to the surrounding tissue can cause the nerve to become irritated or incorporated into scar tissue at some point along its course. There is little clarity as to which nerve in the groin is most likely to be involved, and several investigators have incriminated and therefore divided or released the genital branch of the genitofemoral,[7,43] the ilioinguinal,[44] the iliohypogastric,[45] or the obturator[46] nerves in the treatment of chronic lower abdomen and groin pain during a laparoscopic or open repair for sports hernia. Because most series, with or without nerve division or release, seem to have equal results, it is improbable in the opinion of these investigators that this maneuver plays a role in the treatment of this syndrome.[3,37] Furthermore, nerve entrapment is a common sequela of conventional groin hernia surgery and the pain syndrome in relation to that phenomenon is entirely different from athletic pubalgia.[47]

WHO IS AFFECTED BY ATHLETIC PUBALGIA?

Athletic pubalgia affects both professional and nonprofessional athletes, and may result in activity-limiting pain, which can shorten a professional athlete's career[48] or jeopardize an athlete's opportunity for a college scholarship or playing time. Typically, athletes who suffer from this condition practice their sport at a high level and engage in high-intensity training. There is a growing trend toward treating recreational yet dedicated athletes who derive tremendous personal satisfaction (or quality of life) from the pursuit of their sport.[5,49]

Chronic lower abdomen and groin pain is more common in athletes who are involved in activities in which there are running, kicking, and cutting movements, or explosive turns and changes in direction related to the sport.[7,23,24,37,44,48] Similarly, some other activities such as pushing hard against resistance, like a lineman in football or a hockey player, when pinning a player against the boards, may be contributing factors. Prevalence data indicate that players of soccer, ice hockey, and American football tend to be most commonly affected in the United States.[3,5,22] However, other sports commonly involved include rugby, Australian Rules football, cricket, martial arts, basketball, baseball, field hockey, tennis, swimming, and long-distance running.[5,24,37,48,50]

Athletic pubalgia is more common in men. However, although it is less prevalent in women, there is evidence that it is becoming more frequent. Garvey and colleagues[48] estimate that currently women represent 10% of their cases, and Meyers and colleagues[49] report that women now comprise 15.2% of the patients they have seen in the last 5 years. The apparent change in this demographic characteristic is likely secondary to an increased number of women training and competing at higher competitive levels than before.[22,37,48] Nonetheless, the prevalence of sports hernias remains lower in women and anatomic differences likely protect women from developing this disorder.[22] The lower prevalence of sports hernias in women is probably explained, in part, by anatomic differences between the male and female pelvis.[51] Men have stronger muscles in the lower abdomen and groin that are capable of generating greater force per unit area of insertion when compared with women. Further, the gynecoid pelvis probably provides a greater span of muscular insertion along the pubis and ilioinguinal ligament, and distributes force along a greater surface area, thereby helping to protect women from this lower abdomen and groin pain syndrome. Furthermore, studies have shown gender differences in lower extremity alignment and muscle activation with activities such as kicking a soccer ball, and this difference may predispose an athlete of 1 gender to 1 type of injury, whereas being protective of another.[51] For example, one might posit that these gender differences in extremity alignment and muscle activation may predispose women to anterior cruciate ligament injury, but might protect them from lower abdomen and groin injury.[51]

PRESENTATION

Athletes typically present with the complaint of exercise-related lower abdomen and groin pain that may radiate to the perineum, inner thigh, and scrotum.[3,48] The pain is typically relieved with rest but returns on resumption of physical activity.[5,22,27,52,53] Often the athlete describes the pain as a deep and intense pain that is unilateral.[5,54,55] Typically, patients with sports hernia describe pain that is insidious in onset but some athletes recall an inciting event that may have been the insult leading to injury.[5] Meyers and colleagues[22] found that 71.3% of 157 athletes who were operated on for sports hernia remembered and identified the distinct injury during physical exertion. The lower abdomen and groin pain is often aggravated by sudden acceleration, twisting and turning, cutting or kicking movements, sit-ups, coughing, or sneezing.[4,5,48,56] Pain is usually present for a day or two after a game and may be associated with stiffness and difficulty getting out of bed the following morning.[48] Often after a period of rest from sport the pain returns immediately on return to activity.[48] Kachingwe and Grech[5] distilled from their experience the cluster of 5 signs and symptoms that they felt most indicate a sports hernia: "(1) a subjective complaint of deep groin/lower abdominal pain, (2) pain that is exacerbated with sport-specific activities such as sprinting, kicking, cutting, and/or sit-ups and is relieved with rest, (3) palpable tenderness over the pubic ramus at the insertion of the rectus abdominis and/or conjoined tendon, (4) pain with resisted hip adduction at 0, 45 and/or 90 degrees of hip flexion, and (5) pain with resisted abdominal curl-up."

In our experience, the athlete with lower abdominal and groin pain usually presents for evaluation after the pain has been present for several months. Sometimes, the athlete can relate the onset of pain to an acute incident and may remember a sensation of sudden tearing, but in our practice, this is not common. When the inciting event occurs, 2 types of pain syndrome emerge: (1) the athlete is unable to participate after the first 5 minutes of exertion because of incapacitating pain, and despite conservative care is unable to rehabilitate and return to play; (2) the athlete can usually play through the pain to finish the game, but often at less than 100% capacity, and again despite conservative care cannot rehabilitate to 100%. Certain movements typically exacerbate the pain, such as sudden acceleration, twisting, and turning. After the activity is completed, the athlete frequently has significant discomfort, may complain of a throbbing sensation in the lower abdominal groin region, and have difficulty getting out of a car or have difficulty getting out of bed in the morning. Over a day or 2, the pain cools down and the athlete returns to his/her baseline of chronic discomfort in the lower abdomen and groin that is exacerbated by certain movements.

Thereafter, the athlete often starts to play, and is able to play through the pain or discomfort, but at less then peak performance for the entire season. The athlete may end up missing practices or having lighter training sessions to allow the discomfort to improve enough so that they can compete at game time. Once the season ends, the athlete rests and anticipates that after a few months the problem resolves completely, only to discover that the issue returns when starting to train for the upcoming season. The problem not only has not improved with rest during the off-season, but the athlete feels immediately on resumption of their sport that they are back to square one.

PHYSICAL EXAMINATION FINDINGS

Physical examination findings include localized tenderness at or just above the pubic tubercle on the affected side, which can be elicited during a resisted sit-up.[3,48] On examination, the patient with a sports hernia does not have a detectable true inguinal hernia but the following findings may be present on examination; inguinal canal tenderness, dilated superficial inguinal ring, pubic tubercle tenderness, and tenderness at the hip adductor origin.[3,37]

When we conduct a physical examination, we examine the patient in both a standing and supine position. There is tenderness at or near the rectus insertion, lateral edge of the rectus, or the conjoined tendon/rectus abdominis interface on the affected side, or both sides, if the disease is bilateral. Typically, no cough impulse is elicited on examination, although when the patient is standing, one can occasionally palpate what seems to be a defect just below the conjoined tendon/rectus abdominis interface. If a defect is present, we can occasionally elicit a cough impulse at this location. Generally, there is not a bulge or cough impulse at the external inguinal ring, and there is no dilatation of the external ring itself.

Supine Provocative Testing

To elicit the pain of athletic pubalgia have the patient perform a supine resisted sit-up first with legs flexed (which takes out the lumbar lordosis) then with legs extended (which restores lumbar lordosis). The examiner palpates the rectus abdominus insertion on the affected pubic ramus. This procedure should reproduce the pain that has caused the patient to come to the office.

It is important to evaluate the adductor longus as a possible source of pain. Active leg adduction against resistance evaluates the adductor longus origin and can exacerbate the rectus abdominus symptoms. This positive finding may indicate that the adductor longus origin needs to be addressed either by a steroid or platelet-rich plasma injection or surgically. A diagnostic injection of local anesthetic may assist with this treatment decision.

IMAGING

The most important diagnostic tool in the evaluation of a patient with chronic lower abdomen and groin pain is the history and physical examination. Several diagnostic tools may be used to help establish the presence of athletic pubalgia, or to rule out another disorder in the differential diagnosis of chronic lower abdomen and groin pain.

Plain radiography (radiograph) or computed tomography scanning may be helpful to rule out bony abnormalities, but MRI is essential to evaluate the entire region, including the hip joint.[29,57] MRI may disclose another pathologic condition as the sole cause of lower abdomen and groin pain, or it may identify another condition in addition to athletic pubalgia such as strains, labral tears, osteitis pubis, iliopsoas bursitis, and occult stress fractures.[29,37,58]

In our experience, MRI is sometimes helpful in showing injury to the muscles of the abdominal wall, and is helpful when present in corroborating the clinical opinion. Although these findings are helpful, a patient with a typical history and physical examination, and no other major injury, is a candidate for a repair, irrespective of the abdominal wall findings on MRI. MRI may have an increasingly more significant role in the diagnosis of athletic pubalgia, although historically it showed injury 10% of the time.[59] However, a recent study comparing surgical findings with those seen on MRI suggests that the MRI sensitivity may be as high as 68% in detecting injury.[60] Omar and colleagues[61] have developed a standardized MRI protocol for athletic pubalgia to enhance its role as a diagnostic tool. These investigators have chronicled the findings on MRI that are associated with athletic pubalgia, which include direct visualization of tears in the rectus abdominis, adductor aponeurosis, or tenoperiosteal disruption, secondary cleft sign (indicating adductor injury), edematous or atrophic rectus abdominis near its pubic tendinous attachment or frank disruption of the rectus abdominis tendon at the symphysis or lateral head, and disruption of the adductor tendons.[61]

Dynamic ultrasound may play a role and is used by some groups to establish the diagnosis. The goal of dynamic ultrasound is to establish posterior inguinal wall deficiency, which can be visualized ultrasonographically. With the ultrasound probe placed over the medial aspect of the inguinal region, the athlete is asked to strain. Initial images are taken along the plane of the inguinal canal and then the images are repeated 90° to this. The test is considered positive if there is abnormal ballooning of the posterior inguinal wall.[42] At our center, we do not use ultrasound for the diagnosis of sports hernia. Although ultrasound may show a bulge in the posterior wall of the inguinal canal, it is operator dependent, and bulges may be common and found in any age group.[3,8,29,57]

Herniography is performed by fluoroscopy with an intraperitoneal injection of contrast followed by the patient performing a Valsalva maneuver before imaging.[29] This study is invasive, has a high complication rate, and should play no role in the diagnosis of athletic pubalgia.[33]

NONSURGICAL TREATMENT

Groin pain related to abdominal wall injury is a frequent occurrence. In many instances the injury goes on to heal and is self-limited. In some cases, chronicity occurs, and this subgroup of patients requires surgery. However, despite typical signs and symptoms, a trial of conservative therapy should be the first treatment plan, and surgery should be reserved for failures of conservative measures. For this reason, it is unusual to perform surgery earlier than 3 months from the onset of symptoms.

For the in-season athlete a 4-week trial of rest, selective steroid or platelet-rich plasma injections to the rectus abdominus insertion or the adductor longus origin, or a short steroid burst with taper are treatment options. Allow closed-chain lower extremity workouts during the rest period. At the completion of the rest period a functional return to sport assessment can be performed to see if the athlete is capable of returning to the season. If the pain persists, we leave it up to the athlete to choose whether to return to the season or not. Playing through pain is not believed to worsen the tear or the surgical results of repair.

SURGICAL TREATMENT

Athletes usually opt for surgery after completion of an athletic season. By the time we see them they have usually run the gamut of therapy, including periodic rest, physiotherapy, steroid injections, and nonsteroidal antiinflammatory drugs, with only temporary improvement and return of symptoms on return to sport. Typically, after 1 or 2 seasons of pain and disability, often increasing in intensity as the season progresses, and recurring despite the off-season, the athlete is left with few options. In our practice we have found that athletes tend to seek consultation many months after the onset of symptoms, and it is important to capitalize on the off-season so that surgery and recovery can occur without interfering with the following regular season.

Several operations have been described for the treatment of athletic pubalgia but they all fall into 3 main categories (**Box 2**). These operations include laparoscopic and open procedures. They are all variations of established operations for conventional groin hernias.

Laparoscopic operations can be performed in 1 of 2 ways that differ only in the way that they approach the preperitoneal space in the groin. In the transabdominal preperitoneal (TAPP) approach, the peritoneal cavity is entered, a flap of peritoneum is raised in the inguinal region, and a piece of mesh is placed in this preperitoneal space to cover the myopectineal orifice in the inguinal region. In the totally extraperitoneal (TEP) approach, the peritoneal cavity is not entered at all, and the dissection is started and maintained entirely in the preperitoneal space and that plane is continuously developed into the groin so that mesh can be appropriately placed in the inguinal region. The TAPP and TEP procedure are absolute analogues of one another in terms of where the mesh is placed.

Both are now well established and have similar results in outcomes such as postoperative pain, return to regular activity, and hernia recurrence when used in the treatment of conventional groin hernias.[62] Both operations place mesh (usually a 10-cm × 15-cm rectangle of woven polypropylene) in a preperitoneal position to cover the entire myopectineal orifice and thereby occlude any defect that may be present in the direct, indirect, or femoral space.[63,64] Current debate centers on the density, specifically the

---

Box 2
Operations performed for repair of sports hernia

1) Laparoscopic mesh placement

   Transabdominal preperitoneal (TAPP) hernia repair

   Totally extraperitoneal (TEP) hernia repair

2) Open sutured repair

3) Open mesh repair

Variations on theme:

Combination open sutured repair with mesh on-lay

Any operation with added nerve release/division

Any operation with added muscle release

weight and porosity of the mesh (heavy, medium, or light, related to pore size, weave, and reported as g/mL), because these characteristics may influence scarring, flexibility in situ, whether the mesh is palpable, the presence of chronic pain, and hernia recurrence. It is generally believed that heavier mesh induces more scarring.[65]

Open operations fit into 1 of 2 categories: sutured repairs (**Fig. 3**) and on-lay mesh repairs. These open mesh repairs represent variations of the Lichtenstein technique,[66] generally use polypropylene mesh, and have become the most popular operation for conventional groin hernia repair in the United States.[67] In general, the operation is easy to perform, but there is debate in conventional groin hernia surgery regarding the type of mesh one should use because heavier mesh may cause a more intense inflammatory response, and therefore more scar-tissue formation and more pain. Heavyweight mesh is less pliable, and can be palpable when used as a muscle on-lay. Therefore, there has been a shift to using lighter mesh for conventional groin hernia surgery.[68]

Sutured repairs are probably the most commonly performed operations for athletic pubalgia.[3,7,22,28,37,61] Sutured repairs are becoming less common for conventional groin hernias, because they create tension when obliterating the hernia defect and therefore cause more pain, require more analgesia, and a have a longer recovery than one sees with mesh-based tension-free repairs.[69,70] However, in athletic pubalgia, sutured repairs satisfy the need of the surgeon to create stability of the anterior pelvis, which is often accomplished by broadening the rectus abdominis insertion, which creates some degree of tension. In addition, most sutured repairs reinforce the posterior inguinal wall, which many investigators report as attenuated. In the treatment of sports hernias, surgeons have performed several conventional open operations, usually with adaptation. These operations include variants of the Shouldice, Bassini, McVay, and Maloney darn repairs, and the range of procedures has been summarized in recent review articles.[3,37] Two recent publications of large series at high-volume centers for this disorder both used an open sutured technique.[7,22,28]

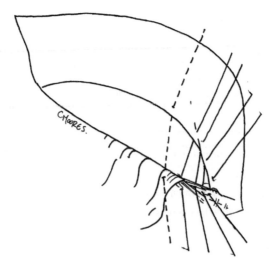

Fig. 3. The repair focuses on reattachment of the rectus primarily, and reinforcement of the posterior wall of the inguinal canal secondarily. The first 2 or 3 sutures bring the rectus abdominis muscle and the edge of rectus down to the pubis, pubic tubercle, and medial aspect of the Cooper ligament. The next 2 or 3 sutures bring the conjoined tendon down to the shelving portion of the ilioinguinal ligament to complete the repair. (*Artwork created by* Craig Moores, Medical Student, Albany Medical College, Albany, NY.)

We too prefer an open sutured technique that is best described as a McVay/Bassini variant. Some investigators report a combination of open sutured repair covered by on-lay mesh,[3] and there is increasing speculation that nerve division/release is an important step in some patients.

Summary of Outcomes

In Nam and Brody's review article published in 2008, 12 series of open repair and 7 series of laparoscopic repair were collected from 1991 until 2007.[3] In the laparoscopic series, TAPP or TEP was performed, and the reported success of return to full activity varied from 87% to 100%. Of the 12 open operations, all were variations of conventional hernia surgery, including Bassini, Shouldice, McVay, Lichtenstein, or darn repairs, and usually described as modified. Patient satisfaction levels with surgery also ranged from 77% to 100%. Jansen and colleagues[71] also reviewed long-standing groin pain in athletes and reported that although good to excellent results were reported in most studies, the level of evidence was low (level 4 evidence, ie, case series). Therefore, no meaningful comparison of operative approaches can be made, and these investigators concluded that there is a compelling need for the rigor of comparative trials.

It is unusual that such disparate surgical approaches would all yield suitable clinical outcomes. Yet, despite the limitations of the data, it seems that success rates are high across the board. This finding may be related to the possibility that surgeons are operating on a wide variety of different lower abdomen and groin issues, many of which get better over time, particularly if an enforced reduction of activity occurs because of the pain and disability from a surgical procedure. However, there may be unifying principles of treatment that are satisfied to some extent by all of these operations. These principles include (1) reinforcement of the posterior wall, and (2) fixation of the rectus abdominis or rectus/conjoined tendon interface. All sutured repairs in some way reinforce the posterior wall, and generally reinforce or broaden the rectus insertion. For example, Mushaweck focuses her repair on the posterior wall, in essence imbricating the transversalis fascia, but finishing her second running suture by capturing the rectus abdominis to lateralize it, in essence broadening its insertion. On the other hand, Meyers focuses his repair on the "surgical reattachment of the inferolateral edge of the rectus abdominis muscle with its fascial investment to the pubis and adjacent anterior ligaments. The operation is similar but not identical to a Bassini hernia repair." So in addition to fixation of the rectus abdominis, there is also extension of the repair in Bassini fashion to tighten (repair) the posterior wall.

Mesh repairs may accomplish the same task, whether placed open or laparoscopically. They all clearly reinforce the posterior wall, and they may broaden the fixation of the rectus abdominis inadvertently by inducing fibrosis and scarring of the rectus abdominis to the mesh, which fixates the muscle.

Adjunctive techniques have been performed to add additional benefit to the laparoscopic operation, such as inguinal ligament tenotomy at its insertion,[72] and ilioinguinal nerve release by performing iliopubic tract division at its origin.[43,73] However, when these maneuvers are performed, standard mesh repairs are still performed, and therefore it is impossible to determine if these adjunctive measures add benefit.

OUR OPERATIVE APPROACH

We prefer to perform an operation that is a McVay/Bassini variant. In our experience, the important elements of surgery are fixation of the rectus abdominis to the pubis as well as stabilization of the conjoined tendon/rectus abdominis interface. Unlike conventional hernia repair, more attention is devoted to the pillar of the rectus muscle by broadening its insertion. The same attention is devoted to the posterior wall of the inguinal canal as one might do in conventional groin hernia surgery, although with less need to extend this to the internal ring.

A short groin incision is made along skin crease lines just above the external ring. This incision is carried down through subcutaneous tissues until the external oblique aponeurosis is reached. It is opened in the direction of its fibers into the external ring, with care to preserve the nerves. The external oblique is separated from underlying structures and the spermatic cord is encircled and retracted inferiorly to expose the posterior wall of the inguinal canal. The important landmarks are the following: lateral edge of rectus, pubic tubercle, conjoined tendon, shelving portion of ilioinguinal ligament, and posterior wall of the inguinal canal. At this point the findings are variable. There is often attenuation and bulging of the posterior wall (however, we do not operate on normal groins, and there is no good comparison group to establish normalcy). There is less frequently disruption of the rectus abdominis or conjoined tendon or both. This condition has usually healed at the time of surgery, but one can see gaps in the muscle or fascial discontinuity. There may be partial detachment of the rectus at its insertion.

Sometimes the groin seems normal. Despite this range of findings, the results are good after repair if the patient has the typical lower abdomen and groin pain syndrome associated with athletic pubalgia. At the beginning of the repair, the pubis/pubic tubercle is roughened with electrocautery to create an inflammatory surface for tendon reinsertion. The lateral edge of rectus is brought down to the periosteum of the tubercle with 1 or 2 stitches using Orthocord (Depuy Orthopaedics, Warsaw, IN, USA), and then the edge of rectus is brought down to the Cooper ligament with 1 stitch, followed by 1 interrupted suture approximating the conjoined tendon/rectus abdominis interface with the shelving portion of the ilioinguinal ligament. At this point, 1 or 2 reinforcing stitches extend laterally, pulling conjoined tendon to shelving portion. It is unusual to use more than 5 sutures. The repair does not obliterate the entire posterior wall and does not extend to the internal ring. All nerves are preserved. The cord is then dropped back into position, and the external oblique aponeurosis closed, as well as the skin and subcutaneous tissues. If the adductor longus is involved it can either be injected with steroid or platelet-rich plasma at the time of surgery or a functional lengthening can be performed by releasing half of the fibers at its origin.

If patients have the typical symptom complex of athletic pubalgia, but have a clear-cut conventional groin hernia, then we perform a laparoscopic TAPP procedure, which is superior to sutured repair for conventional groin hernias.[61,62] Our TAPP technique has been described.[64] Similarly, if we have already opened the groin, and find a clear-cut groin hernia in a patient with the typical athletic pubalgia symptom complex, then our approach is to broaden the rectus insertion with 1 or 2 sutures, but still perform an open mesh repair. Mesh on-lay repairs for conventional hernias have a lower recurrence rate when compared with sutured repairs. However, we believe additional rectus fixation is required to treat athletic pubalgia symptoms.

POSTOPERATIVE REHABILITATION

The operation is performed as an outpatient surgical procedure. We use local anesthesia preemptively in the incision and perform ilioinguinal nerve blocks, give 1 mg Dilaudid subcutaneously in the postanesthesia care unit, and oxycodone as needed for postoperative pain control. We allow weight bearing as tolerated with relative rest for the first 10 days. The wound is then evaluated. For the next 2 weeks gentle hip range of motion and closed-chain lower extremity exercises are permitted. At about week 4 light abdominal core exercises are added, and at about week 5 sport-specific activity is advanced as tolerated. Full return to sport is at about 6 weeks.

SUMMARY

Athletic pubalgia is a distinct syndrome of lower abdomen and groin pain that is found predominantly in high-performance athletes. These individuals tend to have recurring pain, more pronounced with certain activities, and which affects athletic performance. Athletic pubalgia is probably a syndrome caused by muscle injury, because muscle disruption, detachment, or attenuation is frequently found, and muscle injury likely leads to failure of the transversalis fascia, with the resultant formation of a bulge in the posterior wall of the inguinal canal. These patients often require surgical therapy after failure of nonoperative measures. A variety of surgical options have been used, and most patients improve and return to high-level competition. The principles of surgical treatment are (1) fixation of the rectus abdominis, and (2) reinforcement of the posterior wall of the inguinal canal.

REFERENCES

1. Hawkins RD, Hulse MA, Wilkinson C, et al. The association football medical research program: an audit of injuries in professional football. Br J Sports Med 2001;35:43–7.
2. Arnason A, Sigurdsson SB, Gudmundsson A, et al. Risk factors for injuries in football. Am J Sports Med 2004;32:5S–16S.
3. Nam A, Brody F. Management and therapy for sports hernia. J Am Coll Surg 2008;206(1):154–64.
4. LeBlanc KE, LeBlanc KA. Groin pain in athletes. Hernia 2003;7:68–71.
5. Kachingwe AF, Grech S. Proposed algorithm for the management of athletes with athletic pubalgia (sports hernia): a case series. J Orthop Sports Phys Ther 2008; 38(12):768–81.
6. Ziprin P, Prabhudesai SG, Abrahams S, et al. Transabdominal preperitoneal laparoscopic approach for the treatment of sportsman's hernia. J Laparoendosc Adv Surg Tech A 2008;18(5):669–72.
7. Muschaweck U, Berger L. Minimal repair technique of sportsmen's groin: an innovative open-suture repair to treat chronic inguinal pain. Hernia 2010;14:27–33.
8. Campanelli G. Pubic inguinal pain syndrome: the so-called sports hernia. Hernia 2010;14:1–4.
9. Shindle MK. Hockey injuries: a pediatric sport update. Curr Opin Pediatr 2010; 22(1):54–60.
10. Gilmore OJ. Gilmore's groin. Journal of the Society of Sports Therapists 1992; 4(1):12–4.
11. Gilmore OJ. Gilmore's groin: ten years experience of groin disruption–a previously unsolved problem in sportsmen. Sports Med Soft Tissue Trauma 1991;1(3):12–4.
12. Brunet B, Brunet-Geudj E, Genety J, et al. La pubalgie: syndrome "fourre-tout" pur une plus grande riguer diagnostique et therapeutique. Intantanes Medicaux 1978;7(27):2387–90.
13. Ekberg O, Persson NH, Abrahamsson PA, et al. Longstanding groin pain in athletes: a multidisciplinary approach. Sports Med 1988;6:56–61.
14. Renstrom P, Peterson L. Groin injuries in athletes. Br J Sports Med 1980;14:30–6.
15. Smodiaka VN. Groin pain in soccer players. Phys Sports Med 1980;8(8):57–61.

16. Taylor DC, Meyers WC, Moylan JA, et al. Abdominal musculature abnormalities as a cause of groin pain in athletes. Inguinal hernias and pubalgia. Am J Sports Med 1991;19:239–42.

17. Gullmo A. Herniography. The diagnosis of hernia in the groin and incompetence of the pouch of Douglas and pelvic floor. Acta Radiol 1980;361:1–76.

18. Ekberg O, Blomquist P, Olsson S. Positive contrast herniography in adult patients with obscure groin pain. Surgery 1981;89:532–5.

19. Polglase AL, Frydman GM, Farmer KC. Inguinal surgery for debilitating chronic groin pain in athletes. Med J Aust 1991;155:674–7.

20. Malycha P, Lovell G. Inguinal surgery in athletes with chronic groin pain: the 'sportsman's' hernia. Aust N Z J Surg 1992;62:123–5.

21. Williams P, Foster ME. 'Gilmore's groin'–or is it? Br J Sports Med 1995;29:206–8.

22. Meyers WC, Foley DP, Garrett WE, et al. Management of severe lower abdominal or inguinal pain in high-performance athletes. PAIN (performing athletes with abdominal or inguinal neuromuscular pain study group). Am J Sports Med 2000;28:2–8.

23. Werner J, Hagglund M, Walden M, et al. UEFA injury study: a prospective study of hip and groin injuries in professional football over seven consecutive seasons. Br J Sports Med 2009;43:1036–40.

24. Robertson BA, Barker PJ, Fahrer M, et al. The anatomy of the pubic region revisited: implications for the pathogenesis and clinical management of chronic groin pain in athletes. Sports Med 2009;39(3):225–34.

25. Kumar A, Doran J, Matt ME, et al. Results of inguinal canal repair in athletes with sports hernia. J R Coll Surg Edinb 2002;47:561–5.

26. Genitsaris M, Goulimaris I, Sikas N. Laparoscopic repair of groin pain in athletes. Am J Sports Med 2004;32:1238–42.

27. Ingoldby CJ. Laparoscopic and conventional repair of groin disruption in sportsmen. Br J Surg 1997;84:213–5.

28. Meyers WC, Lanfranco A, Castellanos A. Surgical management of chronic lower abdominal and groin pain in high-performance athletes. Curr Sports Med Rep 2002;1:301–5.

29. Swan KG, Wolcott M. The athletic hernia: a systemic review. Clin Orthop Relat Res 2007;455:78–87.

30. Hackney RG. The sports hernia: a cause of chronic groin pain. Br J Sports Med 1993;27:58–62.

31. Srinivasan A, Schuricht A. Long-term follow-up of laparoscopic preperitoneal hernia repair in professional athletes. J Laparoendosc Adv Surg Tech A 2002; 12(2):101–6.

32. Lovell G, Malycha P, Pieterse S. Biopsy of the conjoint tendon in athletes with chronic groin pain. Australian Journal of Science and Medicine in Sport (AJSMS) 1990;22(4):102–3.

33. Yilmazlar T, Kizil A, Zorluoglu A, et al. The value of herniography in football players with obscure groin pain. Acta Chir Belg 1996;3:115–8.

34. Orchard JW, Read JW, Neophyton J, et al. Groin pain associated with ultrasound findings of inguinal canal-posterior wall deficiency in Australian Rules footballers. Br J Sports Med 1998;32:134–9.

35. Joesting DR. Diagnosis and treatment of sportsman's hernia. Curr Sports Med Rep 2002;1:121–4.

36. Zimmerman G. Groin pain in athletes. Aust Fam Physician 1988;17(12):1046–52.

37. Caudill P, Nyland J, Smith C, et al. Sports hernias: a systematic literature review. Br J Sports Med 2008;42:954–64.

38. Schilders E, Bismil Q, Hons MB, et al. Adductor-related groin pain in competitive athletes. J Bone Joint Surg Am Vol 2007;89:2173–8.
39. Laor T. Hip and groin pain in adolescents. Pediatr Radiol 2010;40:461–7.
40. Falvey EC, Franklyn-Miller A, McCrory PR. The groin triangle: a patho-anatomical approach to the diagnosis of chronic groin pain in athletes. Br J Sports Med 2009; 43:213–20.
41. Kavanaugh EC, Koulouris G, Ford S, et al. MR imaging of groin pain in the athlete. Semin Musculoskelet Radiol 2006;10:197–207.
42. Koulouris G. Imaging review of groin pain in elite athletes: an anatomic approach to imaging findings. AJR Am J Roentgenol 2008;191:962–72.
43. Dudai M. Twelve years of experience with laparoscopic treatment of sportsman hernia in 546 groins. How did we improve our treatment and results. Surg Laparosc Endosc Percutan Tech 2006;16(6):454–5.
44. Brown R, Mascia A, Kinnear D, et al. An 18-year review of sports groin injuries in the elite hockey player: clinical presentation, new diagnostic imaging, treatment, and results. Clin J Sport Med 2008;18(3):221–6.
45. Ziprin P, Williams P, Foster ME. External oblique aponeurosis nerve entrapment as a cause of groin pain in the athletes. Br J Surg 1999;86(4):566–8.
46. Bradshaw C, McCrory P, Bell S, et al. Obturator nerve entrapment. A cause of groin pain in athletes. Am J Sports Med 1997;25:402–8.
47. Vuillemier H, Hubner M, Demartines N. Neuropathy after herniorrhaphy: indication for surgical treatment and outcome. World J Surg 2009;33(4):841–5.
48. Garvey JFW, Read JW, Turner A. Sportsman hernia: what can we do? Hernia 2010;14:17–25.
49. Meyers WC, McKechnie A, Philippon MJ, et al. Experience with "sports hernia" spanning two decades. Ann Surg 2008;248(4):656–65.
50. Morales-Conde S, Socas M, Barranco A. Sportsmen hernia: what do we know? Hernia 2010;14:5–15.
51. Brophy RH, Backus S, Kraszewski AP, et al. Differences between sexes in lower extremity alignment and muscle activation during soccer kick. J Bone Joint Surg Am 2010;92:2050–8.
52. Diaco JF, Diaco DS, Lockhart L. Sports hernia. Oper Tech Sports Med 2005;13: 68–70.
53. Van Veen RN, de Baat P, Heijboer MP, et al. Successful endoscopic treatment of chronic groin pain in athletes. Surg Endosc 2007;21:189–93.
54. Moeller JL. Sportsman's hernia. Curr Sports Med Rep 2007;6:111–4.
55. Ahumada LA, Ashruf S, Espinosa-de-los-Monteros A, et al. Athletic pubalgia: definition and surgical treatment. Ann Plast Surg 2005;55;393–6.
56. Anderson K, Strickland SM, Warren R. Hip and groin injuries in athletes. Am J Sports Med 2001;29:521–33.
57. Davies AG, Clarke AW, Gillmore J, et al. Review: imaging of groin pain in the athlete. Skeletal Radiol 2010;39:629–44.
58. Nelson EN, Kassarjian A, Palmer WE. MR imaging of sports-related groin pain. Magn Reson Imaging Clin N Am 2005;13(4):727–42.
59. Albers SL, Spritzer CE, Garrett WE Jr, et al. MR findings in athletes with pubalgia. Skeletal Radiol 2001;30(5):270–7.
60. Zoga AC, Kavanagh EC, Omar IM, et al. Athletic pubalgia and the "sports hernia": MR imaging findings. Radiology 2008;247(3):797–807.
61. Omar IM, Zoga AC, Kavanagh EC, et al. Athletic pubalgia and "sports hernia": optimal MR imaging technique and findings. Radiographics 2008;5: 1415–38.

62. Gong K, Zhang N, Lu Y, et al. Comparison of the open tension-free mesh-plug, transabdominal preperitoneal (TAPP), and totally extraperitoneal (TEP) laparoscopic techniques for primary unilateral inguinal hernia repair: a prospective randomized controlled trial. Surg Endosc 2011;25(1):234–9.

63. Novitsky YW, Czerniach DR, Kercher KW, et al. Advantages of laparoscopic transabdominal preperitoneal herniorrhaphy in the evaluation and management of inguinal hernias. Am J Surg 2007;193(4):466–70.

64. Litwin DE, Pham QN, Oleniuk FH, et al. Laparoscopic groin hernia surgery: the TAPP procedure. Transabdominal preperitoneal hernia repair. Can J Surg 1997; 40(3):192–8.

65. Earle DB, Mark LA. Prosthetic material in inguinal hernia repair: how do I choose? Surg Clin North Am 2008;88(1):179–201.

66. Amid PK, Shulman AG, Lichtenstein IL. Open "tension-free" repair of inguinal hernias; The Lichtenstein technique. Eur J Surg 1996;162:447–53.

67. Rutkow IM. Demographic and socioeconomic aspects of hernia repair in the United States in 2003. Surg Clin North Am 2003;83(5):1045–51.

68. Novitsky YW, Harrell AG, Hope WW, et al. Meshes in hernia repair. Surg Technol Int 2007;16:123–7.

69. Schmedt CG, Sauerland S, Bittner R. Comparison of endoscopic procedures vs Lichtenstein and other open mesh techniques for inguinal hernia repair: a meta-analysis of randomized controlled trials. Surg Endosc 2005;19(2):188–99.

70. Bittner R, Sauerland S, Schmedt CG. Comparison of endoscopic techniques vs Shouldice and other open nonmesh techniques for inguinal hernia repair: a meta-analysis of randomized controlled trials. Surg Endosc 2005;19(5):605–15.

71. Jansen JA, Mens JM, Backx FJ, et al. Treatment of longstanding groin pain in athletes: a systematic review. Scand J Med Sci Reports 2008;18:263–74.

72. Lloyd DM, Sutton CD, Altafa A, et al. Laparoscopic inguinal ligament tenotomy and mesh reinforcement of the anterior abdominal wall. Surg Laparosc Endosc Percutan Tech 2008;18:363–8.

73. Mann CD, Sutton CD, Garcea G, et al. The inguinal release procedure for groin pain: initial experience in 73 sportsmen/women. Br J Sports Med 2009;43: 579–83.

Hip Problems and Arthroscopy: Adolescent Hip as it Relates to Sports

Leah Jacoby, BS[a], Yen Yi-Meng, MD, PhD[b,c], Mininder S. Kocher, MD, MPH[c,d,*]

KEYWORDS

- Hip arthroscopy • Adolescent athletic injuries • Hip disorders
- Sports injury of the hip

Injuries of the hip and pelvis in pediatric athletes are receiving increased attention, which may be due, in part, to the increased participation in competitive sports and focusing on a single sport at younger ages. The majority of injuries are soft tissue injuries, apophyseal injuries, or bony injuries that heal with nonoperative supportive treatment. Unique injury patterns can be seen in patients who have underlying pediatric hip disorders such as hip dysplasia, slipped capital femoral epiphysis (SCFE), and Legg-Perthes disease. With the advent of hip arthroscopy and the development of more advanced imaging of the hip through magnetic resonance imaging (MRI), internal derangements of the hip such as labral tears, loose bodies, femoroacetabular impingement (FAI), and chondral injuries are being diagnosed and treated with increased frequency. This article reviews the more common injuries of the hip and pelvis in pediatric athletes.

SPORTS-RELATED HIP INJURIES

Avulsion Fracture

Avulsion injuries are common among skeletally immature athletes because of the inherent weakness across the open apophysis.[1] The incidence of avulsion fractures

[a] Duke University School of Medicine, Durham, NC 27710, USA
[b] Department of Orthopaedic Surgery, Children's Hospital Boston, 300 Longwood Avenue, Boston, MA 02115, USA
[c] Harvard Medical School, Boston, MA 02115, USA
[d] Division of Sports Medicine, Department of Orthopaedic Surgery, Children's Hospital Boston, 300 Longwood Avenue, Hunnewell 2, Boston, MA 02115, USA
* Corresponding author. Division of Sports Medicine, Department of Orthopaedic Surgery, Children's Hospital Boston, 300 Longwood Avenue, Hunnewell 2, Boston, MA 02115.
E-mail address: Mininder.kocher@childrens.harvard.edu

Clin Sports Med 30 (2011) 435–451
doi:10.1016/j.csm.2011.01.003
0278-5919/11/$ – see front matter © 2011 Elsevier Inc. All rights reserved.

sportsmed.theclinics.com

is increasing, especially among 14- to 17-year-olds, as a result of the growth in competitive sports participation.

Avulsion fractures result from indirect trauma caused by sudden, violent, or unbalanced muscle contraction, and are most commonly associated with sports such as soccer, rugby, ice hockey, gymnastics, and sprinting, that involve kicking, rapid acceleration and deceleration, and jumping. Whereas in adults this mechanism of injury typically causes a muscle or tendon strain, in skeletally immature athletes the consequences are more severe, because of the inherent biomechanical weakness and subsequent separation of the apophyseal region. Intensive training exposes the epiphyseal plate to repetitive tensile stress while simultaneously enhancing muscle contractility and power. The inherent weakness at the epiphyseal plate, combined with the increased functional demands placed on the musculature, may predispose athletes to subsequent avulsion injury. Once the injury has occurred, the degree of bony displacement is restricted by the periosteum and surrounding fascia.

Although avulsion fractures can occur at any major muscle attachment, the 3 most common sites of avulsion injuries include the anterior superior iliac spine (ASIS), the anterior inferior iliac spine (AIIS) (**Fig. 1**), and the ischial tuberosity, because of violent contraction of the sartorius, rectus femoris, and the hamstring muscles, respectively. In addition, avulsion fractures of the lesser trochanter can also occur from the iliopsoas.

Clinical presentation typically follows a traumatic incident or strenuous exercise, and is characterized by acute onset of localized pain and swelling that is exacerbated on palpation and by passive stretching of the involved muscle. Patients will characteristically assume a position that places the least amount of tension on the involved muscle. Although clinical presentation is often diagnostic, radiological imaging is useful in determining the size of the avulsed fragment and degree of bony displacement.

Controversy exists regarding the optimal management of avulsion fractures, particularly those involving the ischial tuberosity.[1] Avulsion fractures at the ischial tuberosity are especially problematic if they are large fragments that are widely displaced, because they can cause difficulty with sitting and hamstrings function, and can irritate the sciatic nerve. The initial management typically will be conservative, including rest and ice, followed by protected weight bearing with crutches until symptoms resolve.

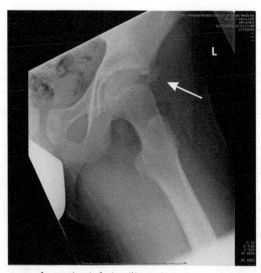

Fig. 1. Avulsion fracture of anterior inferior iliac spine. Arrow denotes fragment.

Thereafter, progression to light isometric stretching and full weight bearing is indicated, and return to full sports participation can occur once full strength and a pain-free range of motion is achieved. The need for surgical intervention is rare, and is typically based on ongoing symptoms and the degree of bony displacement. As a general rule, large displaced fragments greater than 2 cm may require surgical fixation; however, the optimal timing of surgical intervention remains unclear.

Hip Bursitis

Causes of bursitis include chronic microtrauma, arthritis, regional muscle dysfunction, overuse, and acute injury.[2,3] Hip bursitis is most commonly caused from activities involving repetitive motion of the hip such as running or cycling, or from a direct injury to the hip such as a fall or tackle.

In the hip, the 2 major bursae are the iliopsoas bursa and the trochanteric bursa. Iliopsoas bursitis is reported in all ages whereas trochanteric bursitis is more commonly seen in adults, although runners and ballet dancers are at increased risk of developing deep trochanteric bursitis from overuse. The iliopsoas bursa is the largest synovial bursa in the body and is located between the iliopsoas tendon (**Fig. 2**A) and the lesser trochanter, extending upward into the iliac fossa beneath the iliacus muscle.[4] The trochanteric bursa is located on the lateral side of the greater femoral trochanter and provides cushioning for the gluteus tendons, iliotibial band, and tensor fascia latae.[3] Less commonly affected is the iliopectineal bursa, which is situated between the iliopsoas muscle and femoral head at the place where the iliopsoas inserts onto the lesser femoral trochanter.

Clinical symptoms of hip bursitis depend on the bursa affected. Symptoms of iliopsoas bursitis include pain in the anterior groin, tenderness to palpation over the area of the lesser trochanter, and pain that is aggravated by resisted hip flexion. Symptoms of trochanteric bursitis include pain on the lateral aspect of the hip and thigh, pain when lying on the affected side, tenderness to palpation on the lateral hip, increased pain with transition from sitting to standing, and pain when walking up stairs. Pain may be able to be reproduced clinically by abducting and externally rotating the hip.[5] In both cases, other symptoms typical of inflammation such as erythema, swelling, and warmth may also be present over the joint.

Diagnosing hip bursitis is primarily clinical, and radiologic imaging is often unnecessary. Iliopsoas bursitis is not usually seen on a radiograph unless some bony pathology such as osteoarthritis is involved. In the case of a trochanteric bursitis, plain films may show linear or round calcifications that are isolated or clustered adjacent to

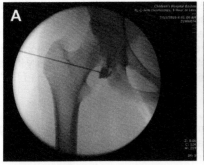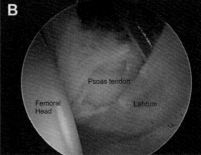

Fig. 2. (*A*) Intraoperative fluoroscopy of psoas tendon injection. (*B*) Intraoperative arthroscopy of psoas tendon.

the greater trochanter.[3] Bone scans, ultrasonography, MRI, and computed tomography (CT) may also be used to localize the area of inflammation.

Treatment of hip bursitis is usually nonsurgical and includes rest, ice, gentle stretching, avoidance of excessive hip motion, nonsteroidal anti-inflammatory drugs (NSAIDs), and physical therapy to strengthen rotational hip muscles. Steroid injections may help to alleviate painful symptoms of the bursitis (**Fig. 2**B). Some refractory cases may require surgical intervention including a bursectomy, bony prominence resection, or tendon release.[5]

Stress Fracture

Stress fractures of the hip in adolescents occur most commonly in distance runners who are putting constant tension on the pelvis and femur. These fractures originate from either abnormal forces on normal bones (fatigue fractures) or normal forces on abnormal bones (insufficiency fractures).[6] Female athletes are more likely than their male counterparts to develop stress fractures, particularly if they also suffer from amenorrhea, disordered eating, and low bone density—a condition known as female athlete triad. Other possible causes of stress fractures include chronic glucocorticoid use, smoking, hyperparathyroidism, hyperthyroidism, malabsorption syndromes, and calcium deficiencies.

The most common sites of stress fractures in the hip are the femurs, pubic rami, iliac crests, and sacroiliac joints. Whereas older runners may suffer from tension surface femoral neck stress fractures and are at increased risk of nonunion, deformity, malunion, or avascular necrosis, the young runner is more likely to suffer from compression surface femoral neck stress fractures, which are more likely to resolve without significant consequences.[7] Distance runners are also the most likely to develop stress fractures at the inferior pubic ramus.

Stress fractures of the hip often present with subtle clinical symptoms, making diagnosis difficult. For an early stress fracture, hip pain may be described as vague, insidious, and persistent, which worsens with activity and is relieved by rest.[8] As the fracture worsens, the pain may occur earlier or at rest. On physical examination, pain may be reproduced by extreme range of motion, particularly with internal rotation, adduction, and flexion.[9] Pain may also be increased with weight bearing (standing sign) or hopping (hop test) on the affected leg.[10] Plain radiographs have low sensitivity for detecting stress fractures in an acute setting because visible changes are usually not present until some periosteal healing has begun. Bone scans, CT, or MRI can be more helpful in diagnosing a stress fracture and should be considered if plain films are nondiagnostic (**Fig. 3**).

Management of hip stress fractures differs depending on the location, chronicity, and causative factors.[6] In most adolescents conservative treatment, which includes non–weight bearing on the affected leg, NSAIDs, regional muscular strengthening, and non–weight-bearing range of motion exercises, should be the first line of treatment. If healing is not occurring within 4 to 8 weeks, the use of an electrical bone growth stimulator may be tried. Surgical management is usually a last resort for the treatment of nonhealing stress fractures, and may include open reduction and internal fixation, especially if avascular necrosis, nonunion, malunion, or progressive varus deformity is suspected.[11,12]

Impingement

One of the most common causes of hip pain in athletes is femoroacetabular impingement, also known as hip impingment.[13] Anatomically this impingement is caused by the contact between the proximal femur and the rim of the acetabulum. If there is an excessive overhang of the acetabulum causing the labrum to be impinged between the acetabulum and the femoral head with hip flexion, it is called a pincer mechanism.

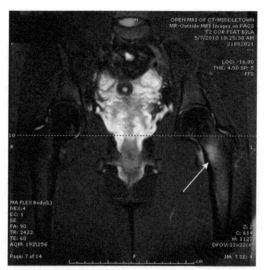

Fig. 3. T2-weighted MRI of pelvis showing edema and femoral neck stress fracture on the left hip. Arrow denotes edema.

If the impingement is caused by bony overgrowth of the femoral head, it is called a cam mechanism.[14]

Most often, the impingement is anterior and occurs with hip flexion or rotation. Sports involving multiple pivoting movements, such as football, soccer, lacrosse, basketball, ice hockey, and dance, are the most aggravating to the hip.[14] Impingement symptoms can be reproduced in the clinic with the flexion, adduction, and internal rotation (FADIR) test. Radiographic imaging (**Fig. 4**) is very helpful in visualizing any

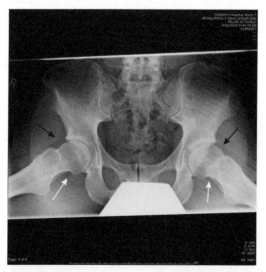

Fig. 4. Dunn lateral view of pelvis showing cam impingement. Black arrows indicate the cam lesions that cause the femoral head-neck junction to become convex. White arrows show the posterior femoral head-neck junction, which is concave and normal.

anatomic abnormalities that might be causing the impingement. MRI can be especially helpful for assessing the presence of labral and chondral injuries.

The progression of impingement is gradual, but has potential for severe injury to the labrum and articular cartilage of the hip and osteoarthritis if left untreated. Physical therapy to improve hip muscle flexibility and strength may help with the painful symptoms of the impingement, but treatment often requires arthroscopy or open surgery with surgical dislocation to relieve the impingement and restore bony alignment.[14]

Labral Tear

The acetabular labrum is a ring of fibrocartilage that runs around the acetabulum of the hip joint, and both deepens the acetabulum and stabilizes the femoral head. Injuries to the acetabular labrum occur as a result of mechanical stresses or excessive twisting in sports such as football, soccer, ballet, ice hockey, rugby, running, and cycling. Disorders such as hip dysplasia and FAI increase the risk of labral tears, due to the mechanical shearing of the labrum.

Although tears can occur in any part of the labrum, tears in the anterior portion seem more prevalent. This prevalence may be because the anterior labrum is subjected to greater stresses due to the anterior orientation of the acetabulum and femoral head, and the fact that the femoral head relies on the labrum, joint capsule, and ligaments for anterior stability.[15]

Most often, labral tears present as anterior hip or groin pain, although it can also present as lateral or deep buttock pain. Patients often report a variety of mechanical symptoms including clicking, locking or catching, or giving way.[15] While the pain can be caused by an acute injury, more often it is of gradual onset and increases in severity over time. The pain can be reproduced in the clinical setting with tests such as the flexion-abduction-external rotation (FABER) test or other manipulations of the hip, depending on the location of the tear. The most widely used imaging for diagnosing labral tears is an MR arthrogram, which uses contrast dye to visualize any disruption in the labrum.

The gold standard for both diagnosing and treating labral tears is arthroscopy (**Fig. 5**). Although conservative management may be sufficient to decrease pain, surgical repair or debridement of the torn labral fragment is the most definitive treatment. Success rates with surgical repairs are good, and arthroscopy has been shown to be a safe and effective procedure in the pediatric population as well as in adults.[16]

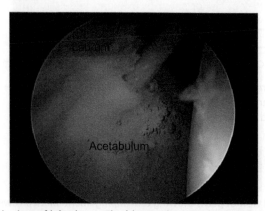

Fig. 5. Arthroscopic view of labral tear. The blue probe is in the tear that separates the labral from the chondral surface.

Hip Dislocation

Hip dislocation in children and adolescents is most commonly the result of an underlying hip disorder (discussed later). Traumatic hip dislocation in children differs from that in adults, as it requires less force to dislocate the joint and has fewer associated injuries.[17] This difference is caused by increased joint laxity in children, making dislocation possible with relatively minor trauma. The most common causes of traumatic hip dislocation in children and adolescents are falls, motor vehicle accidents, and high-velocity impact sports such as rugby and football.

While the femoral head in children may dislocate in any direction, posterior dislocations occur more frequently. Patients with a posterior hip dislocation present with classic lower limb deformity and shortening of the affected limb. The hip is usually held in flexion, adduction, and internal rotation. The femoral head may also be palpated posteriorly (**Fig. 6**).[18]

The treatment for a traumatic hip dislocation is immediate reduction by closed manipulation performed under general anesthesia. Imaging to confirm correct reduction of the joint is essential.

The most serious complications of a dislocated hip in children are avascular necrosis of the femoral head. Risk factors for the development of avascular necrosis include delayed reduction, increased severity of trauma, and older age. Other potential complications of hip dislocation include late posttraumatic osteoarthritis, coax magna, heterotopic ossification, and recurrent dislocation.[17]

INJURY DUE TO UNDERLYING HIP DISORDER

While hip injury in the pediatric athlete is not uncommon, often the cause in this age group is an underlying disorder of the hip. Previously discussed injuries such as impingement and dysplasia are some of the common problems in pediatric hips that stem from anatomic or mechanical abnormalities. Two other hip disorders unique to pediatric and adolescent patients are SCFE and Legg-Perthes disease.

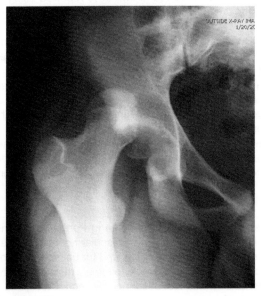

Fig. 6. Posterior hip dislocation.

Slipped Capital Femoral Epiphysis

SCFE involves the posterior slippage of the proximal femoral epiphysis caused by mechanical shearing forces, with concomitant extension and external rotation of the femoral neck and shaft. SCFE is regarded as the most common hip disorder of adolescence, with an increased prevalence among males, and with peak onset around 11 years of age.[1] Increased body mass index is a significant risk factor for the development of SCFE, with both biomechanical and endocrinological factors implicated.[19]

Classification of SCFE has traditionally been based on acuity of symptoms and severity of the slip; however, a greater emphasis is now being placed on mechanical stability because of its greater prognostic value. A mechanically stable slip will allow weight bearing, whereas a patient who has an unstable SCFE typically represents an acute physeal fracture with concomitant microscopic instability, resulting in pain and an inability to bear weight.

Accurate, early diagnosis of SCFE is important in preventing both short-term complications, including chondrolysis and avascular necrosis of the femoral head, and longer-term problems such as hip dysfunction and osteoarthritis. The insidious and often ambiguous onset of symptoms combined with the absence of radiological changes early in the condition is the common cause of delayed diagnosis. Symptoms associated with a stable slip typically involve a dull ache that is exacerbated by exercise, but can be localized anywhere from the groin to medial aspect of the knee. The delayed onset of significant pain and dysfunction may allow for the progression from a stable to unstable slip, with major implications for long-term prognosis.[20]

Management of SCFE is fraught with challenges, especially for severe slips caused by significant deformity of the femoral head, and there is an inherent risk of iatrogenic avascular necrosis and subsequent osteoarthritis. Several potential risk factors of avascular necrosis have been reported, including the use of multiple pins, pin position and penetration, complete or partial reduction, and the stability and severity of slip. Unfortunately, at present there is little in the literature regarding the optimal management of acute, unstable SCFE. A recent survey of Pediatric Orthopaedic Society of North America (POSNA) members found that 57% reported using a single threaded screw for fixation for unstable SCFE, whereas 40.3% recommended 3 threaded screws.[1]

There is a clear relationship between the stability and severity of the slip and subsequent postoperative risk of osteonecrosis. Patients who had stable lesions showed no increase in risk of osteonecrosis, whereas those who had unstable lesions demonstrated an increased level of risk that was proportional to the grade or severity of the slip. In situ pinning without reduction using a single cannulated screw was associated with the lowest risk of iatrogenic osteonecrosis of the femoral head, irrespective of stability or severity of slip (Fig. 7).[1]

Bilateral SCFEs have been recently reported to occur in around 50% of cases, though simultaneous presentation is unusual.[1] Despite this high incidence, the optimal management of the contralateral hip when presented with a unilateral SCFE remains controversial.[1,19]

Legg-Perthes

Legg-Calve-Perthes disease, also known as Legg-Perthes or Perthes disease, is an idiopathic, self-limiting condition involving avascular necrosis of the femoral head.[1,2] It typically presents in the first decade of life, and for unknown reasons predominates among males aged 4 to 8 years, with a male to female gender ratio averaging 5:1.[21-24] In the past 95 years, since it was first described by Legg, Calve, and Perthes, we have gained little insight into the etiology and pathophysiology of this complex condition.[25]

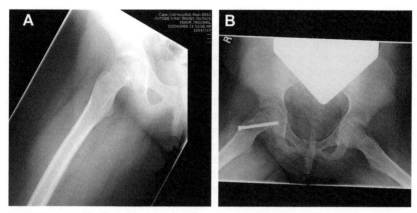

Fig. 7. (*A*) Preoperative frog-leg lateral radiograph of mild slipped capital femoral epiphysis. (*B*) Postoperative frog-leg lateral view after in situ fixation with a single threaded screw.

Pathogenesis appears complex, and involves avascular necrosis, followed by resorption, collapse, and subsequent repair of the capital femoral epiphysis, resulting in impaired growth and development of the hip joint.[26] The natural history of the disease in variable, and is largely dependant on the age of onset and the degree of femoral head involvement, but is also greatly influenced by intervention.[25,27,28] The younger a child is at the onset of the disease, the greater the time he has for subsequent growth and remodeling.[29] Moreover, in the long term, 50% of those who had childhood Perthes disease who did not receive treatment developed subsequent osteoarthritis in the fifth decade of life.[2]

Femoral head biopsies from patients who had the disease have demonstrated lesions with varying degrees of necrosis and repair, indicating that repetitive injury to the circumflex arteries rather than a single traumatic event may be responsible for the pathological findings in Perthes disease.[1] Several hypotheses have been formulated to explain this hypovascularity. Two thrombophilic risk factors, factor-V Leiden mutation and anticardiolipin antibodies, which enhance intravascular clotting and increase blood viscosity, are significantly associated with the disease.[30,31] Also postulated is intermittent increases in intra-capsular pressure, causing a tamponade effect and subsequent compression of the retinacular vessels as they course through the restricted intracapsular space.[1] Unfortunately, the literature remains conflicting, and there is a lack of evidence to support either of these hypotheses at present.

Perthes disease is specific to the hip joint, and typically present as an insidious, unilateral, painless limp.[1] If pain is present, it is usually mild, is exacerbated by exercise, and is frequently referred to the knee. The most consistent examination finding includes reduced internal rotation and abduction of the hip, and these are important prognostic indicators. In the early stages of the disease, this attributable to muscle spasm and synovitis, whereas later on in the disease, bony impingement of the femoral head on the acetabulum results in restricted hip motion. The prevalence of bilateral cases reported in the literature ranges from 8% to 24%, and interestingly they are more common in girls.[32,33] Development and outcome of the disease in each hip appears to be an independent event, with endocrinological etiologies such as hypoparathyroidism or skeletal dysplasia playing a role.[26]

A large number of radiological classification systems have been developed that attempt to stratify patients according to the severity of their disease, predict prognosis, and provide parameters for instituting treatment.[26] The two most commonly used classification systems include the Catterall classification, which defines four groups based on the involvement of the epiphysis (25%, 50%, 75%, or 100% involvement), and the Herring classification, which defines three groups according to the degree of collapse in the lateral epiphyseal pillar during the fragmentation stage **(Fig. 8)**.[34,35] The Herring classification system is a more accurate predictor of long-term outcome.

The treatment of Perthes disease remains highly controversial regarding conservative versus surgical intervention.[29] The primary goals of intervention include maintenance of hip motion, pain relief, and containment. At present there is a lack of conclusive data in the literature regarding the indications for; and the benefits of specific treatment modalities and as a result surgical intervention largely reflects the physician's personal preference. For patients who have severe disease, surgical intervention appears preferable to non-operative treatment, because it improves the sphericity of the femoral head and provides greater acetabular coverage."[1] The two most common surgical methods for containment include the femoral varus osteotomy and the Salter innominate osteotomy.[36]

Herring and colleagues, who devised the Herring lateral pillar classification system, conducted one of the largest studies on the topic to date, and concluded that patients over the age of 8 years at the time of onset that have a Herring classification of B or B/C border have a better outcome with surgical treatment (femoral osteotomy or innominate osteotomy) than they do with non-operative treatment (brace treatment or range of motion exercises). Children that fit into group B and were less than 8 years old at the time of onset were shown to have favorable outcomes irrespective of treatment, whereas group C, children of all ages frequency had poor outcomes regardless of treatment modality.[37,38]

ARTHROSCOPY
History

Described originally by Burman[39] in 1931, arthroscopy of the hip has more recently become an established procedure.[40-44] Arthroscopic surgery of the hip may offer potential advantages over traditional open arthrotomy and surgical dislocation in terms of limited invasiveness and diminished morbidity. The most recognized indications of hip arthroscopy are for the management of labral tears[45-49] and loose bodies[46,50]; however, hip arthroscopy has been described for a variety of other hip disorders, including osteoarthritis,[46] osteonecrosis,[46] osteochondral fracture,[51]

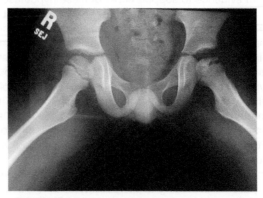

Fig. 8. Legg-Perthes disease.

chondral injury,[46] hip dysplasia,[52] septic arthritis,[53–55] inflammatory arthritis,[45,56] synovial chondromatosis,[57,58] foreign bodies,[59] ligamentum teres tears,[60–62] and complications after total joint arthroplasty.[63–66]

Most of the experience in hip arthroscopy has been with hip disorders in adults. The indications and results of hip arthroscopy in children and adolescents have been less well characterized.[51,56,67–70] Pediatric hip conditions include Legg-Perthes disease, slipped capital femoral epiphysis, developmental dysplasia of the hip, septic arthritis, coxa vara, juvenile rheumatoid arthritis, and chondrolysis.[1,71] Gross described his early experience with hip arthroscopy in patients who had congenital dislocation of the hip, Legg-Perthes disease, SCFE, and neuropathic subluxation. Bowen and colleagues[51] described arthroscopic chondroplasty of unstable osteochondral lesions of the femoral head as sequelae after skeletal maturity in patients who had Legg-Perthes disease as children. Other indications in the pediatric population have included labral tears, loose bodies, chondral lesions, juvenile rheumatoid arthritis, and septic arthritis.[56,67,68] In a review of 24 hip arthroscopies performed in 21 patients aged 11 to 21 years, Schindler and colleagues[69] concluded that hip arthroscopy was effective for synovial biopsy and loose body removal; however, as a diagnostic procedure, the arthroscopy failed to correlate with the presumptive cause of symptoms in 11 hips (46%).

A review of current literature supports hip arthroscopy for many pediatric pathologies including septic arthritis, labral disorders, SCFE, and Legg-Perthes disease.[48,49,67–69,72] DeAngelis and Busconi[68] note that the advantages of pediatric hip arthroscopy include less invasiveness than arthrotomy, quicker return to activities, and avoidance of femoral head dislocation, which Schindler and colleagues[69] note to be a known cause of femoral head necrosis that can lead to joint degeneration and premature physeal closure. A study done by the primary author (M.S.K.) of 54 hip arthroscopies in 42 patients showed overall significant improvement in the modified Harris hip score after arthroscopy in subjects ages 18 years and younger. Specifically, there was significant improvement after arthroscopy in patients with isolated labral tears, Legg-Perthes disease, developmental dysplasia of the hip, and inflammatory arthritis.[72]

Specific Indications for Hip Arthroscopy in Children and Adolescents

Multiple epiphyseal dysplasia
Multiple epiphyseal dysplasia (MED) is a genetic disorder in cartilage formation and deposition that specifically affects the epiphyses. In general, it is inherited in an autosomal dominant pattern, although recessive inheritance is seen as well. MED can involve multiple epiphyses in the body with variable phenotypes. Previous studies have suggested a prevalence of 9 to 16 cases per 100,000 births.[73,74]

Whereas the autosomal recessive form presents at birth with abnormalities such as clubfoot, cleft palate, cystic ear swelling, and clinodactyly, the autosomal dominant form of this disorder presents in late childhood with a variety of symptoms. Symptoms range from mild (often undiagnosed or misdiagnosed) to more severe cases. A patient with this disorder may present with some or all of the following symptoms: pain in the hips, early fatigue after exercise, gait abnormalities, and angular deformities in the lower extremity such as coxa vara, genu varum, or valgus deformity at the distal tibia.

In addition to clinical presentation, MED can be diagnosed based on both genetic testing and radiographic imaging. Radiographs may show a delay in the appearance of ossification centers in the long tubular bones as well as epiphyses that are small, fragmented, and irregular.[75] Treatment of painful and/or subluxed hip joints in skeletally immature patients involves surgical intervention. An acetabular shelf procedure can be done for coverage. Preexisting coxa vara often precludes femoral varus-producing osteotomy.[76] In addition, patients with MED are at higher risk of developing early-onset osteoarthritis. This condition usually becomes symptomatic in the second or third decade of life and in advanced cases may necessitate total joint arthroplasty.[76]

Developmental dysplasia of the hip

Intra-articular pathology is often associated with developmental dysplasia of the hip.[21,71,77] Hip dysplasia may present in adolescence or young adulthood as hip pain from a degenerative labral tear or chondral lesion. Anterior labral tears may also occur as a result of anterior impingement from a post-SCFE deformity or pistol-grip deformity.[70,78–83] Although favorable results have been reported from the arthroscopic management of intra-articular pathology in dysplastic hips,[49] the authors' preferred approach is to address the underlying dysplasia with periacetabular osteotomy, with or without proximal femoral osteotomy.[1,71] After periacetabular osteotomy, some patients may present with increasing hip pain and mechanical symptoms caused by a degenerative labral tear. In the authors' series, improvement was found in symptoms with arthroscopic debridement in 6 of 8 patients; however, the 2 patients who had full-thickness degenerative joint disease did not improve after arthroscopic debridement, questioning its efficacy in patients who have advanced degenerative joint disease.

Loose bodies

Loose bodies of the hip may occur from traumatic injury or as sequelae of hip disorders such as Legg-Perthes disease, spondyloepiphyseal dysplasia, chondrocalcinosis, or avascular necrosis. In patients who have Legg-Perthes disease, an unstable osteochondral fragment in the central portion of the femoral head may persist after the healing phase, particularly in patients who have a flattened, aspherical head. Patients may present with pain and mechanical symptoms such as catching or locking. The loose osteochondral lesions may be visible on radiographs, CT scan, or MRI. Arthroscopic excision has yielded excellent results with minimal morbidity.[46,50] In the authors' series, loose bodies were associated with Legg-Perthes disease, spondyloepiphyseal dysplasia, and traumatic osteochondral fracture, and excision typically resulted in resolution of pain and mechanical symptoms during this period of follow-up; however, the longer-term prognosis in patients who have Legg-Perthes disease remains guarded if there is substantial asphericity of the femoral head (**Fig. 9**).[1,71]

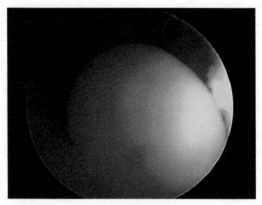

Fig. 9. Loose body in the hip joint after traumatic hip injury.

Septic arthritis

Arthroscopic synovectomy of the hip in cases of inflammatory arthritis has been suggested to improve pain and function.[56] In the cited series, 3 patients who had inflammatory arthritis underwent arthroscopic synovectomy for hip pain and dysfunction that was recalcitrant to medical therapy, and all 3 patients demonstrated improvement.

Arthroscopic irrigation and debridement of septic arthritis of the hip in children has been reported.[53–55] The authors' preference is for open arthrotomy through a limited anterior approach to the hip, because this allows for capsulectomy, drilling of the femoral neck to rule out associated osteomyelitis, thorough debridement of infected tissue, and placement of a drain.

Complications

Complications associated with arthroscopy of the hip include all of those for adults, such as pudendal nerve irritation and recurrent injury, as well as potential complications that are unique to the pediatric population including proximal femoral physeal separation, osteonecrosis, and growth disturbances. In a review of 218 pediatric hip arthroscopies, Kocher and colleagues[72] reported an overall complication rate of 1.8%, which included transient pudendal nerve palsy, instrument breakage, and suture abscess, but no cases of proximal femoral physeal separation, osteonecrosis, or growth disturbance were noted. In addition, both Kocher and colleagues[72] and Schindler and colleagues[69] showed complete pudendal nerve functional return and relatively low recurrence rates for most pediatric hip arthroscopies.

SUMMARY

Hip arthroscopy offers potential advantages over traditional open arthrotomy and surgical dislocation in terms of limited invasiveness and diminished morbidity. Most of the experience in hip arthroscopy has been with hip disorders in adults; the indications and results of hip arthroscopy in children and adolescents have been less well characterized. The pediatric hip has unique conditions, including Legg-Perthes disease, SCFE, developmental dysplasia of the hip, septic arthritis, coxa vara, juvenile rheumatoid arthritis, and chondrolysis. Hip arthroscopy in children and adolescents may be efficacious for certain indications, including isolated labral tears, loose bodies and chondral flaps associated with Legg-Perthes disease or spondyloepiphyseal dysplasia, labral tears associated with hip dysplasia after prior periacetabular osteotomy, and inflammatory arthritis. Further development of hip arthroscopy in children and adolescents is necessary to refine indications, evaluate longer-term results, and develop pediatric-specific instrumentation.

REFERENCES

1. Millis MK, Kocher MS. Hip, pelvis, femur: pediatric aspects. In: Koval KJ, editor. Othopaedic knowledge update 7. Chicago: American Academy of Orthopaedic Surgeons; 2002. p. 387–94.
2. Johnston CA, Wiley JP, Lindsay DM, et al. Iliopsoas bursitis and tendinitis. A review. Sports Med 1998;25:271–83.
3. Shbeeb MI, Matteson EL. Trochanteric bursitis (greater trochanter pain syndrome). Mayo Clin Proc 1996;71:565–9.
4. Butcher JD, Salzman KL, Lillegard WA. Lower extremity bursitis. Am Fam Physician 1996;53:2317–24.

5. Bird PA, Oakley SP, Shnier R, et al. Prospective evaluation of magnetic resonance imaging and physical examination findings in patients with greater trochanteric pain syndrome. Arthritis Rheum 2001;44:2138–45.

6. Paluska SA. An overview of hip injuries in running. Sports Med 2005;35: 991–1014.

7. Bergman AG, Fredericson M. MR imaging of stress reactions, muscle injuries, and other overuse injuries in runners. Magn Reson Imaging Clin N Am 1999;7: 151–74, ix.

8. Brukner P. Exercise-related lower leg pain: bone. Med Sci Sports Exerc 2000;32: S15–26.

9. Browning KH, Donley BG. Evaluation and management of common running injuries. Cleve Clin J Med 2000;67:511–20.

10. Noakes TD, Smith JA, Lindenberg G, et al. Pelvic stress fractures in long distance runners. Am J Sports Med 1985;13:120–3.

11. Boyd KT, Peirce NS, Batt ME. Common hip injuries in sport. Sports Med 1997;24: 273–88.

12. Kneeland JB. MR imaging of sports injuries of the hip. Magn Reson Imaging Clin N Am 1999;7:105–15, viii.

13. Ganz R, Parvizi J, Beck M, et al. Femoroacetabular impingement: a cause for osteoarthritis of the hip. Clin Orthop Relat Res 2003;417:112–20.

14. Kuhlman GS, Domb BG. Hip impingement: identifying and treating a common cause of hip pain. Am Fam Physician 2009;80:1429–34.

15. Lewis CL, Sahrmann SA. Acetabular labral tears. Phys Ther 2006;86:110–21.

16. Siparsky PN, Kocher MS. Current concepts in pediatric and adolescent arthroscopy. Arthroscopy 2009;25:1453–69.

17. Zrig M, Mnif H, Koubaa M, et al. Traumatic hip dislocation in children. Acta Orthop Belg 2009;75:328–33.

18. Herring J. Tachdjian's pediatric orthopaedics. Philadelphia: WB Saunders; 2002.

19. Loder RT, Aronsson DD, Weinstein SL, et al. Slipped capital femoral epiphysis. Instr Course Lect 2008;57:473–98.

20. Kocher MS, Bishop JA, Weed B, et al. Delay in diagnosis of slipped capital femoral epiphysis. Pediatrics 2004;113:e322–5.

21. Fabry G. Clinical practice: the hip from birth to adolescence. Eur J Pediatr 2010; 169:143–8.

22. Wiig O, Terjesen T, Svenningsen S, et al. The epidemiology and aetiology of Perthes' disease in Norway. A nationwide study of 425 patients. J Bone Joint Surg Br 2006;88:1217–23.

23. Kim WC, Hiroshima K, Imaeda T. Multicenter study for Legg-Calve-Perthes disease in Japan. J Orthop Sci 2006;11:333–41.

24. Wang NH, Lee FT, Chin LS, et al. Legg-Calve-Perthes disease: clinical analysis of 57 cases. J Formos Med Assoc 1990;89:764–71.

25. Terjesen T, Wiig O, Svenningsen S. The natural history of Perthes' disease. Acta Orthop 2010;81:708–14.

26. Kim HK. Legg-Calve-Perthes disease. J Am Acad Orthop Surg 2010;18:676–86.

27. Catterall A. The natural history of Perthes' disease. J Bone Joint Surg Br 1971;53: 37–53.

28. McAndrew MP, Weinstein SL. A long-term follow-up of Legg-Calve-Perthes disease. J Bone Joint Surg Am 1984;66:860–9.

29. Wall EJ. Legg-Calve-Perthes' disease. Curr Opin Pediatr 1999;11:76–9.

30. Balasa VV, Gruppo RA, Glueck CJ, et al. Legg-Calve-Perthes disease and thrombophilia. J Bone Joint Surg Am 2004;86A:2642–7.

31. Kenet G, Ezra E, Wientroub S, et al. Perthes' disease and the search for genetic associations: collagen mutations, Gaucher's disease and thrombophilia. J Bone Joint Surg Br 2008;90:1507–11.
32. Guille JT, Lipton GE, Tsirikos AI, et al. Bilateral Legg-Calve-Perthes disease: presentation and outcome. J Pediatr Orthop 2002;22:458–63.
33. Salter RB, Thompson GH. Legg-Calve-Perthes disease. The prognostic significance of the subchondral fracture and a two-group classification of the femoral head involvement. J Bone Joint Surg Am 1984;66:479–89.
34. Catterall A. Natural history, classification, and x-ray signs in Legg-Calve-Perthes' disease. Acta Orthop Belg 1980;46:346–51.
35. Herring JA, Neustadt JB, Williams JJ, et al. The lateral pillar classification of Legg-Calve-Perthes disease. J Pediatr Orthop 1992;12:143–50.
36. Kim JR, Shin SJ. Severe Perthes' disease or late avascular necrosis after successful closed reduction of developmental dysplasia of the hip. J Pediatr Orthop B 2010;19:155–7.
37. Herring JA, Kim HT, Browne R. Legg-Calve-Perthes disease. Part II: prospective multicenter study of the effect of treatment on outcome. J Bone Joint Surg Am 2004;86-A:2121–34.
38. Herring JA, Kim HT, Browne R. Legg-Calve-Perthes disease. Part I: classification of radiographs with use of the modified lateral pillar and Stulberg classifications. J Bone Joint Surg Am 2004;86-A:2103–20.
39. Burman MS. Arthroscopy or the direct visualization of joints: an experimental cadaver study. 1931. Clin Orthop Relat Res 2001;390:5–9.
40. Byrd JWT. Indications and contraindications. In: Byrd JWT, editor. Operative hip arthroscopy. New York: Thieme; 1998. p. 7–24.
41. Frich LH, Lauritzen J, Juhl M. Arthroscopy in diagnosis and treatment of hip disorders. Orthopedics 1989;12:389–92.
42. Ide T, Akamatsu N, Nakajima I. Arthroscopic surgery of the hip joint. Arthroscopy 1991;7:204–11.
43. McCarthy JC. Hip arthroscopy: applications and technique. J Am Acad Orthop Surg 1995;3:115–22.
44. Parisien JS. Arthroscopy of the hip. Present status. Bull Hosp Jt Dis Orthop Inst 1985;45:127–32.
45. Byrd JW. Labral lesions: an elusive source of hip pain case reports and literature review. Arthroscopy 1996;12:603–12.
46. Byrd JW, Jones KS. Prospective analysis of hip arthroscopy with 2-year follow-up. Arthroscopy 2000;16:578–87.
47. Dorrell JH, Catterall A. The torn acetabular labrum. J Bone Joint Surg Br 1986;68: 400–3.
48. Suzuki S, Awaya G, Okada Y, et al. Arthroscopic diagnosis of ruptured acetabular labrum. Acta Orthop Scand 1986;57:513–5.
49. Byrd JW, Jones KS. Hip arthroscopy in the presence of dysplasia. Arthroscopy 2003;19:1055–60.
50. Byrd JW. Hip arthroscopy for posttraumatic loose fragments in the young active adult: three case reports. Clin J Sport Med 1996;6:129–33 [discussion: 133–4].
51. Bowen JR, Kumar VP, Joyce JJ 3rd, et al. Osteochondritis dissecans following Perthes' disease. Arthroscopic-operative treatment. Clin Orthop Relat Res 1986;209:49–56.
52. Noguchi Y, Miura H, Takasugi S, et al. Cartilage and labrum degeneration in the dysplastic hip generally originates in the anterosuperior weight-bearing area: an arthroscopic observation. Arthroscopy 1999;15:496–506.

53. Blitzer CM. Arthroscopic management of septic arthritis of the hip. Arthroscopy 1993;9:414–6.
54. Bould M, Edwards D, Villar RN. Arthroscopic diagnosis and treatment of septic arthritis of the hip joint. Arthroscopy 1993;9:707–8.
55. Chung WK, Slater GL, Bates EH. Treatment of septic arthritis of the hip by arthroscopic lavage. J Pediatr Orthop 1993;13:444–6.
56. Holgersson S, Brattstrom H, Mogensen B, et al. Arthroscopy of the hip in juvenile chronic arthritis. J Pediatr Orthop 1981;1:273–8.
57. Okada Y, Awaya G, Ikeda T, et al. Arthroscopic surgery for synovial chondromatosis of the hip. J Bone Joint Surg Br 1989;71:198–9.
58. Witwity T, Uhlmann RD, Fischer J. Arthroscopic management of chondromatosis of the hip joint. Arthroscopy 1988;4:55–6.
59. Goldman A, Minkoff J, Price A, et al. A posterior arthroscopic approach to bullet extraction from the hip. J Trauma 1987;27:1294–300.
60. Delcamp DD, Klaaren HE, Pompe van Meerdervoort HF. Traumatic avulsion of the ligamentum teres without dislocation of the hip. Two case reports. J Bone Joint Surg Am 1988;70:933–5.
61. Gray AJ, Villar RN. The ligamentum teres of the hip: an arthroscopic classification of its pathology. Arthroscopy 1997;13:575–8.
62. Kashiwagi N, Suzuki S, Seto Y. Arthroscopic treatment for traumatic hip dislocation with avulsion fracture of the ligamentum teres. Arthroscopy 2001;17:67–9.
63. Mah ET, Bradley CM. Arthroscopic removal of acrylic cement from unreduced hip prosthesis. Aust N Z J Surg 1992;62:508–10.
64. Nordt W, Giangarra CE, Levy IM, et al. Arthroscopic removal of entrapped debris following dislocation of a total hip arthroplasty. Arthroscopy 1987;3:196–8.
65. Shifrin LZ, Reis ND. Arthroscopy of a dislocated hip replacement: a case report. Clin Orthop Relat Res 1980;146:213–4.
66. Vakili F, Salvati EA, Warren RF. Entrapped foreign body within the acetabular cup in total hip replacement. Clin Orthop Relat Res 1980;150:159–62.
67. Berend KR, Vail TP. Hip arthroscopy in the adolescent and pediatric athlete. Clin Sports Med 2001;20:763–78.
68. DeAngelis NA, Busconi BD. Hip arthroscopy in the pediatric population. Clin Orthop Relat Res 2003;406:60–3.
69. Schindler A, Lechevallier JJ, Rao NS, et al. Diagnostic and therapeutic arthroscopy of the hip in children and adolescents: evaluation of results. J Pediatr Orthop 1995;15:317–21.
70. Snow SW, Keret D, Scarangella S, et al. Anterior impingement of the femoral head: a late phenomenon of Legg-Calve-Perthes' disease. J Pediatr Orthop 1993;13:286–9.
71. Millis MK, Kocher MS. Hip and pelvic injuries in the young athlete. 2nd edition. Philadelphia: WB Saunders Co; 2002.
72. Kocher MS, Kim YJ, Millis MB, et al. Hip arthroscopy in children and adolescents. J Pediatr Orthop 2005;25:680–6.
73. Andersen PE Jr, Hauge M. Congenital generalised bone dysplasias: a clinical, radiological, and epidemiological survey. J Med Genet 1989;26:37–44.
74. Wynne-Davies R, Gormley J. The prevalence of skeletal dysplasias. An estimate of their minimum frequency and the number of patients requiring orthopaedic care. J Bone Joint Surg Br 1985;67:133–7.
75. Makitie O, Mortier GR, Czarny-Ratajczak M, et al. Clinical and radiographic findings in multiple epiphyseal dysplasia caused by MATN3 mutations: description of 12 patients. Am J Med Genet A 2004;125:278–84.

76. Ranade AS, McCarthy JJ. Multiple epiphyseal dysplasia, vol. 2010: Medscape; 2009. Avaliable at: http://www.emedicine.medscape.com/article/1259038-overview. Accessed December 29, 2010.
77. Cooperman DR, Wallensten R, Stulberg SD. Acetabular dysplasia in the adult. Clin Orthop Relat Res 1983;175:79–85.
78. Byrd JW. Hip arthroscopy utilizing the supine position. Arthroscopy 1994;10: 275–80.
79. Czerny C, Hofmann S, Neuhold A, et al. Lesions of the acetabular labrum: accuracy of MR imaging and MR arthrography in detection and staging. Radiology 1996;200:225–30.
80. Funke EL, Munzinger U. Complications in hip arthroscopy. Arthroscopy 1996;12: 156–9.
81. Klaue K, Durnin CW, Ganz R. The acetabular rim syndrome. A clinical presentation of dysplasia of the hip. J Bone Joint Surg Br 1991;73:423–9.
82. Petersilge CA, Haque MA, Petersilge WJ, et al. Acetabular labral tears: evaluation with MR arthrography. Radiology 1996;200:231–5.
83. Byrd JWT. Complications associated with hip arthroscopy. In: Byrd JWT, editor. Operative hip arthroscopy. New York: Thieme; 1998. p. 171–6.

The Mature Athlete with Hip Arthritis

James A. Browne, MD

KEYWORDS

• Mature athlete • Hip arthritis • Arthroscopy

Recent years have seen a growth in participation in sport among older athletes. From elite competitors to weekend recreational warriors, sport remains an important pursuit for many into the middle decades of life. Despite the inevitable decline in athletic performance with age, mature athletes often strive to maintain or improve their performance over time. Masters competitions are now a fixture in most team and individual sports previously thought to be the exclusive pursuit of youth.

The differential diagnosis for sports injuries of the hip in mature athletes is diverse and includes the same potential etiologies seen in their younger counterparts. The key consideration in this population is the potential presence of arthritis. As with other joints, an acute injury may lead to the discovery that the previously asymptomatic hip has pre-existing degenerative changes. The athlete, aware only of the acute injury and interested in quick return to participation, may find this revelation to be emotionally troubling and difficult to accept. An acute injury can also accelerate the onset of arthritic symptoms and lead to significant disability.

Treatment of the injured mature hip without arthritis largely proceeds as outlined elsewhere in this issue with an emphasis on physiologic instead of chronologic age. When arthritis is present, however, the patient and surgeon face difficult decisions when considering surgical options. This article examines the etiology of hip arthritis as well as nonoperative and operative considerations in this patient population.

SPORTS AND HIP ARTHRITIS

It is well known that the prevalence of hip osteoarthritis increases with age.[1] A recent systematic review reported the mean radiographic prevalence of hip osteoarthritis to be 1.6% in patients 35 to 39 years of age, with a mean interval increase in prevalence of 1.2% every 5 years culminating in a mean prevalence of 14.0% at 85 years and older.[2]

Most authors agree that there is insufficient evidence to support a causal role for physical activity in precipitating hip osteoarthritis.[3,4] While athletes are known to be at an increased risk of osteoarthritis in the joints they use most, this is likely explained

The author has nothing to disclose.

Department of Orthopaedic Surgery, University of Virginia, PO Box 800159, Charlottesville, VA 22908-0159, USA

E-mail address: jab8hd@virginia.edu

by the risk of chronic and acute joint injury followed by post-traumatic degenerative changes.[3,5] One large prospective analysis of 16,961 patients found that high levels of physical activity (running 20 or more miles per week) were associated with osteoarthritis among men under age 50, although the study was limited in relying on self-reported data and did not assess occupational physical activity.[6] The literature contains numerous other studies with conflicting results, reporting either an increased risk[7] or no association between sporting activities and osteoarthritis of the hip.[8,9] Interpretation of these studies is limited by their retrospective designs, small numbers, and varying definitions of arthritis. In patients with normal joints and neuromuscular function, lifelong participation in sports with minimal joint impact and torsional loads likely presents minimal risk for the development of osteoarthritis.[10]

Increasing evidence suggests that structural factors play a role in the development of hip arthritis. Both hip dysplasia[11,12] and femoroacetabular impingement[13–15] have been associated with degenerative changes in the hip joint. In both cases, morphologic osseous abnormality is theorized to result in abnormal contact stresses and loading of the articular cartilage, accompanying soft tissue injuries (labral), and ultimately premature degeneration of the joint.[16] In dysplastic hips, reduced surface area for load transmission leads to increased contact stresses on the cartilage, whereas impingement results in bony abutment of the proximal femur and acetabulum with subsequent chondrolabral injury and cartilage degeneration.[15,17,18]

The rate at which degeneration develops in patients with femoroacetabular impingement or mild dysplasia is unknown. While some proponents have suggested that surgical intervention may preserve the hip joint and prevent or delay osteoarthritis,[14,19] there is no high-level evidence to confirm the prophylactic utility of hip arthroscopy in altering the natural history of these structural problems.

NONOPERATIVE MANAGEMENT

Treatment of the injured hip in a mature athlete typically follows a stepwise progression beginning with over-the-counter analgesics and temporary restriction of activities. Resting the joint can decrease pain and swelling in the acute phase following injury. Physical therapy will not improve any underlying mechanical or structural problems and may exacerbate symptoms in patients with femoroacetabular impingement; extremes of motion and passive stretching should thus be avoided. Permanent activity and behavioral modification, including cessation of certain sporting activities that require supraphysiologic motion or high impact, should be considered in patients with clear underlying abnormal bony morphology consistent with femoroacetabular impingement.[15,20]

Intra-articular corticosteroid injection also may be beneficial in the mature athlete with degenerative changes in the hip joint. At least four randomized controlled trials exist that support transient relief of pain and improvement in function in the majority of patients with hip arthritis treated with intra-articular steroid injection compared with placebo.[21–24] Fairly consistent in these small studies is the observation of good pain relief and improved hip motion for approximately 1 month followed by rapid subsequent decline and no residual benefit past 3 months. The best clinical results are typically seen in patients with mild hip disease only; steroid injections have been reported as efficacious in 75% to 90% of patients with mild arthritis compared with only 9% to 20% of patients with severe arthritis.[23,25] Ultrasound data suggest that the steroid also may have a benefit in reducing synovitis.[26] An intra-articular hip injection thus appears to be best suited for transient reduction of pain in mature athletes with mild arthritis and may be useful depending upon the short-term goals of the patient.

In addition to affording pain relief and facilitating return to activity, intra-articular corticosteroid injection can have diagnostic utility in excluding extra-articular sources of pain. Multiple studies examining the response to total hip arthroplasty have reported sensitivity and specificity of intra-articular injections in excess of 90% in identifying intra-articular sources of pain.[27–29] The injection typically is performed using ultrasound or fluoroscopic guidance to ensure accurate placement.

Viscosupplementation is not approved by the US Food and Drug Administration (FDA) for treating coxarthrosis. However, it has been used for more than 20 years for hip arthritis in Europe. A recent randomized trial reported that a single intra-articular injection of hyaluronic acid was no more effective than placebo for treating the symptoms of hip osteoarthritis.[30] Complications of the injection included exacerbation of pain, flares, pruritus, and hematoma at the injection site, all of which seemed to outweigh any potential placebo benefit. This confirmed the findings of a previous randomized placebo-controlled study that also demonstrated no significant benefit to hip injection with hyaluronic acid at final follow-up.[24] Given the best data currently available, viscosupplementation cannot be widely recommended for the treatment of hip osteoarthritis.

HIP ARTHROSCOPY IN THE MATURE ATHLETE
Indications

Surgical options that preserve the hip joint have inherent appeal for older athletes with early arthritis that have failed conservative treatment. Arthroscopy is a minimally invasive option that is generally well tolerated and holds the promise of returning to sporting activities that may be inappropriate following total hip arthroplasty (THA). It may also be seen as a way to delay THA and reduce the need for future revision procedures. Potential arthroscopic interventions for osteoarthritis in the hip include joint lavage, debridement of synovium and osteophytes, capsular release, labral resection, osteoplasty, and removal of loose bodies.

Early experience with hip arthroscopy in the setting of osteoarthritis has suggested that careful selection and narrow indications are important in ensuring a good outcome. The literature contains several reports of hip arthroscopy in the setting of osteoarthritis (**Table 1**). Universal to these studies is the finding of increasingly poor outcomes, regardless of primary diagnosis, as the severity of arthritis increases. Once arthritis is apparent on plain radiographs, the outcome of hip arthroscopy becomes somewhat unpredictable and unreliable with unclear durability.[35,36] Reported success rates differ significantly between studies depending upon the surgical technique, quantification of cartilage damage, and outcome measure reported. However, the presence of mechanical symptoms has been shown to be a good prognostic factor.[37] Removal of loose bodies has also been shown to be reliable in the absence of significant radiographic arthritis.[35,37]

The largest long-term study in the literature, consisting of 106 hips treated with debridement and microfracture, revealed age and Outerbridge classification to be predictive of eventual need for THA.[36] A multivariate analysis at 10 years of follow-up suggested that patients over 40 with any grade 3 or 4 changes in the joint had at least a 90% chance of progressing to hip replacement. THA occurred in 78% of patients with grade 3 and 4 changes compared with 20% in grades normal through 2. The authors urged caution in treating patients older than 40 with articular cartilage damage. Other long-term studies have confirmed the limited role and poor prognosis of simple debridement in patients with arthritis, noting very similar high rates of conversion to THA.[35]

Table 1
A review of the literature of hip arthroscopy outcomes in patients with osteoarthritis

Study	Procedure	Number of Hips	Mean Patient Age (Range)	Follow-Up (Range)	Results	Conclusions
Farjo et al,[31] 1999	Debridement	28	41 y (14–70)	34 mo (13–100)	3 of 14 (21%) good results in patients with radiographic osteoarthritis, 6 of 14 underwent total hip arthroplasty (THA) at average 14 mo	Patients with radiographic arthritis less likely to have good outcome
Walton et al,[32] 2004	Debridement	39	47 y (22–87)	Minimum 4 mo	28 of 39 (72%) with chondral degeneration had poor clinical outcome	Osteoarthritis on plain films and chondromalacia observed intraoperatively associated with poor outcome ($P<.0001$)
Kim et al,[33] 2007	Debridement	43	40 y (18–68)	Average 50 mo	74% of patients with Tonnis 0 or 1 showed some improvement	Poor results in patients with underlying femoroacetabular impingement
Philippon et al,[34] 2009	Treatment of FAI	112	41 y	Average 2.3 y (2.0–2.9)	<2 mm of joint space corresponded to worse outcomes and satisfaction and were 39 times more likely to progress to THA	Joint space narrowing predictive of worse outcome
Byrd and Jones,[35] 2010	Debridement	52	38 y (14–84)	10 y	79% of patients with arthritis required conversion to THA	Arthritis (major predictor) and age associated with negative outcome
McCarthy et al,[36] 2010	Debridement/ microfracture	106	39 y (± 13)	10 y	Age >40 and Outerbridge grades III and IV independently predictive of THA	Caution should be used in older patients with cartilage changes

It is noteworthy that many of these reports predate the current understanding of femoroacetabular impingement. Some of the poor reports reported for arthroscopic isolated labral debridement may be explained by a lack of understanding of the underlying impingement phenomenon. Kim and colleagues,[33] in reviewing their experience with hip arthroscopy in 43 patients with early osteoarthritis, discovered significantly worse results following debridement of a labral tear in patients with previously undetected femoroacetabular impingement. Scrutiny for femoroacetabular impingement seems warranted before hip arthroscopy in patients with early arthritis.

The reported results in the literature are also based upon labral debridement. Recent work has suggested that an intact labrum plays a role in the biomechanical stability of the hip joint, implying that preservation and repair of the labrum may minimize the risk or progression of premature arthritis.[38] Labral repair after treating femoroacetabular impingement has been shown to be predictive of improved outcomes.[39] Although degenerative tears are typically not amenable to repair, Philippon and colleagues[34] reported that they saw no association between the condition of the articular cartilage and their ability to repair or debride the labrum. This would suggest that repair may be possible in many patients with early arthritic changes. Furthermore, their multivariate analysis of 112 patients treated arthroscopically for femoroacetabular impingement suggested that labral repair versus debridement was an independent predictor of a higher postoperative modified Harris Hip Score.[34]

Relevant information also can be gleaned by extrapolating from lessons learned in the knee. More extensive and longer-term experience with knee arthroscopy has led to the conclusion that arthroscopic lavage does not result in a relevant benefit for patients with generalized knee osteoarthritis in terms of pain relief or improvement of function.[40–43] However, certain subgroups of patients with knee arthritis may benefit from targeted arthroscopic intervention for specific indications. Clinical practice guidelines released by the American Academy of Orthopedic Surgery recommends arthroscopic partial meniscectomy or loose body removal as an option in patients with symptomatic osteoarthritis of the knee who also have primary signs and symptoms of a torn meniscus and/or a loose body.[41] Other patient factors that have been associated with good outcomes following arthroscopic debridement include those with only mild degenerative changes, mechanical symptoms, symptoms of short duration, and history of a specific injury.[43–45]

Imaging

Qualifying and quantifying the amount of arthritis are important when considering a patient for a hip preserving procedure (**Fig. 1**). Joint space narrowing is felt to be the most useful and robust way to radiographically assess early osteoarthritis on radiographs.[46] A minimum joint space width less than 2.0 mm is probably the most widely used indicator of pathology,[1,47] and this has been shown to correlate significantly with pain in the hip from degenerative changes.[48] Philippon and colleagues[34] reported that patients with a preoperative joint space less that 2 mm had lower outcome scores and decreased satisfaction, and were 39 times more likely to progress to THA following arthroscopy for femoroacetabular impingement. However, joint space narrowing has been reported in asymptomatic patients as they age, and it is not entirely clear whether joint space loss at the hip is a feature of normal aging or an indication of the arthritic process.[1]

Magnetic resonance imaging (MRI) has been shown to be a more sensitive indicator of early cartilage damage than plain radiographs. Kim and colleagues[33] noted better relief of symptoms following arthroscopic labral debridement in patients with normal plain films and degenerative changes of the cartilage evident only on MRI (Tonnis

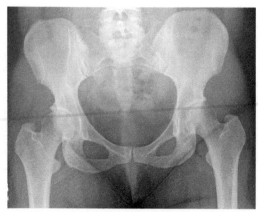

Fig. 1. A 47-year-old female professional golfer with right groin pain. Note the dysplastic features of the acetabulum with joint space narrowing.

grade 0) compared with those with evidence of early arthritis on simple radiographs (Tonnis grade 1). More advanced MRI techniques, such as the delayed gadolinium-enhanced MRI of cartilage (dGEMRIC) technique, ultimately may prove useful in selecting candidates for hip arthroscopy as has been reported with acetabular osteotomies.[49]

Labral disruption is felt by many to be part of the continuum of hip degenerative joint disease.[50] However, a high prevalence of tears has been identified in cadaver studies, suggesting that labral pathology may be part of the natural process of aging.[51,52] Furthermore, significant variability of the MRI appearance of the labrum exists in asymptomatic patients and increases with age.[53,54] All labral tears or abnormalities identified on MRI may not be symptomatic or the primary source of a patient's pain.[55] This underscores the utility of an intra-articular injection to rule out extra-articular pain sources and help accurately identify whether the labral abnormality seen on imaging is the primary pain generator in these patients.

HIP RESURFACING

Hip resurfacing is a hip arthroplasty that preserves the bone in the proximal femur. The femoral head is capped and articulates with the native cartilage or an acetabular component. The concept has been around since before stemmed prostheses. The advantages of resurfacing include bone preservation, avoiding stress shielding of the proximal femur, less risk of dislocation, and possible easier revision to a stemmed prosthesis. The disadvantages include its lack of modularity and the fact that it cannot be used for hips with decreased bone stock of the femoral head–neck junction. Complications include femoral neck fracture and aseptic loosening. For metal-on-metal implants, local and systemic reactions to metal ions are a risk. For metal-on-polyethylene implants, osteolysis can lead to failure.[56,57]

Several factors have limited the enthusiasm for this procedure. The metal ions, especially in women of child bearing age, and the steep learning curve with increased failure in the initial patients are concerning. Many engineering issues, such as failure of uncemented femoral components, have also hampered this procedure, although many have been resolved. It remains an appealing option in selected young patients as a bone-conserving solution.

THA AND RETURN TO SPORT

The limitations of THA, both inherent to the procedure and imposed by the surgeon, are relevant when considering older athletes for hip arthroscopy. Although implants, fixation methods, and bearing options continue to improve, a hip replacement remains a mechanical construct and is subject to breakage, periprosthetic fracture, and dislocation. Wear of the bearing surface, which continues to be a major limiting step in the durability of many joint replacements, has been shown to be a direct function of use.[58]

Traditionally, most arthroplasty surgeons have advocated that patients avoid high-impact activity following hip replacement.[59,60] There is little in the way of evidence to guide patients in regards to appropriate activity levels and sport participation; most recommendations are based upon expert opinion. Klein and colleagues[61] surveyed members of the American Academy of Hip and Knee Surgeons to develop consensus guidelines for return to athletics following hip replacement. High-impact activities were generally not allowed (racquetball, jogging, contact sports, baseball, high-impact aerobics) whereas low-impact activities were typically permitted (golf, swimming, walking, treadmill, stationary bicycle, elliptical machine). Most arthroplasty surgeons also allowed hiking, bowling, road cycling, dancing, and doubles tennis. Cross-country and downhill skiing were typically allowed with experience.

Return to athletics following hip replacement should ultimately be an individual decision between the patient and his or her surgeon. Numerous variables come into play, including surgical technique, implant factors, the patient's abilities and interests, and the demands of individual sports.

SUMMARY

Hip arthroscopy is a relatively recent addition to the armamentarium of surgeons taking care of the mature athlete with hip pathology. While this tool has many appealing features, its role in the care of the older patient with early hip arthritis has yet to be precisely defined. The current literature suggests that narrow indications and limited goals are important in successful patient outcomes. Patients should be counseled regarding expectations and anticipated long-term results. While arthroscopic debridement may relieve mechanical symptoms in a patient with early arthritis, it seems unlikely that it will significantly delay the arthritic process once it has been established. The long-term outcome of arthroscopic hip debridement is guarded in patients with radiographic evidence of degenerative joint disease and narrowing of the joint space.

REFERENCES

1. Lanyon P, Muir K, Doherty S, et al. Age and sex differences in hip joint space among asymptomatic subjects without structural change: implications for epidemiologic studies. Arthritis Rheum 2003;48(4):1041–6.
2. Dagenais S, Garbedian S, Wai EK. Systematic review of the prevalence of radiographic primary hip osteoarthritis. Clin Orthop Relat Res 2009;467(3):623–37.
3. Cymet TC, Sinkov V. Does long-distance running cause osteoarthritis? J Am Osteopath Assoc 2006;106(6):342–5.
4. Willick SE, Hansen PA. Running and osteoarthritis. Clin Sports Med 2010;29(3):417–28.
5. Baker P, Coggon D, Reading I, et al. Sports injury, occupational physical activity, joint laxity, and meniscal damage. J Rheumatol 2002;29:557–63.

6. Cheng Y, Macera CA, Davis DR, et al. Physical activity and self-reported, physician-diagnosed osteoarthritis: is physical activity a risk factor? J Clin Epidemiol 2000;53(3):315–22.

7. Marti B, Knobloch M, Tschopp A, et al. Is excessive running predictive of degenerative hip disease? Controlled study of former elite athletes. BMJ 1989;299:91–3.

8. Panush RS, Schmidt C, Caldwell JR, et al. Is running associated with degenerative joint disease? JAMA 1986;255:1152–4.

9. Lane N, Oehlert J, Block D, et al. The relationship of running to osteoarthritis of the knee and hip and bone mineral density of the lumbar spine: a 9-year longitudinal study. J Rheumatol 1998;25:334–41.

10. Buckwalter JA, Martin JA. Sports and osteoarthritis. Curr Opin Rheumatol 2004; 16(5):634–9.

11. Jacobsen S, Sonne-Holm S. Hip dysplasia: a significant risk factor for the development of hip osteoarthritis. A cross-sectional survey. Rheumatology 2005;44(2): 211–8.

12. Reijman M, Hazes JM, Pols HA, et al. Acetabular dysplasia predicts incident osteoarthritis of the hip: the Rotterdam study. Arthritis Rheum 2005;52:787–93.

13. Leunig M, Beaulé PE, Ganz R. The concept of femoroacetabular impingement: current status and future perspectives. Clin Orthop Relat Res 2009;467:616–22.

14. Ganz R, Parvizi J, Beck M, et al. Femoroacetabular impingement: a cause for osteoarthritis of the hip. Clin Orthop Relat Res 2003;417:112–20.

15. Ganz R, Leunig M, Leunig-Ganz K, et al. The etiology of osteoarthritis of the hip: an integrated mechanical concept. Clin Orthop Relat Res 2008;466:264–72.

16. Mavcic B, Iglic A, Kralj-Iglic V, et al. Cumulative hip contact stress predicts osteoarthritis in DDH. Clin Orthop Relat Res 2008;466:884–91.

17. Johnston TL, Schenker ML. Relationship between offset angle alpha and hip chondral injury in femoroacetabular impingement. Arthroscopy 2008;24:669–75.

18. Wagner S, Hofstetter W, Chiquet M, et al. Early osteoarthritic changes of human femoral head cartilage subsequent to femoroacetabular impingement. Osteoarthritis Cartilage 2003;11:508–18.

19. Kuhlman GS, Domb BG. Hip impingement: identifying and treating a common cause of hip pain. Am Fam Physician 2009;80:1429–34.

20. Parvizi J, Leunig M, Ganz R. Femoroacetabular impingement. J Am Acad Orthop Surg 2007;15:561–70.

21. Flanagan J, Casale FF, Thomas TL, et al. Intra-articular injection for pain relief in patients awaiting hip replacement. Ann R Coll Surg Engl 1988;70:156–7.

22. Jones A, Regan M, Ledingham J, et al. Importance of placement of intra-articular steroid injections. Br Med J 1993;307:1329–30.

23. Lambert RG, Hutchings EJ, Grace MG, et al. Steroid Injection for osteoarthritis of the hip: a randomized, double-blind, placebo-controlled trial. Arthritis Rheum 2007;56:2278–87.

24. Qvistgaard E, Christensen R, Torp-Pedersen S, et al. Intra-articular treatment of hip osteoarthritis: a randomized trial of hyaluronic acid, corticosteroid, and isotonic saline. Osteoarthritis Cartilage 2006;14:163–70.

25. Margules KR. Fluoroscopically directed steroid instillation in the treatment of hip osteoarthritis: safety and efficacy in 510 cases. Arthritis Rheum 2001;44:2449–50.

26. Micu MC, Bogdan GD, Fodor D. Steroid injection for hip osteoarthritis: efficacy under ultrasound guidance. Rheumatology 2010;49:1490–4.

27. Deshmukh AJ, Thakur RR, Goyal A, et al. Accuracy of diagnostic injection in differentiating source of atypical hip pain. J Arthroplasty 2010;25(Suppl 6): 129–33.

28. Faraj AA, Kumaraguru P, Kosygan K. Intra-articular bupivacaine hip injection in differentiation of coxarthrosis from referred thigh pain: a 10-year study. Acta Orthop Belg 2003;69(6):518–21.
29. Crawford RW, Gie GA, Ling RS, et al. Diagnostic value of intra-articular anaesthetic in primary osteoarthritis of the hip. J Bone Joint Surg Br 1998;80(2): 279–81.
30. Richette P, Ravaud P, Conrozier T, et al. Effect of hyaluronic acid in symptomatic hip osteoarthritis: a multicenter, randomized, placebo-controlled trial. Arthritis Rheum 2009;60(3):824–30.
31. Farjo LA, Glick JM, Sampson TG. Hip arthroscopy for acetabular labral tears. Arthroscopy 1999;15:132–7.
32. Walton NP, Jahromi I, Lewis PL. Chondral degeneration and therapeutic hip arthroscopy. Int Orthop 2004;28:354–6.
33. Kim KC, Hwang DS, Lee CH, et al. Influence of femoroacetabular impingement on results of hip arthroscopy in patients with early osteoarthritis. Clin Orthop Relat Res 2007;456:128–32.
34. Philippon MJ, Briggs KK, Yen YM, et al. Outcomes following hip arthroscopy for femoroacetabular impingement with associated chondrolabral dysfunction: minimum two-year follow-up. J Bone Joint Surg Br 2009;91(1):16–23.
35. Byrd JW, Jones KS. Prospective analysis of hip arthroscopy with 10-year follow-up. Clin Orthop Relat Res 2010;468(3):741–6.
36. McCarthy JC, Jarrett BT, Ojeifo O, et al. What factors influence long-term survivorship after hip arthroscopy? Clin Orthop Relat Res 2011;469(2):362–71.
37. O'Leary JA, Berend K, Vail TP. The relationship between diagnosis and outcome in arthroscopy of the hip. Arthroscopy 2001;17(2):181–8.
38. Crawford MJ, Dy CJ, Alexander JW, et al. The 2007 Frank Stinchfield Award. The biomechanics of the hip labrum and the stability of the hip. Clin Orthop Relat Res 2007;465:16–22.
39. Espinosa N, Beck M, Rothenflug DA, et al. Treatment of femoroacetabular impingement: preliminary results of labral refixation: surgical technique. J Bone Joint Surg Am 2006;88:925–35.
40. Reichenbach S, Rutjes AW, Nüesch E, et al. Joint lavage for osteoarthritis of the knee. Cochrane Database Syst Rev 2010;5:CD007320.
41. American Academy of Orthopaedic Surgery Treatment of Osteoarthritis (OA) of the Knee Recommendation Summary. Available at: http://www.aaos.org/research/guidelines/OAKrecommendations.pdf. Accessed August 10, 2010.
42. Moseley JB, O'Malley K, Petersen NJ, et al. A controlled trial of arthroscopic surgery for osteoarthritis of the knee. N Engl J Med 2002;347:81–8.
43. Baumgaertner MR, Cannon WD Jr, Vittori JM, et al. Arthroscopic debridement of the arthritic knee. Clin Orthop Relat Res 1990;253:197–202.
44. Stuart MJ, Lubowitz JH. What, if any, are the indications for arthroscopic debridement of the osteoarthritic knee? Arthroscopy 2006;22:238–9.
45. Aaron RK, Skolnick AH, Reinert SE, et al. Arthroscopic débridement for osteoarthritis of the knee. J Bone Joint Surg Am 2006;88:936–43.
46. Croft P, Cooper C, Wickham C, et al. Defining osteoarthritis of the hip for epidemiologic studies. Am J Epidemiol 1990;132:514–22.
47. Nevitt M. Definition of hip osteoarthritis for epidemiological studies. Ann Rheum Dis 1996;55:652–5.
48. Jacobsen S, Sonne-Holm S, Soballe K, et al. The relationship of hip joint space to self reported hip pain: a survey of 4151 subjects of the Copenhagen City Heart Study: the Osteoarthritis Substudy. Osteoarthritis Cartilage 2004;12:692–7.

49. Cunningham T, Jessel R, Zurakowski D, et al. Delayed gadolinium-enhanced magnetic resonance imaging of cartilage to predict early failure of Bernese peri-acetabular osteotomy for hip dysplasia. J Bone Joint Surg Am 2006;88:1540–8.
50. McCarthy JC, Noble PC, Schuck MR, et al. The Otto E. Aufranc Award: the role of labral lesions to development of early degenerative hip disease. Clin Orthop Relat Res 2001;393:25–37.
51. McCarthy JC, Noble PC, Schuck MR, et al. The watershed labral lesion: its relationship to early arthritis of the hip. J Arthroplasty 2001;16:81–7.
52. Seldes RM, Tan V, Hunt J, et al. Anatomy, histologic features, and vascularity of the adult acetabular labrum. Clin Orthop Relat Res 2001;382:232–42.
53. Abe I, Harada Y, Oinuma K, et al. Acetabular labrum: abnormal findings at MR imaging in asymptomatic hips. Radiology 2000;216:576–81.
54. Cotton A, Boutry N, Demondion X, et al. Acetabular labrum: MRI in asymptomatic volunteers. J Comput Assist Tomogr 1998;22:1–7.
55. Martin RL, Irrgang JJ, Sekiya JK. The diagnostic accuracy of a clinical examination in determining intra-articular hip pain for potential hip arthroscopy candidates. Arthroscopy 2008;24:1013–8.
56. Amstutz HC, Le Duff MJ. Hip resurfacing results for osteonecrosis are as good as for other etiologies at 2 to 12 years. Clin Orthop Relat Res 2010;468:375–81.
57. Mont MA, Ragland PS, Etienne G, et al. Hip resurfacing arthroplasty. J Am Acad Orthop Surg 2006;14(8):454–63.
58. Schmalzried TP, Shepherd EF, Dorey FJ, et al. The John Charnley Award. Wear is a function of use, not time. Clin Orthop Relat Res 2000;381:36–46.
59. Clifford PE, Mallon WJ. Sports after total joint replacement. Clin Sports Med 2005; 24:175–86.
60. McGrory BJ, Stuart MJ, Sim FH. Participation in sports after hip and knee arthroplasty: review of literature and survey of surgeon preferences. Mayo Clin Proc 1995;70:342–8.
61. Klein GR, Levine BR, Hozack WJ, et al. Return to athletic activity after total hip arthroplasty. Consensus guidelines based on a survey of the Hip Society and American Association of Hip and Knee Surgeons. J Arthroplasty 2007;22:171–5.

Rehabilitation After Hip Femoroacetabular Impingement Arthroscopy

Michael Wahoff, PT, SCS*, Mark Ryan, MS, ATC, CSCS

KEYWORDS

- Rehabilitation • Circumduction
- Femoroacetabular impingement • Return to sport

More than 30,000 hip arthroscopies were performed in 2008. This number is expected to grow at a rate of 15% over the next 5 years, resulting in more then 70,000 hip arthroscopies performed each year by 2013.[1] Hip arthroscopic techniques to repair labral tears and address femoroacetabular impingement (FAI) continue to evolve. Multiple published studies have reported positive surgical outcomes.[2–8] Although there is evidence to support arthroscopic procedures to address labral tears and FAI, there are few published evidence-based rehabilitation studies dedicated to postoperative rehabilitative care.[9–11]

Pain, loss of motion, changes in muscle strength and motor control, loss of stability, and loss of function can be caused by FAI and labral tear.[12–14] Hip arthroscopic procedures are used to correct the bony geometry and provide an intact labral complex and ligamentous structure for improved hip congruency. A thorough postoperative rehabilitation program must protect the integrity of these healing tissues, control pain and inflammation, allow for early range of motion (ROM), reduce muscle inhibition, restore neuromuscular control and proprioception, normalize gait, and improve strength. For the athlete, power, speed, and agility are recommended for optimal return to competition. A positive outcome is not necessarily how quickly patients return to their preinjury level of function or sport but the overall longevity and patient satisfaction.

PRINCIPLES OF HIP ARTHROSCOPY REHABILITATION

The following are the key principles of rehabilitation after hip arthroscopy: (1) rehabilitation is an individualized and evaluation-based (not time-based) program designed

The authors have no conflicts of interest.
Howard Head Sports Medicine, 181 West Meadow Drive, Vail, CO 81657, USA
* Corresponding author.
E-mail address: Wahoff@vvmc.com

to be able to address specific findings of the surgeon, the procedures performed, and the patient's individual characteristics; (2) circumduction is critical for early mobility to provide an environment in and around the joint to reduce the risk of scar tissue; and (3) sport-specific functional rehabilitation should be provided.

Rehabilitation is considered individualized, with specific time lines for weight bearing and ROM restrictions determined by the specific procedures performed on the patient. Compliance with these restrictions by patients and therapists is critical to allow for soft tissue healing. Rehabilitation is done in phases and should be comprehensive, be easy to understand, and err on the side of safety. Exercise progressions used are similar in all patients during the early and mid phases. Specific objective criteria to advance are used to progress to the next phases. Such advancement allows for differences in a patient's age, genetics, nutrition, concomitant injuries, symptom onset, goals, and sport-specific demands.[15] The 4 phases of rehabilitation include maximum protection and mobility (phase 1), controlled stability (phase 2), strengthening (phase 3), and return to sport (phase 4) (**Fig. 1**).

REHABILITATION PROTOCOLS

Phase 1 of the rehabilitation program is shown in **Table 1**. Hip arthroscopy is a package of several to all procedures listed in **Table 2**. Patients who undergo a microfracture for the treatment of full-thickness chondral injuries are restricted to foot-flat weight bearing (FFWB, 9 kg) for 6 to 8 weeks.[2,16] Patients who do not undergo a microfracture are restricted to FFWB for 3 weeks to decrease postoperative inflammation and reduce the risk of a stress fracture due to the osteoplasty. Patients are restricted to 50% weight bearing for another week to allow time for restoration of motor control. Hip extension past neutral is restricted for 21 days because it has been shown to increase anterior hip forces and place stress on the anterior labrum and capsule.[17] ROM restrictions also include no external rotation (ER) for 17 to 21 days, depending on the viability of the tissue, capsular closure technique, and overall joint laxity; flexion up to 120°; and abduction up to 45°. A hip hinge brace assists in limiting extension and ER and is worn when ambulating for 17 to 21 days. Patients wear calf pumps while at rest as a preventative measure for blood clots.

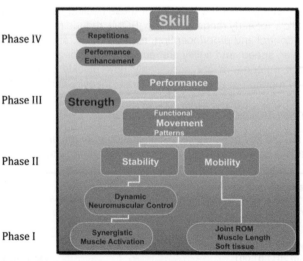

Fig. 1. The 4 phases of rehabilitation as shown in a motor control diagram.

Table 1
Phase 1 of rehabilitation program

Phase 1: Maximum Protection and Mobility

Goals	1. Protect the integrity of the repaired tissues 2. Diminish pain and inflammation 3. Restore ROM within the restrictions 4. Prevent muscular inhibition
Restrictions	See **Table 2**
Treatment Strategies	1. CPM: 30°–70° placed in 10° abduction 　4–6 h/d × 3 d, then 1–2 h/d × 2 wk (non-Mfx patients) 　4–6 h/d × 6–8 wk (Mfx patients)[16] 2. Ice and compression: as needed in phase 1 3. Nonresistant stationary bicycle: 20 min 1–2 times/d × 6 wk 4. Circumduction (passive ROM): 2 times/d × 2 wk, 　then daily through 10 wk 5. Laying prone for a minimum of 2 h/d: phases 1 and 2 6. Lymphatic massage/soft tissue: as needed in phases 1 and 2 7. Pain-free gentle muscle stretching 8. Isometrics 9. Active ROM: emphasis on gluteus medius and deep rotators 10. Aquatic pool program 11. Cardiovascular and upper body exercises (see **Table 5**)
Minimum Criteria To Advance	1. Minimal complaints of pain with all phase 1 exercises 2. Proper muscle firing pattern with all phase 1 exercises 3. Minimal complaints of "pinching" sensation in the 　hip before 100° of flexion 4. Full weight bearing is allowed and tolerated

Abbreviations: CPM, continuous passive motion; Mfx, microfracture.

Table 2
Restrictions and precautions per surgical procedures performed

Procedure	PROM	WB	CPM	Brace
Osteoplasty Rim Trimming	No limits	FFWB × 21 d then 50% × 1 wk	4–6 h × 3 d then 1–2 h × 2 wk	21 d
Chondroplasty	No limits	WBAT	4–6 h × 3 d then 1–2 h × 2 wk	No
Microfracture	No limits	FFWB × 6–8 wk	4–6 h × 6–8 wk	No
Labral Repair	Flexion up to 120°, abduction up to 45° No external rotation × 17–21 d, Ext to 0 × 1 wk but no ext > 0 x 17–21 d	—	4–6 h × 3 d then 1–2 h × 2 wk	17–21 d
Capsule Plication and Capsule Closure	Flexion up to 120°, abduction up to 45° No external rotation for 17–21 d, Ext to 0 × 1 wk but no ext >0 x 17–21 d	—	4–6 h × 3 d then 1–2 h × 2 wk	17–21 d

Abbreviations: CPM, continuous passive motion; FFWB, foot-flat weight bearing; PROM, passive range of motion; WB, weight bearing; WBAT, weight bearing as tolerated.

POSTOPERATIVE THERAPY MODALITIES

Pain and inflammation is decreased with ice, compression, and lymphatic massage. As the initial swelling decreases, other soft tissue techniques are used, including effleurage, petrissage, myofascial release, and active release techniques. Emphasis is placed on the tensor fasciae latae (TFL), gluteus medius, iliotibial band, adductors, iliopsoas, and lumbar spine.

Mobility within the ROM restrictions is achieved with the continuous passive motion machine, stationary bike, aquatic therapy, and passive ROM, with emphasis on circumduction (**Fig. 2**). Patients are instructed to lay prone for a minimum of 2 h/d to keep the hip flexors from shortening.

MUSCULATURE RESTORATION

Restoration of normal muscle performance is critical to reestablish dynamic hip joint congruency after surgery. Correct motor function is achieved through careful selection of exercises for muscular strength (capacity to actively develop tension), work (force × distance), power (rate of work output), or endurance (ability to delay onset of fatigue).[18] Isometric (static), isotonic (eccentric or concentric), slow- and fast-speed dynamic, and functional exercises are used depending on the phase of rehabilitation and the goal of the exercise. Goals of these exercises can include preventing muscle inhibition, regaining neuromuscular control and proprioception, or increasing strength, power, and/or endurance. It is critical that the exercises selected are based not only on the muscles recruited and the amount of force they will produce but also on the fact that they can be performed while maintaining the surgical precautions and with consideration to the joint reaction forces that they may place on the joint.

Quadriceps, gluteus maximus, and transverse abdominis (TA) pain-free isometrics are initiated on day 1. Active prone hamstring curls are used to facilitate early motor control, active prone terminal knee extensions (**Fig. 3**) are used to facilitate glutes and quads to neutral hip extension, and active prone and hook-lying internal rotations (**Fig. 4**) are used to facilitate active rotation within safe ROM. Quad rocking facilitates patient-controlled hip flexion and can be used to facilitate spine mobility or stability. Stool rotations (**Fig. 5**) are used after week 3.

It has been shown that the gluteus medius muscle is a key stabilizer of the hip during gait.[19] Gluteus medius strength when compared with the maximum voluntary contraction from the smallest amount of force produced to the highest is achieved with supine abduction, non–weight-bearing standing abduction, side-lying abduction,

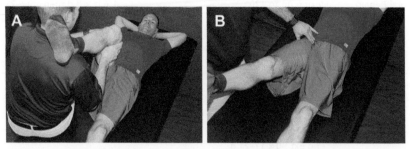

Fig. 2. Circumduction. (*A*) Passive clockwise and counter-clockwise ROM at the hip at ~70 degrees flexion. (*B*) Passive clockwise and counter-clockwise ROM at the hip with the leg straight.

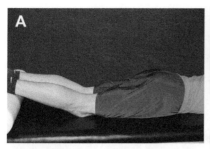
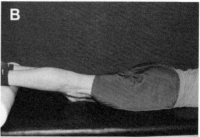

Fig. 3. Prone terminal knee extensions. (*A*) Start position. (*B*) Extend knee and hip to neutral with quad and glutes.

weight-bearing opposite hip abduction, flexed hip weight bearing opposite hip abduction, and pelvic drop exercises, respectively.[20] This progression to strengthen the gluteus medius is used with the exception of side-lying abduction, which should be avoided because of the increased acetabular joint forces.[21] Standing abduction in internal rotation (**Fig. 6**) is emphasized throughout rehabilitation because it can be performed early to activate the gluteus medius within the ER restrictions and because of the low flexor activation with this exercise.

Gentle stretching of the iliopsoas is performed early by bringing the patient's opposite knee to the chest in supine position. Gentle Thomas stretch can be used when tolerated after week 4 and kneeling stretch when the patient can tolerate weight bearing. Patient can gently stretch the quads and hamstrings when pain free. The piriformis can be stretched in side-lying position with support. Stretching of the adductors is not recommended to protect the surgical area; however, soft tissue work seems to reduce the patient's complaint of tightness usually brought on by hypertonicity in this muscle group. Aquatic therapy is highly recommended throughout rehabilitation. Protection of the incisions is achieved with op-site waterproof dressings (Smith and Nephew, London, UK).

Daily circumduction is continued, whereas ER and extension are initiated by the physician's orders. Active assisted FABER slides (**Fig. 7**) and active butterfly exercise (**Fig. 8**) allow the patient to control the amount of ER.

REHABILITATION PROGRESSION

Weaning off crutches depends on the patient's tolerance to the gradual increase in weight bearing and demonstration of proper firing of the gluteal muscles without

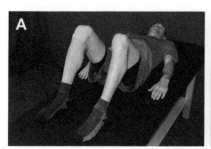
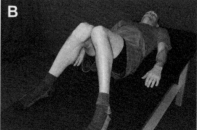

Fig. 4. Active reverse butterflies. (*A*) Start in hook-lying position with feet slightly wider than shoulder width apart and toes pointed inward. (*B*) Rotate thighs inward to touch knees and hold 5 seconds then bring knees outward.

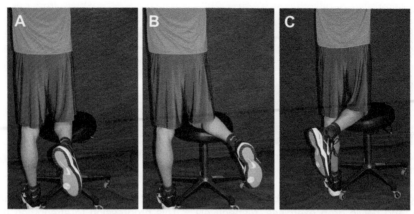

Fig. 5. Stool rotations. (*A*) Knee flexed to 90 degrees placed on spinning stool and lightly weighted with hip in neutral. (*B*) Actively rotate hip inward controlling pelvis with core muscles then return to neutral. (*C*) When external rotation allowed, actively rotate hip outward.

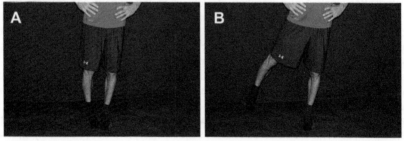

Fig. 6. Standing abduction in internal rotations. (*A*) Start position with knee straight and toes pointed slightly inward. (*B*) Slowly bring your leg straight out to the side keeping toes slightly pointed inward and your pelvis level.

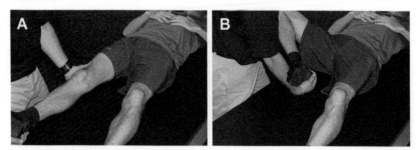

Fig. 7. FABER slides. (*A*) Start position with heel resting on hand which is resting on table and opposite hand behind knee. (*B*) Active assisted flexion, abduction, and external rotation supporting and assisting as needed.

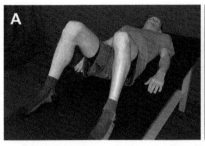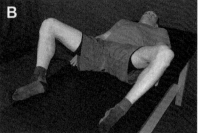

Fig. 8. Active butterflies. (*A*) Start position hook-lying with feet shoulder width apart. (*B*) Slowly allow knees to fall out and hold 5 seconds then return.

a Trendelenburg gait (phase 2 as listed in **Table 3**). Progressive increases in weight bearing of 10% to 25% every 1 to 3 days or slower is recommended. Aquatic therapy may assist in the patient's ability to wean off crutches. Restoring normal gait without using a standard or underwater treadmill is recommended because the authors think that a sheer stress is placed on the anterior aspect of the hip when ambulating on the moving tread of the treadmill.

Table 3	
Phase 2 of the rehabilitation program	
Phase 2: Controlled Stability	
Goals	1. Normalize gait
	2. Restore full ROM
	3. Improve neuromuscular control, balance, proprioception
	4. Initiate functional exercises maintaining core and pelvic stability
Precautions	1. Recommend no treadmill use
	2. Avoid hip flexor and adductor irritation
	3. Avoid joint irritation: too much volume, force, or not enough rest
	4. Avoid ballistic or aggressive stretching
Treatment Strategies	1. Wean off crutches as per weight-bearing guidelines
	2. Gait training with emphasis on gluteal firing and core control
	3. Nonresistant stationary bicycle until a minimum of 6 wk
	4. Circumduction, prone lying, and soft tissue and muscle stretching as before
	5. Full passive ROM including ER and extension
	6. Active ROM, core stability, weight bearing, and movement preparation exercises
	7. Progress aquatic pool program
	8. Progress cardiovascular and upper body exercises (see **Table 4**)
	9. Initiate functional exercises in late phase 2
Minimum Criteria to Advance	1. Gait is pain free and normalized
	2. Full ROM with mild stiffness into ER
	3. No joint inflammation, muscular irritation, or pain
	4. Successfully initiated functional exercises without pain and good neuromuscular control

MUSCULATURE BALANCE

Assessment of the entire lumbar-pelvic-hip complex and lower extremity kinetic chain helps to address muscle imbalances, sacroiliac joint, lumbar spine articular dysfunctions, and restrictions in the fascial planes. Treatments to facilitate normal mechanics of these functional units include manual mobilization and/or manipulations of the thoracic or lumbar spine, sacroiliac joint, and soft tissue work as previously described.[22–25] Manual mobilization of the hip capsule is performed only as needed after week 6.

During this phase, improvement of neuromuscular control is critical using sensorimotor exercises for balance and proprioception. Endurance is emphasized while using weight-shifting exercises including reverse lunge static holds (**Fig. 9**) and double knee bends with weight shift. Standing abduction in internal rotation (SAIR) is performed bilaterally, and exercises emphasizing the gluteus maximus and medius, including prone hip extensions off the edge of tables, bridges, and clams, and manually resisted exercises are performed. Core exercises such as supine heel slides, supine marching, or standing knee to chest are used to facilitate the iliopsoas muscle. These exercises should be performed with proper firing of the TA in core neutral position while avoiding overfiring of the TFL. Emphasis is placed on correct muscle firing patterns while not allowing patients to work beyond their ability. A dynamic movement preparation group of exercises including toe touches, standing knee to chest (**Fig. 10**), standing knee to chest with rotation (**Fig. 11**), walk outs (**Fig. 12**), lateral lunges, and scorpions (**Fig. 13**) can be initiated. Pilates as an adjunct to rehabilitation is recommended versus yoga.

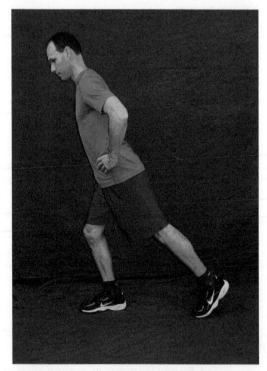

Fig. 9. Reverse lunge static hold. Start with surgical leg forward with hip and knee flexed and opposite leg straight behind. Slowly shift your weight onto the forward leg by coming up on the toes of the back foot while bending at the ankle of the forward foot.

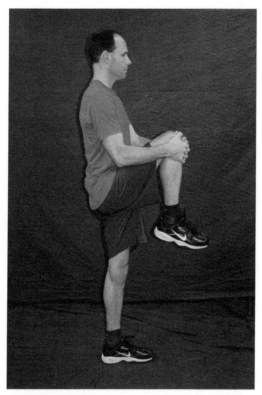

Fig. 10. Standing knee to chest.

REHABILITATION: MIND AND BODY

Rehabilitation after hip arthroscopy can be a challenge for many patients who are otherwise very active individuals. The long period of inactivity after surgical procedures can be difficult on the athlete/patient both mentally and physically. There are many options available for athletes that concurrently address the rehabilitation of the hip while maintaining or minimizing the loss of fitness. These activities can be performed in compliance with all weight-bearing and ROM restrictions. Incorporating a philosophy of focusing not only on the surgically repaired hip and each phase individually (as seen in **Fig. 14**) but also on the athlete or patient as a whole (as seen in **Fig. 15**) keeps the athletes engaged mentally and physically and should allow for an easier transition to their respective sport when the injured hip is healed. Athletes can take pride in maintaining fitness or even improving on weaknesses that otherwise go unaddressed in their sport training (**Table 4**).

ADVANCING REHABILITATION BEYOND THE HIP

Cardiovascular fitness activities are generally started during phase 1 after postoperative day 7. Intensity and duration can be progressed throughout phase 1 and can continue into phase 2 of the hip rehabilitation program.

Upper extremity strengthening is efficiently, effectively, and safely performed during phase 1 using suspension-type training. This setup allows the patient to perform a multitude of exercises using body weight resistance rather than attempt to carry

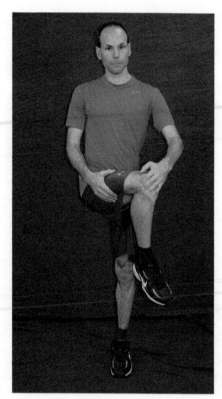

Fig. 11. Standing knee to chest with rotation.

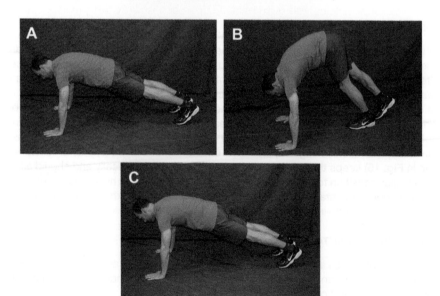

Fig. 12. Walk out. (*A*) Start in standing then bend forward and touch the floor keeping the knees straight and walk the hands out. (*B*) Keeping the knees straight and hands in one spot while walking the feet up. (*C*) Walk hands out again.

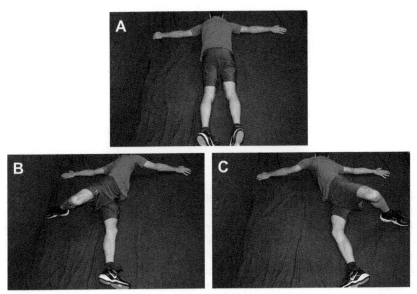

Fig. 13. Scorpions. (*A*) Start position on stomach with arms straight out in a T. (*B*) Keeping the shoulders as flat to the floor as possible bring the leg and hip up and across the opposite leg rotating from the hip, pelvis, and spine. (*C*) Return and perform with the opposite leg.

dumbbells or other weights while on crutches. Minimal movement is required, and resistance can easily be altered with small changes in foot position. Bodyweight can be distributed as dictated by weight-bearing restrictions. Cord resistance exercises can be used in late phase 1, whereas sitting on a Swiss ball and/or kneeling for proprioceptive training as the patient is weaning off crutches (**Fig. 16**).

During the later stages of phase 2, nonmicrofracture patients may be cleared to begin running in the pool in chest-deep water progressing to waist-deep water. This exercise is done in preparation for the land running progression at the beginning of phase 3. Running is delayed as long as possible for patients who have undergone a microfracture, but pool running should be initiated several weeks in advance of land running if necessary for the running athlete. Skating athletes are allowed to return to the ice at this time. Cycling resistance can be added at week 6.

Phase 2 sees more mobility of the patient and allows a return to the athlete's presurgery upper extremity strength regimen. Returning to the gymnasium to use dumbbells, barbells, and/or machines, athletes can achieve previous levels of upper body strength. Core conditioning can be advanced as well, with consideration to type and intensity of forces placed on the hip with particular attention to iliopsoas overuse.

The athletes are allowed to initiate their sport progressions during phase 3, provided they have restored a normal gait and established the necessary strength and stability around the hip joint. This initiation will allow athletes to load the entire system (heart, lungs, muscles, joints) similar to the loading requirements of their sport to maximize

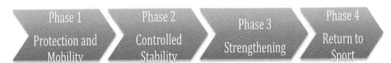

Fig. 14. Rehabilitation as separate phases.

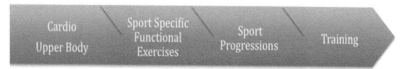

Fig. 15. Rehabilitation as a continuum.

motor control and metabolic demands as the overall strength of the hip increases. Following the 3 *P*'s principle, the program is pain-free, progressive, and predictable.

RETURN TO PLAY

Sport progressions during this stage are performed within a pain-free ROM, with a duration and intensity that does not result in an increase in soreness of the joint or musculature. A progressive plan involves beginning with simple, slow, and short-duration activities. As the athlete gains strength, endurance, and confidence in the hip, more complex and faster movements of increasing volume can be performed. A predictable plan means beginning only with movements that are known to the athlete. It is not a time to explore a new running, cycling, or skating form or a route that may have unknown distances or uneven surfaces or require reactive movements such as defending someone.

Running progression on land and skating progressions with specific drills and speeds are initiated. The athlete can now swim without the pull buoy, and cycling resistance can be further added. Athletes are allowed to shoot a basketball, throw

Table 4		
Cardiovascular fitness and conditioning		
	Cardiovascular Fitness	**Upper Body/Sport Specific Conditioning**
Phase 1	55%–70% of maximum heart rate up to 30 min 1. Upper body ergometry 2. Single well–leg rowing 3. Swimming with pull buoy	1. Suspension-type training (see **Fig. 16**) 2. Cord resistance exercise training
Phase 2	85% for phase 1 cardiovascular exercises; 55%–70% for phase 2 exercises 1. Swimming with pull buoy 2. Easy return to ice for skating sports 3. Resistance on bicycle	1. Presurgery upper body regimen: dumbbells, barbells, machines at lower resistance 2. Core conditioning: planks, crunches, avoiding hip flexor dominant exercises
Phase 3	1. Swimming without pull buoy 2. Running progression in pool (non-Mfx patients) 3. Running, skating, cycling progressions 4. Strength days emphasizing PAQ with minimum rest between sets in late phase 3	1. Shooting, swinging, hitting, dribbling, kicking, throwing sport–specific progressions
Phase 4	1. Maximize presurgery fitness regimen: running, cycling, skating, swimming, strengthening	1. Advanced sport specific drills

Abbreviations: Mfx, microfracture; PAQ, power, agility, quickness.

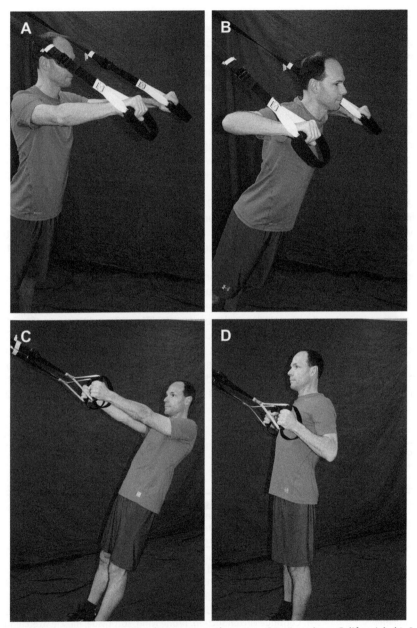

Fig. 16. TRX Suspension Training (Fitness Anywhere, Inc, San Francisco, California). (*A & B*) Push start-end. (*C & D*) Pull start-end.

a baseball, swing a racquet or a bat, or dribble or pass a soccer ball depending on their individual sport. The volumes and intensities at which these sport-specific exercises are performed need to be to be controlled, and rest days are mandatory. A careful plan is best developed to find a balance in strengthening; cardiovascular, aquatic, core, and sport-specific exercises; and rest.

Sport progressions, as previously described, are critical aspects of phases 3 and 4, whereas double leg strengthening is initiated and progressed to single leg strengthening. Phase 3 is shown in **Table 5**. Neuromuscular control emphasized in phase 2 is maintained. Endurance strength is emphasized (15–20 repetitions minimum) throughout phase 3, eventually incorporating power, agility, and quickness training into the program. Depending on the demands of the sport involved and the overall condition of the surgical hip, the athlete's strengthening program is adjusted with focus primarily on progressive endurance strengthening, power and agility movements, or both. Cardiovascular fitness is achieved with the traditional programs (running, bike, elliptical trainer), sport progressions (skating, dance), or metabolic conditioning that is gained from using power and agility exercises with shorter rest periods. Recovery during this training can include balance, coordination, or mobility exercises.

Passive circumduction is continued for 10 weeks and should continue actively for an additional 4 weeks; soft tissue work and gentle stretching should also be done. Glute activation exercises continue using SAIRs, single leg bridges, and manually resisted exercises. Core neutral position with transverse abdominal control should be emphasized with all exercises.

Double leg strengthening includes leg press, double knee bends with resistance, and tuck squats (**Fig. 17**). Olympic lifts are not recommended early because of the quick explosive movements required to perform them correctly. Single leg strengthening progressively added includes balance squats (**Fig. 18**), split squats (**Fig. 19**), reverse lunges, lateral lunges (**Fig. 20**), and single knee bends (**Fig. 21**). Resistance is added with sport cords, dumbbells, or kettlebells. As the patient demonstrates the ability to perform single knee strengthening with adequate endurance and good form, power and agility movements are added, including lateral and diagonal agilities with sport cords. Single knee bend, lateral agility (**Fig. 22**), diagonal agility (**Fig. 23**),

Table 5
Phase 3 of the rehabilitation program

Phase 3: Strengthening	
Goals	1. Restore muscular strength and endurance 2. Optimized neuromuscular control, balance, proprioception 3. Restore cardiovascular endurance 4. Progress sport progressions
Precautions	1. Recommend no treadmill use 2. Avoid hip flexor and adductor irritation 3. Avoid joint irritation: too much volume, force, or not enough rest 4. Avoid ballistic or aggressive stretching 5. Avoid contact and high velocity activities
Treatment Strategies	1. Continue circumduction, prone lying, soft tissue, muscle stretching, gluteal activation, core stabilization, movement prep exercises and aquatic pool program as needed 2. Sport progressions or functional activities 3. Cardiovascular fitness (see **Table 4**) 4. Double leg strengthening 5. Single leg strengthening
Minimum Criteria to Advance	1. Perform all phase 3 exercises pain free and with correct form 2. Pass sport test

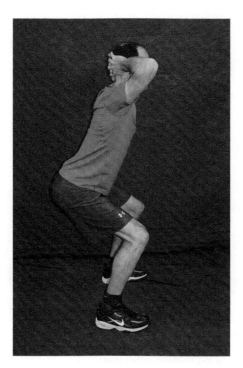

Fig. 17. Tuck squats.

and forward lunge onto a box (**Fig. 24**) are the 4 exercises that comprise the sport test.[10]

Phase 3 should culminate in the passing of a sports test (as shown in **Table 6**) that once completed allows the athlete to return to practice without limitations to train and prepare for competition. The athlete transitions into full training with a dedicated return to sport plan with any specific precautions as recommended by the physician. Specific demands of the sport are addressed with advanced power, plyometrics, performance, and conditioning training. These transitions should occur smoothly not only if hip-specific treatments were applied throughout the phases of rehabilitation

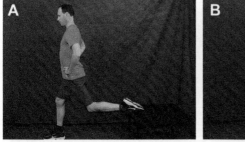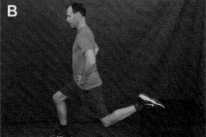

Fig. 18. Balance squat. (*A*) Start position with one leg behind supported on a bench and other leg forward enough to prevent knee from coming out past the toes when squatting. (*B*) Perform squat on forward leg keeping pelvis level.

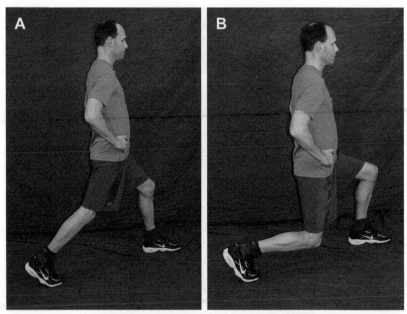

Fig. 19. Split squat. (*A*) Start position with one leg behind on the floor while other leg is forward enough to prevent knee from coming out past the toes when squatting. (*B*) Perform squat on forward leg keeping pelvis level.

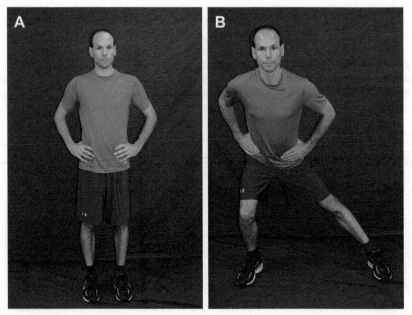

Fig. 20. Lateral lunge. (*A*) Start position. (*B*) Step lateral while squatting keeping the knee straight ahead and the pelvis level.

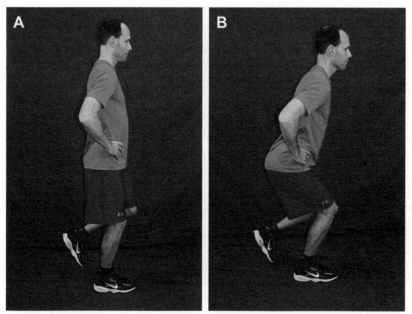

Fig. 21. Single knee bend. (*A*) Start position. (*B*) Keep knee from collapsing into adduction, internal rotation and valgus and hip neutral while performing single leg squat 30–70 degrees knee flexion.

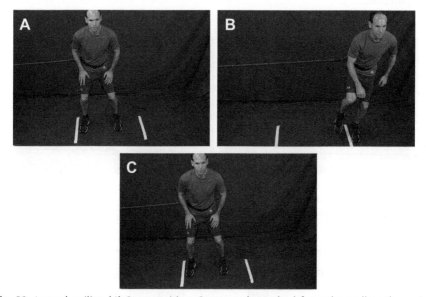

Fig. 22. Lateral agility. (*A*) Start position: Sport cord attached from the wall to the waist. First line placed on floor the distance away from wall where the cord remains taut. Second line is the placed away from the first the distance from the patient's greater trochanter to the floor. (*B*) Patient performs a lateral push-off from the leg nearest the wall with enough force to land with the opposite leg past the second line. (*C*) The increase in cord tension will result in a force that pulls the patient back. The patient should land in front of the first line and absorb the landing with a controlled squat.

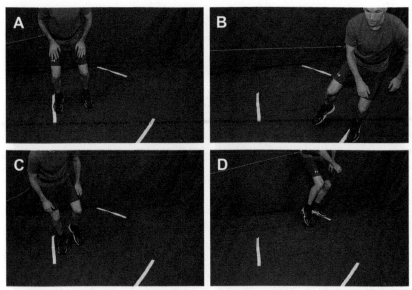

Fig. 23. Diagonal agility. (*A*) Start position: Same as lateral agility except 2 lines are placed at a 45 degree angles forward and backward from the first. (*B*) The patient performs the lateral push-off from the leg nearest the wall as before but lands first rep on forward line. (*C*) The patient returns to the first line landing in a controlled squat. (*D*) The patient performs the next rep landing on the back line and continues alternating forward and backward lines.

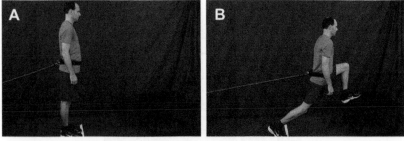

Fig. 24. Forward lunge onto box. (*A*) Start position. Cord attached from wall to back of waist and taut. (*B*) Perform a deep forward lunge onto a box the height of the patient's knees then return and perform with opposite leg.

Table 6 Functional hip sport test		
Exercise	**Goal**	**Points**
Single knee bends	3 min	1 point earned for each 30 s completed
Lateral agility	100 s	1 point earned for each 20 s completed
Diagonal agility	100 s	1 point earned for each 20 s completed
Forward lunge on box	2 min	1 point earned for each 30 s completed

Passing score: 17 of 20.

Table 7	
Phase 4 of the rehabilitation program	
Phase 4: Return to Sport	
Goals	1. Restore power and maximize plyometric strength
	2. Return to play
	3. Independent in maintenance program
	4. Understands proper care for the long-term health of the hip
Precautions	1. No specific precautions unless noted by the physician
Treatment Strategies	1. Develop a return to sport plan
	2. Sport training and conditioning
	3. Power, plyometric, performance training
Minimum Criteria to Advance	1. Cleared by the physician
	2. Completed sport training and conditioning
	3. Full return to nonrestricted practice

but also if cardiovascular fitness, conditioning, and sport progressions were used. Phase 4 is shown in **Table 7**.

SUMMARY

Rehabilitation after FAI arthroscopy is different for different patients. By following the restrictions set by the physician while performing early circumduction, using the minimal criteria to advance through each subsequent phase, and allowing patients to perform functional sport progressions throughout the rehabilitation athletes will be able to return to sport smoothly and effectively with positive outcomes.

REFERENCES

1. US markets for arthroscopy devices 2009. Report by Millennium Research Group (MRG).
2. Philippon MJ, Briggs KK, Kuppersmith DA. Outcomes following hip arthroscopy with microfracture. Arthroscopy 2007;23:211.
3. Philippon MJ, Schenker M, Briggs KK, et al. Femoroacetabular Impingement in 45 professional athletes: associated pathologies and return to sport following arthroscopic decompression. Knee Surg Sports Traumatol Arthrosc 2007;15: 908–14.
4. Philiipon MJ, Briggs KK, Yen YM, et al. Outcomes following hip arthroscopy for femoroacetabular impingement with associated chondrolabral dysfunction: minimum two-year follow-up. J Bone Joint Surg Br 2009;91:16–23.
5. Byrd JW, Jones KS. Prospective analysis of hip arthroscopy with 2-year follow-up. Arthroscopy 2000;16:578–87.
6. Hartmann A, Gunther KP. Arthroscopically assisted anterior decompression for femoroacetabular impingement: technique and early clinical results. Arch Orthop Trauma Surg 2009;129:1001–9.
7. Philippon MJ, Yen YM, Briggs KK, et al. Early outcomes after hip arthroscopy for femoroacetabular impingement in the athletic adolescent patient: a preliminary report. J Pediatr Orthop 2008;28:705–10.
8. Bardakos NV, Vasconcelos JC, Villar RN. Early outcome of hip arthroscopy for femoroacetabular impingement: the role of femoral osteoplasty in symptomatic improvement. J Bone Joint Surg Br 2008;90:1570–5.

9. Stalzer S, Wahoff M, Scanlan M. Rehabilitation following hip arthroscopy. Clin Sports Med 2006;25:337–57.

10. Wahoff MS, Briggs KK, Philippon MJ. Hip arthroscopy rehabilitation: evidence-based practice. In: Kibler B, editor. Orthopedic knowledge update: sports medicine 4. Lexington (Kentucky): AAOS; 2008. p. 273–81, 23.

11. Enseki KR, Martin RL, Draovitch P, et al. The hip joint: arthroscopic procedures and postoperative rehabilitation. J Orthop Sports Phys Ther 2006;36:516–25.

12. Philippon MJ, Maxwell BR, Johnston TL, et al. Clinical presentation of femoroacetabular impingement. Knee Surg Sports Traumatol Arthrosc 2007;15:1041–7.

13. Clohisy JC, Knaus ER, Hunt DM, et al. Clinical presentation of patients with symptomatic anterior hip impingement. Clin Orthop Relat Res 2009;467:638–44.

14. Sink EL, Gralla J, Ryba A, et al. Clinical presentation of femoroacetabular impingement in adolescents. J Pediatr Orthop 2008;288:806–11.

15. Noyes FR, DeMaio M, Mangine RE. Evaluation-based protocols: a new approach to rehabilitation. Orthopedics 1991;14:1383–5.

16. Crawford K, Philippon MJ, Sekiya JK, et al. Microfracture of the hip in athletes. Clin Sports Med 2006;25:327–35.

17. Lewis CL, Sahrmann SA, Moran DW. Anterior hip joint force increases with hip extension, decreased gluteal force, or decreased iliopsoas force. J Biomech 2007;40:3725–31.

18. Sapega AA. Current concepts review: muscle performance evaluation in orthopaedic practice. J Bone Joint Surg Am 1990;72:1562–74.

19. Torry MR, Schenker ML, Martin HD, et al. Neuromuscular hip biomechanics and pathology in the athlete. Clin Sports Med 2006;25:179–97.

20. Bolgla LA, Uhl TL. Electromyographic analysis of hip rehabilitation exercises in a group of healthy subjects. J Orthop Sports Phys Ther 2005;35:487–94.

21. Krebs DE, Elbaum L, Riley PO, et al. Exercise and gait effects on in vivo hip contact pressures. Phys Ther 1991;71:301–9.

22. Kendall FP, McCreary EK, Provance PG. Muscle testing and function. 4th edition. Baltimore (MD): Lippincott Williams and Wilkins; 1996.

23. Lewit K. Manipulative therapy in rehabilitation of the locomotor system. London: Butterworth-Heinemann; 1991.

24. Sahrmann SA. Diagnosis and treatment of movement impairment syndrome. St Louis (MO): Mosby; 1990. p. 345–94.

25. Jull GA, Janda V. Muscles and motor control in low back pain: assessment and management. In: Twomey LT, Taylor JR, editors. Physical therapy of the low back. New York: Churchill and Livingstone; 1987. p. 253–78.

Index

Note: Page numbers of article titles are in **boldface** type.

A

Abductor muscle, injuries of, 274–275, 276, 277, 278
   tears of, in greater trochanteric pain syndrome, 394–396
Acetabulum, cartilage of, damage to, classification of, 337, 340
     treatment of, outcomes of, 347–348
   debridement of, 333–334, 335
   locations on, 336–337
   zone system of, 337, 338
Adolescent(s), avulsion fracture and, 435–437
   femoroacetabular impingement in, 438–440
   hip dislocation in, 441
   hip injury in, due to underlying hip disorder, 441–444
   hip problems of, related to sports, arthroscopy in, **435–462**
   labral tear in, 440
   stress fracture of hip in, 438
Apophyseal avulsion injuries, of anterior superior and inferior iliac spines, 410
Apprehension testing, in hip instability, 358
Arthritis, of hip, mature athlete with, **453–462**
     nonoperative management of, 454–455
     sports and, 453–454
   septic, arthroscopy of, 447
Arthrography, magnetic resonance, 301–302
Arthroplasty, total hip, and return to sport, 459
Arthroscopy, in femoroacetabular impingement. See *Femoroacetabular impingement.*
   in multiple epiphyseal dysplasia, 445–446
   of hip, 305
     anesthesia for, 286–287
     arthroscopic portals for, 287–288
     challenges of, 331–347
       and opportunities in, **217–224**
     complications of, 291–292, 347, 447
     experience with, 288–290
     history of, 285, 444–445
     in mature athlete, imaging for, 447–458
       indications for, 445–457
     indications for, in children and adolescents, 445–447
     joint preservation in, 332
     mechanics of, 285–292
     patient positioning for, 287
     postoperative therapy modalities after, 466
     rehabilitation after, principles of, 463–464
     rehabilitation protocols after, 464–465

Clin Sports Med 30 (2011) 483–489
doi:10.1016/S0278-5919(11)00014-7
0278-5919/11/$ – see front matter

sportsmed.theclinics.com

Moving?

Make sure your subscription moves with you!

To notify us of your new address, find your **Clinics Account Number** (located on your mailing label above your name), and contact customer service at:

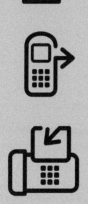

Email: journalscustomerservice-usa@elsevier.com

800-654-2452 (subscribers in the U.S. & Canada)
314-447-8871 (subscribers outside of the U.S. & Canada)

Fax number: 314-447-8029

Elsevier Health Sciences Division
Subscription Customer Service
3251 Riverport Lane
Maryland Heights, MO 63043